Dysphagia Following Stroke

DATE DUE

OC30 08			

Clinical Dysphagia Series

Jay C. Rosenbek
Series Editor

Dysphagia Following Stroke by Stephanie K. Daniels
and Maggie-Lee Huckabee

Dysphagia Following Stroke

A Volume in the Clinical Dysphagia Series

Stephanie K. Daniels
Maggie-Lee Huckabee

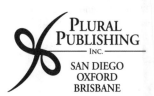
PLURAL
PUBLISHING
INC.

SAN DIEGO
OXFORD
BRISBANE

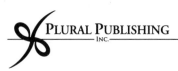

5521 Ruffin Road
San Diego, CA 92123

e-mail: info@pluralpublishing.com
Web site: http://www.pluralpublishing.com

49 Bath Street
Abingdon, Oxfordshire OX14 1EA
United Kingdom

Typeset in 10/13 Garamond by Flanagan's Publishing Services, Inc.
Printed in the United States of America by Bang Printing

Library of Congress Cataloging-in-Publication Data:
Daniels, Stephanie K.
  Dysphagia following stroke / Stephanie K. Daniels and Maggie-Lee Huckabee.
      p. ; cm. — (Dysphagia series)
  Includes bibliographical references and index.
  ISBN-13: 978-1-59756-196-9 (alk. paper)
  ISBN-10: 1-59756-196-7 (alk. paper)
  1. Deglutition disorders. 2. Cerebrovascular disease—Complications.
  [DNLM: 1. Deglutition Disorders—etiology. 2. Stroke—complications. WI 250
D186d 2008] I. Huckabee, Maggie Lee. II. Title. III. Dysphagia series (Plural Pub.)
  RC815.2.D36 2008
  616.3'23—dc22

                                                            2008000330

Contents

Foreword

Drs. Maggie-Lee Huckabee and Stephanie Daniels are rehabilitation scientists of the first order. They have spent portions of their entire professional lives in both the laboratory and the clinic. For them, the person with dysphagia is not merely a set of structures and muscles working in disharmony. Treatment is not merely an array of mechanical manipulations. Evidence-based practice is not merely the data. Swallowing, they know, is influenced by the sight and smell of food; by affect, experiences, and expectations; by companions, environment, and need. Treatment is a human interaction. Evidence-based practice rests equally on evidence, clinical acumen, and what each patient wants and needs.

Their book, *Dysphagia Following Stroke*, reflects who they are and what they want for their profession and the patients it serves. This book displays clinical gems on every page. These gems were hardened by the pressure of their scientific rigor and cut and polished by their clinical experience.

Huckabee and Daniels end their preface with a fond and firm warning to me, "never again." If they continue to feel that way after the very real anguish writing a book produces begins to dissipate, I'll certainly respect their wishes. I and the profession will have to be content with this last, infinitely useful "practical source book." If, however, they ultimately decide that the pain was not so bad, then we may have other books to guide our steadily growing practice in dysphagia. Until that time, we have this book and that's not bad.

Jay Rosenbek, Ph.D.
Editor, Clinical Dysphagia Series

Preface

This text is geared toward the clinician working with stroke patients in all settings: hospitals, rehabilitation centers, outpatients, and long-term care. It is intended as a practical sourcebook, and although many areas have been addressed in other texts, this book focuses specifically on evaluation and management of stroke. The clinician may wish to refer to other texts for more in-depth but nonpopulation specific coverage of specific issues or techniques. We recognize that the stroke patient can present as a patient with complex needs. The full range of clinical encounters cannot be addressed; thus, we focus specifically on the effects of stroke and not the potential complicating features of the critically or chronically ill patient.

Acknowledgments

Writing a book is no easy task and many people are called on for assistance. Carol Stach reviewed many versions of the book. She provided keen attention to detail and grammar, helped us keep content clinically relevant, and provided excellent moral support. Gina Tillard kept the fires going in Hawea, New Zealand during cold winter days and nights and proved an excellent sounding board concerning matters of content and clinical application. Joe Murray provided the key endoscopy figure and reviewed the endoscopy text to ensure that it was on target. He is always good for lively discussion. Thanks to Phoebe Macrae for assistance in the final frenzy of last minute editing. Adrienne and Tom shared their beautiful Lake Hawea and the pups, Jock and Archie, providing us with the best environment for initiating this undertaking-Cheerio! And last, but certainly not least, we must acknowledge Jay Rosenbek, our mentor and friend. Jay, to you we very fondly and very firmly say "never again."

Abbreviations

A-P = anterior-posterior

BA = Brodmann's area

BOT = base of tongue

CAD = coronary artery disease

CEA = carotid endarterectomy

CIMT = constraint-induced motor therapy

CN = cranial nerve

CSE = clinical swallowing examination

CT = computed tomography

DWI = diffusion-weighted imaging

E-E = expiration-expiration

E-I = expiration-inspiration

EMG = electromyography

EMST = expiratory muscle strength training

ES = electrical stimulation

FEESST = fiberoptic endoscopic evaluation of swallowing with sensory testing

FIM = functional independence measure

HLC = hyolaryngeal complex

I-E = inspiration-expiration

I-I = inspiration-inspiration

IOPI = Iowa Oral Pressure Instrument

LAR = laryngeal adductor reflex

LHD = left hemisphere damage

LMN = lower motor neuron

LMS = lateral medullary syndrome

LSVT = Lee Silverman Voice Treatment

MASA = Mann Assessment of Swallowing Ability

MEP = maximum expiratory pressure

MRI = magnetic resonance imaging

NA = nucleus ambiguous

NGT = nasogastric feeding tube

NIH-SSS = National Institutes of Health-Swallowing Safety Scale

NMES = neuromuscular electrical stimulation

NPO = nothing by mouth

NTS = nucleus tractus solitarius

NZIMES = the New Zealand Index for the Multidisciplinary Evaluation of Swallowing

OTT = oral transit time

P-A = penetration-aspiration

PEG = percutaneous endoscopic gastrostomy

PPW = posterior pharyngeal wall

PTT = pharyngeal transit time

PVWM = periventricular white matter

PWI = perfusion-weighted imaging

RAS = reticular activating system

RHD = right hemisphere damage

SA = swallowing apnea

SAD = swallowing apena duration

sEMG = submental electromyography

SMA = supplementary motor area

STD = stage transit duration

tPA = tissue plasminogen activator

TPN = total parenteral nutrition

TTS = thermal-tactile stimulation

TVF = true vocal folds

UES = upper esophageal sphincter

UMN = upper motor neuron

VFSS = videofluoroscopic swallow study

VPMpc = parvicellular component of the ventroposterior medial nucleus

1 Introduction to Dysphagia and Stroke

OVERVIEW OF STROKE

Epidemiology of Stroke

Stroke affects 2000 people per million worldwide each year and approximately 700,000 individuals in the United States annually (Broderick et al., 1998). Stroke risk increases with age and is higher in non-whites compared to whites (Broderick et al., 1998; Sacco et al., 1998). The incidence of stroke has shown a significant decline in the United Kingdom (Rothwell et al., 2004) and New Zealand (Carter et al., 2006) over the past 20 years; however, no change in incidence was reported in the United States during the 1990s (Klein-dorfer et al., 2006).

Eighty percent of strokes are secondary to ischemia, whereas hemorrhage accounts for 20%. Ischemia implies reduced blood flow to the brain and generally is caused by atherosclerosis, which is a buildup of plaque along the lining of the artery. The buildup of plaque leads to stenosis, narrowing of the artery, and formation of a thrombosis, or stationary clot. Thrombotic infarction generally involves large vessels but can also occur in small vessels (lacunar infarction). The plaque may dislodge yielding an embolism, which travels in the bloodstream until it becomes lodged and disrupts blood flow. Embolisms frequently arise from the heart. Hemorrhagic strokes may result from hypertension that weakens the wall of vessel, rup-tured aneurysm, or bleeding from an arteriovenous malformation.

1

Risk factors for stroke include increased age, hypertension, heart disease, diabetes mellitus, hypercholesterolemia, family history of stroke, physical inactivity, smoking, alcohol abuse, and cocaine use.

Neurologic Evaluation

Assessment of the acute stroke patient begins when the patient presents to the emergency room. The neurologist will obtain a history from the patient (or family if the patient cannot respond) concerning previous medical conditions, medications, and the nature of the stroke event: time of onset, activity surrounding event, initial deficits, progression and duration of deficits, and other related events. A neurologic examination is completed to determine the exact deficits and consists of evaluation of elemental and higher cortical functions. Elemental functions include examination of cranial nerves, reflexes, and motor and sensory systems. Higher cortical function assessment involves evaluation of attention and memory, affect, language, praxis, visuospatial processing, and neglect. Table 1–1 presents an example of a neurologic examination. Diagnostic testing is completed within the first few days of admission in attempt to uncover the source of the stroke, that is, cardiac embolism, carotid stenosis. Carotid vertebral duplex ultrasound, and/or angiography may be completed to identify arterial stenosis. Evaluation for potential cardiac sources of an embolism may include 2-D and transesophageal echocardiography.

Neuroimaging

Computed tomography (CT) scanning is completed upon admission to identify the presence of a hemorrhagic stroke. If the stroke is an acute ischemic event and the lesion is relatively small, the CT scan initially will be normal as x-ray transmission depends on tissue density, and tissue density is without change in acute stroke. Figure 1–1 shows a large acute ischemic stroke. Diffusion-weighted imaging

Table 1–1. Neurologic Examination

I. Mental Status
  A. Appearance and Behavior
  B. Mood and Affect—depression, anxiety, paranoid, vigilant, distracted, circumstantial, tangential, suspicious
  C. Level and State of Consciousness
      i. Level of consciousness—alert, lethargic, obtunded, stuporous, comatose
      ii. State of consciousness—normal, manic, minimally reactive
  D. Orientation—person, place, time, event
  E. Memory—can be assessed in terms of time course and/or function
      i. Time course
          1. Immediate (digit span, serial 7's, immediate recall of three objects)
          2. Short-term (three objects recall at 5 minutes)
          3. Long-term (presidents 5/5, autobiographical)
      ii. Function
          1. Declarative
              a. Episodic (questions relative to recent/remote event: most recent meal, current events in the news, major life events)
              b. Semantic (general knowledge, e.g., capital of Louisiana)
          2. Procedural (describe/demonstrate overlearned tasks such as swinging a golf club)
          3. Working (digit span backwards, serial 7's, oral arithmetic)
  F. Frontal Lobes
      i. Dorsolateral (verbal fluency: F-A-S, categories; abstract reasoning)
      ii. Medial Frontal (energy level-apathy, anxiety, depression)
      iii. Orbitofrontal (response inhibition-tactile, visual; social inappropriateness)
  G. Language
      i. Spontaneous speech (fluency)
          1. Nonverbal aspects of language-aprosodia
      ii. Naming (confrontation—high-frequency and low-frequency words)
      iii. Repetition (single words, phrases)
      iv. Comprehension
      v. Reading/Writing
  H. Praxis (ideomotor, ideational, limb-kinetic, buccofacial)
  I. Constructional Ability/Neglect
      i. Visuospatial
          1. Copy complex figure (intersecting pentagon)
          2. Mapping (topographic abilities)
          3. Clock drawing (spontaneous, copy)

continues

Table 1–1. *continued*

ii. Neglect
  1. Anosognosia (awareness of deficits)
  2. Hemispatial neglect (cancellation, line bisection)
  3. Extinction (auditory, visual, tactile)
  4. Emotional-Affective processing (expressive, receptive aprosodia)
J. Calculations

II. Cranial Nerves (CN)
  A. CN I—Olfactory (tested only when indicated by history)
  B. CN II—Optic (visual acuity, visual fields, pupil size, regularity, equality, reaction to light, optic fundi)
  C. CN III, IV, VI—Extraocular muscle function (tracking, saccadic eye movements)
  D. CN V—Trigeminal (jaw movement against resistance, jaw jerk reflex, facial sensation, corneal reflex)
  E. CN VII—Facial (symmetry at rest and with movement, corneal reflex, taste anterior 2/3 of tongue, lacrimation and salavation)
  F. CN VIII—Auditory (Webers and Rinne tests, vestibular)
  G. CN IX, X—Glossopharyngeal, Vagus (palatal elevation, uvula position, gag reflex)
  H. CN IX—Spinal Accessory (sternocleidomastoid and trapezius muscle strength)
  I. CN X—Hypoglossal (symmetry of tongue protrusion, lateralization)

III. Somatosensory
  A. Pain and Temperature
  B. Touch, Position, Vibration, Romberg sign
  C. Cortical Sensory (graphesthesia, stereognosis, double simultaneous stimulation)

IV. Motor
  A. Bulk (atrophy, fasciculations)
  B. Tone (hypotonia, rigidity, spasticity)
  C. Strength—Gross Motor
    i. Formal testing (grading 0-5)
    ii. Localization of deficits (flexor-extensor, proximal-distal)
    iii. Drift
  D. Strength—Fine Motor
    i. Pincer, grasp
    ii. Finger tapping

Table 1–1. *continued*

    E. Adventitious (involuntary) Movements
       i. Localization (axial-appendicular, distal-proximal, symmetric-asymmetric)
      ii. Type of dyskinesia
         1. Hypokinetic (parkinsonism)
         2. Hyperkinetic (dystonia, chorea, athetosis, tremor, myoclonus, hemiballism)
      iii. Presence (at rest, suspension, intention)
    F. Cerebellar
       i. Finger-to-nose (dysmetria, past-pointing), heel-to-shin
      ii. Rapid alternating hand movement (dysdiadokinesia)
      iii. Ataxia-axial/appendicular
    G. Gait and Station
       i. Gait
         1. Spontaneous (base, arm swing, associated movements, posture)
         2. Directed (tandem, on toes, on heels)
      ii. Station (Romberg, retropulsion)

V. Reflexes
    A. Deep Tendon Reflexes—muscle stretch reflexes (normal = +2, clonus = +4, hypoactive = 0,1)
    B. Superficial Reflexes
       i. Signs of increased reflexes (Hoffman's crossed adductor, triple flexor, clonus, Babinski response)
      ii. Abdominal reflex, cremasteric reflex, bulbocavernosus, anal wink)
    C. Frontal Release Signs (Glabellar, root, suck, snout, grasp)

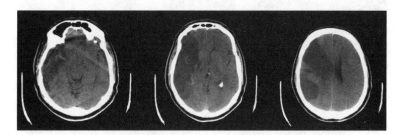

Figure 1–1. Computed tomography scan of a large right middle cerebral artery stroke. The right hemisphere is on the reader's left side.

(DWI) acquisition as part of the magnetic resonance imaging (MRI) scan allows identification of small acute infarcts. Within minutes of symptom onset, DWI detects water diffusion changes related to cytotoxic edema and represents the anatomic extent of the lesion (Figure 1–2). Another relatively new MRI sequence is perfusion-weighted imaging (PWI). PWI details areas of the brain that are hypoperfused, that is, brain regions with restricted blood flow. These early changes in the brain correspond to the full functional extent of the lesion. If blood flow can be restored with therapeutic intervention in a timely fashion, the brain tissue identified on PWI can be salvaged.

Medical Management

Identifying the exact time of stroke onset is critical as it will determine if the stroke patient is eligible for thrombolytic therapies such as tissue plasminogen activator (tPA), which may break up or dissolve blood clots. If administered within the first three hours of symptom onset, these therapies may help limit the stroke damage and severity of disability. Antithrombotic agents, such as aspirin and

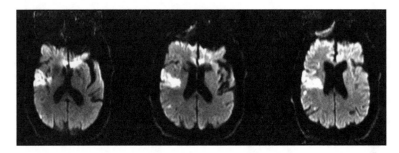

Figure 1–2. Diffusion-weighted imaging scan of an acute right hemisphere stroke. The scan was obtained within 72 hours of admission. The right hemisphere is on the reader's left side.

other antiplatelet drugs and warfarin (Coumadin), are generally used for stroke prevention, but they may also be used in the treatment of acute ischemic stroke. Carotid endarterectomy (CEA) is the primary surgical treatment for stroke prevention. It reduces blockage of the internal carotid arteries, which supply blood to the brain. Greatest benefit of CEA is in patients with greater than 70% symptomatic stenosis. Carotid angioplasty and stenting also may be used in case of stenosis. These may be options in patients for whom the surgical procedure of CEA is too great a risk.

DYSPHAGIA IN STROKE

Incidence

Dysphagia is a common morbidity following acute stroke. Table 1-2 provides a summary of studies detailing the incidence of dysphagia following stroke. Wide discrepancy is evident, as demonstrated in this table, with the incidence of dysphagia ranging from 25% (Gottlieb, Kipnis, Sister, Vardi, & Brill, 1996) to 81% (Meng, Wang, & Lien, 2000). The variability in the incidence of dysphagia following stroke is due, in part, to patient selection methods (e.g., consecutive patients, case series), evaluation methods (e.g., questionnaire, clinical swallowing examination, instrumental evaluation), time post-onset (e.g., 1 week, 1 month) and definition of dysphagia.

The reader will notice in Table 1-2 a wide range of detail concerning the evaluation method and the criteria used to define dysphagia. All of these studies consisted of consecutive stroke patients, which provide a more robust inclusion pool from which to determine epidemiology. The incidence of dysphagia may be underestimated if only stroke patients with complaints of dysphagia or patients referred to speech pathology are evaluated, as it is likely that many stroke patients may not be aware of swallowing problems

Table 1–2. Epidemiology of Dysphagia in Stroke

Study	N	Stroke Detail	Evaluation
Barer (1989)	357	Consecutive, hemispheric	Clinical
Chua & Kong (1996)	53	Consecutive, brainstem	Clinical
Daniels et al. (1998)	55	Consecutive, ischemic, all brain regions, single and multiple strokes, no prior dysphagia	VFSS
DePippo, Holas, & Reding (1994)	139	Consecutive, single and multiple strokes, all brain regions, no prior dysphagia	Clinical
Gordon, Hewer, & Wade (1987)	91	Consecutive, hemorrhagic and ischemic, all regions, single and multiple strokes	Clinical
Gottlieb et al. (1996)	180	Consecutive, all brain regions, single and multiple strokes	Clinical
Hamdy et al. (1997)	20	Consecutive, single hemisphere	Clinical
Hamdy et al. (1998)	28	Consecutive, single hemisphere	VFSS

Poststroke Time of Evaluation	Evaluation Details	Dysphagia Criteria	Incidence
2 days	10 ml water	Marked delay or coughing	29%
N/A	Gag reflex, volitional and reflexive cough, swallowing, vocal quality	Required nasogastric tube	40%
5 days	Two trials of multiple volumes and consistencies	Decreased oral transfer, delayed pharyngeal swallow (>.45 sec), decreased laryngeal elevation, postswallow residual, or penetration, aspiration	Dysphagia 65% Aspiration 38%
5 weeks	Feeding and 3-oz water	Coughing	45%
Within 2 weeks	50 ml water	Inability to drink the volume or choking while drinking	37%
2 weeks	50 ml clear liquids	Single instance of coughing	25%
5–40 days	3 ml, 5 ml, 50 ml water	Coughing, water pooling in mouth, >2 sec delayed swallow, reduced laryngeal elevation, signs of distress or respiratory difficulties, voice change	40%
1 week	10 ml liquid ×13	At minimum: uncoordinated swallow with delayed pharyngeal transit or residual	71%

continues

Table 1–2. *continued*

Study	N	Stroke Detail	Evaluation
Hinds & Wiles (1998)	115	Consecutive, all brain regions	Clinical
Kidd, Lawson, Nesbitt, & MacMahon (1993)	60	Consecutive, first stroke, all brain regions	Clinical; VFSS
Mann, Hankey, & Cameron (1999)	128	Consecutive, first stroke	Clinical; VFSS

Poststroke Time of Evaluation	Evaluation Details	Dysphagia Criteria	Incidence
3 days	5–10 ml, Timed 150 ml	Speed or volume per swallow were outside normative range or evidence of cough or wet hoarseness	67%
3 days	Clinical—5 ml water ×10; VFSS—Multiple volumes and consistencies	Clinical-coughing, voice change VFSS-Not defined	Dysphagia: Clinical 42% VFSS 90% Aspiration: VFSS 42%
Median: 3–10 days	Clinical—saliva, 5 ml–20 ml water; VFSS—5–10 ml thin and thick liquids and semisolids, 20 ml liquid	Disorder of at least one aspect of swallowing Clinical: oral preparation (saliva control, oral hygiene, lip seal, tongue strength and movement, oral preparation, respiration, respiratory disease), oral (gag, palatal function, oral transit time, bolus clearance), pharyngeal: control, pooling, laryngeal elevation, reflexive and volitional cough, voice quality, tracheostomy VFSS: bolus control, operationally defined transit times, pharyngeal wall movement, residue	Dysphagia: Clinical 51% VFSS 64% Aspiration: Clinical 50% VFSS 22%

continues

Table 1–2. *continued*

Study	N	Stroke Detail	Evaluation
Meng et al. (2000)	36	Consecutive, brainstem	Clinical
Odderson, Keaton, & McKenna (1995)	124	Consecutive, ischemic	Clinical
Parker et al. (2004)	70	Consecutive, single hemisphere	Clinical
Sala et al. (1998)	187	Consecutive	Clinical
Schelp, Cola, Gatto, Silva, & Carvalho (2004)	102	Consecutive ischemic and hemorrhagic	Clinical
Sharma, Fletcher, Vassalo, & Ross (2001)	202	Consecutive, ischemic and hemorrhagic, all brain regions, single and multiple strokes	Clinical

Poststroke Time of Evaluation	Evaluation Details	Dysphagia Criteria	Incidence
Rehab, N/A	5–10 ml water swallow	Difficulty swallowing, coughing	81%
24 hours		Alert, follows directions, strong voice and volitional cough, swallows saliva, ice chips and water without problems, intact laryngeal elevation, clear voice, no cough after swallow	39%
3 days	Teaspoon, sips, 30 ml	Throat clear or cough, oral residue, delayed swallow, reduced laryngeal elevation	39%
24 hours	25 ml water, 2 tablespoons semisolid	Slow deglutition, cough, impossible to swallow or coma	30%
6 days	N/A	N/A	76%
3 days	Liquids and semisolids starting with a spoonful of water	Coughing, choking, change in respiratory rate, eyes watering, pocketing, oral leakage, extended time to eat, development of chest symptoms, impaired consciousness	51%

continues

Table 1–2. *continued*

Study	N	Stroke Detail	Evaluation
Smithard, O'Neill, Parks, & Morris (1996)	121	Consecutive, ischemic and hemorrhagic	Clinical (VFSS to subgroup)
Teasell, Foley, Fisher, & Finestone (2002)	20	Consecutive, brainstem	Clinical
Wade & Hewer (1987)	452	N/A	Clinical

N = number, N/A = not available; VFSS = videofluoroscopic swallowing study.

Poststroke Time of Evaluation	Evaluation Details	Dysphagia Criteria	Incidence
48 hours	5 ml water ×3, 60 ml water ×2–3	Risk of aspiration-not stated which measure(s) determined aspiration risk: dribbles water, reduced or repeated laryngeal movement, cough, weak, wet, or absent laryngeal function after swallow, unable to finish 60mL, aspiration present	51%
Rehab, N/A	Consciousness level, voice quality, coughing or choking, oral motor control, bolus control, pharyngeal swallow delay	N/A	55%
7 days	Water from cup	Choking, obvious difficulty or abnormal swallowing patterns, slow speed that was determined by patient judgment	43%

or that only those patients with overt signs of aspiration risk, such as cough, are referred to speech pathology. Conversely, this same pool of patients may arrive equally at an overestimation of dysphagia incidence, as stroke patients without swallowing problems are not evaluated. Identification of dysphagia based on results from the clinical swallowing examination (CSE) generally may underestimate the incidence. As discussed in later chapters, the CSE frequently focuses on overt signs of aspiration, for example, cough, or voice change, which may miss silent aspiration. Use of these results to determine the incidence of dysphagia is problematic as patients may have dysphagia without aspiration. Even when using an instrumental evaluation, the incidence of dysphagia may be overestimated if the identification of dysphagia is based on laryngeal penetration or single occurrences of aspiration (e.g., Daniels & Foundas, 1999) as healthy adults may exhibit laryngeal penetration and infrequent occurrences of aspiration (Robbins, Coyle, Rosenbek, Roecker, & Wood, 1999).

In determining the incidence of dysphagia, Mann, Hankey, and Cameron (2000) provide the most detailed account for the CSE and videofluoroscopic swallow study (VFSS) and include fairly descriptive operational definitions. However, they did not utilize a group of healthy participants in which to compare results from the stroke patients. As discussed in Chapter 3, increasing knowledge of the variability in swallowing, particularly in regard to aging, has greatly expanded our definition of "normal." Thus, without a control group from which to base an acceptable range of normal for transit times, structural timing and movement, and airway invasion, the incidence of dysphagia may be inflated.

The best determination of the incidence of dysphagia and recovery of function would involve: (1) consecutive acute stroke patients followed longitudinally, (2) a cohort of age-matched healthy participants, (3) instrumental assessment, (4) reliably defining dysphagia from multiple measures, for example, bolus flow, structural movement, patient perception, and (5) stability in findings over multiple trials, consistencies, and volumes. Development of a standard method to define dysphagia and recovery of swallowing in stroke patients based on multiple measures of bolus flow has been initiated with a small sample of stroke patients and healthy age-matched participants (Daniels et al., 2006). However, until studies are rigorous in implementing all five of the listed aspects in a large cohort study, determining the incidence of dysphagia and recovery of function will remain elusive.

Lesion Location

Initial notions concerning the occurrence of dysphagia following stroke were based on the assumption that either brainstem or bilateral supratentorial (i.e., cerebral hemispheres, subcortical areas) infarcts were required to produce disturbances in swallowing. The advent of in vivo brain and swallowing imaging techniques has allowed for expansion of our understanding of dysphagia following stroke. It is now widely understood that a single cortical or subcortical infarct may produce dysphagia (Daniels & Foundas, 1999; Robbins, Levine, Maser, Rosenbek, & Kempster, 1993). Lesions anterior to the central sulcus are associated with dysphagia and risk of aspiration more than posterior lesions (Daniels & Foundas, 1999; Robbins et al., 1993). Strokes involving large vessels (e.g., middle cerebral artery) are associated with aspiration more than small vessels (e.g., deep white matter disease). Specific sites that have been associated with dysphagia in stroke patients include: brainstem, premotor and primary motor cortices, primary somatosensory cortex and the insula, as well as the periventricular white matter, which disrupts cortical-subcortical connectivity when lesioned (Alberts, Horner, Gray, & Brazer, 1992; Daniels & Foundas, 1997, 1999; Daniels, Foundas, Iglesia, & Sullivan, 1996; Robbins et al., 1993).

MULTIDISCIPLINARY MANAGEMENT OF DYSPHAGIA IN STROKE

Given the complexity inherent in swallowing and the vast range of skills involved in meticulous diagnostics, a multidisciplinary approach to identification, diagnosis, and management of swallowing impairment is imperative. The unidimensional view inherent in a single discipline requires the diversity in background provided by other various medical disciplines in order to illuminate the multidimensional picture of impaired swallowing pathophysiology. Although the lead clinician in the dysphagia management team is frequently a speech pathologist, assumption of the lead role does not imply that the contribution of the speech pathologist is of greater value to dysphagia management than others.

This text cannot define specific roles or responsibilities; much of that task lies within the individual medical facility and may be guided by professional practice guidelines. However, caution is expressed that the establishment of a team without recognition of input from all related specialties is to the detriment of the patient care. A dysphagia management approach that relies only on patient screening by nursing without the expertise of speech pathology is not in the best interest of the patient. Likewise, an approach by speech pathology without the expertise and contributions of nutrition or others is shortsighted.

2 The Neural Control of Swallowing:

From Central to Peripheral

Swallowing is mediated by a distributed neural network that includes cortical and subcortical structures with descending input to the brainstem. This neural network is composed of multiple levels along the neural axis (cortical, subcortical, brainstem). Specific neural systems (sensory, motor) that cross these levels and interconnect with cortical, subcortical, and brainstem regions are involved in swallowing. Based on anatomic and functional imaging studies, as well as animal models, a neuroanatomic model of swallowing is proposed (Figure 2–1).

It is important that clinicians understand the complexity of the neural network involved in swallowing and appreciate that an infarct when strategically placed along this neural axis can produce acute and protracted dysphagia. In order to advocate for prompt consultation and evaluation of stroke patients, the clinician must understand basic fundamentals of the neural control of swallowing. With further research, we may be able to determine specific stroke locations or combinations of stroke locations, neurocognitive deficits, and/or comorbidities that more accurately predict acute and protracted dysphagia. Until that time, based on our current understanding of the neural control of swallowing, clinicians have a strong argument promoting the evaluation of swallowing in all acute stroke patients. Moreover, an understanding of innervation patterns is paramount when completing a clinical swallowing examination (CSE). Specific sensory or motor impairment on the cranial nerve

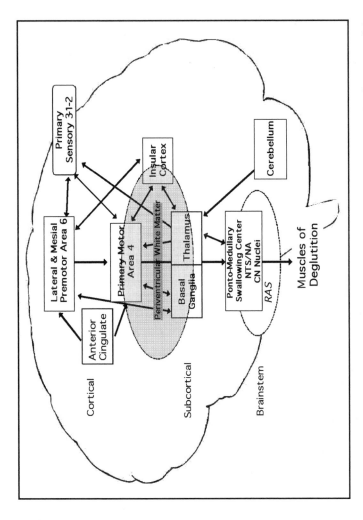

Figure 2–1. Proposed model of the neural networks of swallowing. CN = cranial nerve nuclei, NA = nucleus ambiguus, NTS = nucleus tractus solitarius, RAS = reticular activating system.

examination has a direct impact on swallowing function. Following is an overview of the neurology of swallowing, which is particularly relevant in the stroke population.

METHODS FOR UNDERSTANDING NEURAL CONTROL

Various paradigms have been employed to facilitate our understanding of the neural organization of swallowing. Interestingly, even though methodologies are different, results from studies in animals, healthy adults, and stroke patients have been generally uniform in suggesting a distributed neural network for swallowing.

Animal models formed our initial basis of knowledge concerning deglutition. Reciprocal translational research, that is, research that moves from animal models to humans and vice versa, continues to play an important role in our understanding of normal and abnormal swallowing, especially as more is learned of the potential of neural reorganization following stroke. Animal research has included direct stimulation of specific parts of the brain, ablation, that is, lesioning of specific brain regions, and neuroanatomic tracing with anterograde and retrograde labeling that is used to identify neural pathways in the central and peripheral nervous systems. These techniques have facilitated identification of specific regions of the brain involved with swallowing as well as neural pathways in the central nervous system that are related to deglutition.

In humans, localization of swallowing has been based on ablation paradigms, which utilize anatomic imaging (computed tomography, magnetic resonance imaging) of focal lesions in stroke patients, and functional imaging studies that detail activation of brain regions during the actual act of swallowing. Table 2–1 provides a summary of the various techniques used to study the neural control of swallowing.

Table 2–1. Techniques to Study the Neural Control of Swallowing in Humans

Technique	Procedure	Results	Advantages	Disadvantages
Anatomic Imaging				
Computed Tomography Magnetic Resonance Imaging	Brain images obtained while a person is lying quietly performing no activity. Best if contiguous thin slices.	Lesions are identified and mapped out to determine specific sites. Relationship between lesion size and dysphagia can be made if scans are obtained with limited to no gap between slices.	If obtained at the same time as the instrumental swallowing study, can correlate stroke location with dysfunction.	Patient cannot perform any activity. The computed tomography scan does not immediately show ischemic infarction.
Functional Imaging				
Positron Emission Tomography	Radioactive tracers are injected into the bloodstream. They circulate and diffuse in cerebral tissue. Generally a block design is used where subjects repeatedly swallow (water, saliva) for a specified time alternated with rest periods.	Identifies areas activated during swallowing.	Low susceptibility to motion artifact.	Radiation exposure. Expensive. Reduced temporal resolution.

Technique	Procedure	Results	Advantages	Disadvantages
Functional Magnetic Resonance Imaging	Blood oxygenation level dependent effects are mapped. That is, a task (swallowing) yields increased neuronal activity and metabolism in specific brain regions that yield increased blood flow and volume. Generally an event-related paradigm is used where multiple single swallows are completed over multiple trials.	Identifies areas activated during swallowing.	No radiation exposure. Excellent spatial resolution.	Susceptible to motion; this is mitigated by event-related paradigm. Reduced temporal resolution.
Other Functional Methods				
Transcranial Magnetic Stimulation	Focal magnetic stimulation of specific cortical surfaces is completed using an external coil.	Identifies neural circuitry in swallowing with good temporal resolution.	Cortical regions involved with normal swallowing and recovery of function can be identified.	The effect of stimulation is limited to superficial cortical structures.

continues

23

Table 2–1. *continued*

Technique	Procedure	Results	Advantages	Disadvantages
Transcranial Magnetic Stimulation (*continued*)	Stimulation of these regions yields contraction of specific swallowing musculature that is measured with electromyography. Areas yielding activation are reconstructed on anatomic templates.			An actual swallow cannot be stimulated due to risk of seizure.
Magneto-encephalography	Similar to electroencephalography except that a magnetic versus electric signal is recorded during an activity(i.e., swallowing). Similar to transcranial magnetic stimulation as areas yielding activation are reconstructed on anatomic templates.	Detects postsynaptic magnetic fields generated by neurons activated with swallowing.	Excellent temporal resolution that allows for determination of the onset of activation of specific brain regions during swallowing.	Easy to overinterpret isolated tongue movement as swallowing related movement.

The focus of functional imaging studies has been on swallowing in healthy adults. The use of positron emission tomography and functional magnetic resonance imaging to study stroke patients with dysphagia has proven challenging as patients must swallow with minimal extraneous movement while lying flat on their back. Although other imaging methodologies can be obtained with a person seated, they each have their own advantages and disadvantages in the study of dysphagia in clinical populations.

HIGHER NERVOUS SYSTEM CONTROL

The cerebral cortex and subcortical structures are important in swallowing with evidence that supratentorial regions modify brainstem swallowing responses as well as directly modulate swallowing (Miller & Bowman, 1977; Sumi, 1969). Until recently, it was thought that a stroke must involve the brainstem or both cerebral hemispheres; however, research over the last three decades has revealed that a single unilateral stroke can produce dysphagia. Many physicians are aware of this, but some are not. It is important that the clinician have a good understanding of the role of cortical and subcortical regions in swallowing in order to advocate for obtaining a clinical swallowing examination in all acute stroke patients, not just patients with brainstem or bilateral strokes.

The supratentorial network for swallowing involves a sensory system, motor system, and white matter pathways. Despite methodological differences, anatomic and functional imaging studies have identified similar areas critical for swallowing. These regions include the primary motor cortex, premotor cortex, supplementary motor area (SMA), primary somatosensory cortex, insula, thalamus, basal ganglia, and anterior cingulate (e.g., Daniels & Foundas, 1997, 1999; Hamdy, Mikulis, et al., 1999; Hamdy, Rothwell, et al., 1999; Huckabee, Deecke, Cannito, Gould, & Mayr, 2003; Kern, Jaradeh, Arndorfer, &

Shaker, 2001; Martin, Goodyear, Gati, & Menon, 2001; Mosier & Bereznaya, 2001; Toogood et al., 2005).

Sensory input has parallel ascending and descending input affecting brainstem pathways and cortical pathways. Ascending sensory input is processed by the thalamus (subcortical level) then proceeds to the primary somatosensory cortex (Brodmann's area [BA] 3-1-2, cortical level). Corticocortical connections run along an anterior-posterior axis with sensory input feeding forward to the primary motor cortex (BA 4) and lateral and mesial premotor cortices (BA 6). The lateral premotor cortex integrates input from the prefrontal cortex and cerebellum and is critical for the selection of appropriate movements (Passingham, 1993). The mesial premotor cortex, also referred to as the SMA, is the main cortical target of the basal ganglia (Wise & Strick, 1984) and is critical in the preparation and programming of voluntary movement sequences (Roland, Larsen, Lassen, & Skinhoj, 1980). The anterior cingulate is important for attention as well as the selection of volitional actions and sends output to the primary motor and premotor cortices. The primary motor cortex has descending connections through subcortical regions to sensory and motor cranial nerve nuclei (Kuypers, 1958a, 1958b). Descending input proceeds through subcortical regions. The periventricular white matter (PVWM), which is the white matter adjacent to the body of the lateral ventricles, is important in these swallowing pathways, as it is composed of ascending somatosensory and descending motor fibers as well as intrahemispheric cortico-cortical connections (Schulz, 1994). Descending corticospinal fibers from the mouth/face representation within the ventrolateral precentral gyrus (motor cortex) are located anterolaterally in the PVWM. The anterior insula, in addition to being the primary gustatory cortex (Benjamin & Burton, 1968) has parallel connections with many cortical and subcortical regions that mediate swallowing. These regions include motor and premotor cortices (Mesulam & Mufson, 1985) and the parvicellular component of the ventroposterior medial nucleus of the thalamus (VPMpc) (Mufson & Mesulam, 1984). The VPMpc contains the sensory representation for the face and oral cavity and receives projections from the nucleus tractus solitarius (NTS) (Beckstead, Morse, & Norgren, 1980).

The lateralization of swallowing is a controversial notion. Using various imaging modalities, results thus far are inconclusive as to whether swallowing is preferentially mediated by the left or right hemisphere at the cortical level. Some anatomic imaging studies have suggested that oral stage dysfunction is associated with left hemisphere damage and pharyngeal stage dysfunction and aspiration are associated with right hemisphere damage (Robbins & Levine, 1988, 1993; Robbins et al., 1993), whereas others have suggested no difference in dysfunction between hemispheres (Alberts et al., 1992; Daniels & Foundas, 1999). These same discrepancies in results have also been noted with functional studies. Bilateral activation of the sensorimotor cortex has been suggested by some studies (Hamdy, Mikulis, et al., 1999; Martin et al., 2001; Zald & Pardo, 1999). It has been suggested that lateralization may be dependent on the task (Martin et al., 2001) with right hemisphere activation associated with volitional swallowing and left hemisphere activation with reflexive swallowing (Kern et al., 2001). Conversely, others have noted left hemisphere dominance with volitional swallowing (Dziewas et al., 2003). A third hypothesis has been put forth and suggests bilateral but asymmetric activation of swallowing (Hamdy et al., 1997; Hamdy et al., 1996; Hamdy, Rothwell, et al., 1999). That is, both hemispheres are involved in swallowing, but one hemisphere is more dominant and varies across individuals. This notion suggests dysphagia will occur only if the more dominant hemisphere for swallowing is affected by a stroke; thus, perhaps, explaining why dysphagia may be present in some stroke patients but not in other patients with lesions of similar size and location. Using this model, it has been suggested that recovery of swallowing function is associated with cortical reorganization of nondominant hemisphere (Hamdy et al., 1998).

CENTRAL PATTERN GENERATOR/ BRAINSTEM MECHANISMS

Whereas supratentorial regions are critical for the modulation and initiation of ingestive swallowing, brainstem structures are recognized as providing the basic motor plan for pharyngeal swallowing. These more primitive phylogenic structures have been extensively evaluated through early research by Jean, Doty, Car, and others (Amri & Car, 1988; Amri, Car, & Jean, 1984; Car, 1970, 1973; Car & Amri, 1982; Car, Jean, & Roman, 1975; Doty, 1968; Doty, Richmond, & Storey, 1967; Jean, 1984a, 1984b, 1990), who have outlined the critical role of medullary circuitry in the regulation of pharyngeal and esophageal swallowing. More recent work has highlighted the importance of this circuitry in the coordinative interactions between swallowing and respiration (Dick, Oku, Romaniuk, & Cherniack, 1993; Saito, Ezure, Tanaka, & Osawa, 2003; Shiba, Satoh, Kobayashi, & Hayashi, 1999). The compact clustering of cranial nerve nuclei and interneuronal connections in this region are considered to be responsible for the complex sequencing and execution of the neuromuscular events involved in swallowing.

The first evidence of a central swallowing center was provided by Miller and Sherrington (1916). These researchers provided electrical stimulation to the exposed cortex and brainstem to identify which regions would result in observable swallowing behavior. Although many cortical and subcortical regions elicited swallowing upon stimulation, a study of decerebrated animals revealed that the medullary brainstem appeared to be the lowest common denominator, with stimulation of this area eliciting pharyngeal and esophageal swallowing in the absence of cortical input. Additionally, Miller (1972) reported that stimulation of specific brainstem cranial motor nuclei would not elicit the complex neuromuscular process of pharyngeal swallowing, although the muscles supplied by these motor nuclei are involved in swallowing. This suggests that there is a more complex interdependent circuitry for the act of deglutition.

Central to our current understanding of brainstem mechanisms is the construct of a *central pattern generator*. Rossignol and Dubuc (1994) define this term as "an operational expression to designate an ensemble of neural elements whose properties and connectivity can give rise to characteristic patterns of rhythmic activity in the absence of external feedback" (p. 895). The construct of a central pattern generator for swallowing was initially posed by Doty (1968) subsequent to a study by Doty and Bosma (1956), which documented that swallowing was a sequential and repeatable activation of muscles that occurs even in the presence of impaired peripheral feedback mechanisms.

There are two regions of the brainstem medulla that are considered to represent the anatomic foundation for the swallowing central pattern generator (Kessler & Jean, 1985). The dorsal region of the medulla is anatomically located 1.5 to 4 mm rostral to the obex and consists of the area surrounding and including the NTS and adjacent reticular formation (Jean & Car, 1979). The NTS is the primary sensory nucleus for the facial, glossopharyngeal, and vagus cranial nerves; afferent pathways from the pharynx and larynx, specifically those from the superior laryngeal nerve, travel to the NTS via these cranial nerves (Carpenter, 1978). Additionally, the NTS region receives input from the trigeminal sensory nucleus of the pons. Mucosal receptors in the pharynx respond to touch, pressure, chemicals, and water and facilitate the initiation and repeated activation of pharyngeal swallowing. Muscle spindle receptors, which are embedded in muscles involved in pharyngeal and esophageal swallowing, are considered to trigger interneurons that modify motor output to muscles. Finally, the specific cortical site that evokes swallowing when activated by electrical stimulation sends fibers to synapse in this dorsal medullary region. Subsequently, according to Miller, Bieger, and Conklin (1997), lesions of the dorsal region prevent electrical stimulation of the cortex from evoking swallowing. This suggests that the dorsal region is the initial neural entrance or afferent portal for input that modulates swallowing (Miller et al., 1997). The dorsal group neurons lack direct connection with hypoglossal and trigeminal motoneurons and connect directly only to the nucleus ambiguus (NA) and associated reticular formation. Thus, neurons in the dorsal region are considered the programming interneurons (Amri, Car, & Roman, 1990) that set up the sequential preprogrammed patterns of neuronal activation that are then transmitted to the ventral regions for motor activation.

The second major component of the medullary swallowing center, the ventral region, consists of the area surrounding and including the NA, located 3 to 6 mm rostral to the obex (Jean & Car, 1979). Structurally, the NA is the primary motor nucleus for the glossopharyngeal, vagus, and spinal accessory nerves and has extensive interconnections with other medullary motor nuclei, such as the hypoglossal, facial, and trigeminal motor nuclei (Amri et al., 1990; Jean, Amri, & Calas, 1983). Thus, the neurons and interneurons in this region send out neural commands that control the muscles of the pharynx, larynx, and esophagus (Roman, 1986). Axons in the NA connect with contralateral brainstem regions involved in swallowing (Jean et al., 1983).

The ventral efferent medullary region receives direct input from the dorsal afferent medullary region. Thus, sensory information entering the brainstem via the NTS is intergrated into a swallowing motor plan and then transmitted to the motor nucleus for execution. Interestingly, sensory inputs from the superior laryngeal nerve (vagus), that are known to elicit swallowing upon electrical stimulation, travel to both the dorsal region and directly to NA in the ventral region. However, synaptic pathways to the ventral region are longer than those to the dorsal region suggesting that the superior laryngeal nerve can directly modify motor output during swallowing and provide reflexive laryngeal control for a cough response (Miller et al., 1997). With the exception of connections from the NTS to the NA, there are no other ventral medullary connections to sensory nuclei, supporting the role of a tightly encapsulated neural network underlying swallowing.

Functionally, direct stimulation of the ventral region does not evoke pharyngeal swallowing despite direct motorneuron connection to the muscles of swallowing. Individual contraction of the muscles involved in swallowing occurs but the organized, patterned motor response is absent without the intervening sensory input, and consequent motor plan provided by the dorsal region. Amri and Car (1988), therefore, suggest that the ventral neurons serve to link the sensory input from the dorsal neuron group to the motorneurons involved in swallowing. Given this important link, the ventral neuron group may be referred to as "command interneurons."

In summary, bilateral peripheral afferents from the glossopharyngeal, facial, and vagus nerves enter the afferent portal of the dorsal medullary group. This sensory information is paired with cortical inputs that synapse on the pontine relay nuclei (cortical-subcortical loop), and afferent input from the sensory fibers of the trigeminal nerve. All sensory information is integrated and the appropriate programmed motor response is sent back out to the periphery via the ventral medullary group. The primary structure of this group, the NA, consequently activates sequential efferent cranial nerve fibers from the spinal accessory, vagus, and glossopharyngeal nerves as well as the motor nuclei for the hypoglossal and trigeminal nerves. At its most primitive level of functioning, this functional "central pattern generator" allows for sequential muscle activation in the absence of sensory feedback. However, for ingestive swallowing, this interaction between sensory and motor nuclei via interneuronal fibers modulation of the patterned motor response specific to the incoming sensory input. In functional terms, this allows for differential but safe swallowing of a variety of textures, temperatures, and bolus sizes.

PERIPHERAL NEUROMUSCULAR MECHANISMS

As discussed in the prior section, two regions of the brainstem medulla are involved in the coordinative efforts of accepting incoming sensory input in preparation for swallowing, organizing a swallowing response that is differentiated to that specific sensory input, and engaging that motor plan to execute efficient bolus ingestion. Incoming and outgoing inputs from the brainstem are dependent on activation and efficient transfer of neural information through afferent and efferent cranial nerve (CN) pathways. Thus, elucidation of swallowing neural control demands knowledge of the complex patterns of excitation and inhibition of the cranial nerves that contribute so substantively to swallowing motor control. More importantly, as discussed in Chapter 6, interpretation of CN findings can guide the clinician to more reliable inferences about pharyngeal swallowing behavior. In order to aid clinical application, this section highlights the location of CN nuclei and places cranial nerve excitation and inhibition within the context of neuromuscular contributions to swallowing physiology. Although the following text is accurate based on the authors' research, the clinician is advised that there are discrepancies in the literature regarding some aspects of cranial nerve constitution and innervation.

Although generally considered peripheral organs, the CN have their respective nuclei within the central nervous system. The motor nerves emerge from these nuclei and synapse peripherally at the neuromuscular junction. Sensory nerves initiate in sensory receptors, transverse from the peripheral system, and synapse on cranial nerve nuclei in the central nervous system. In stroke, knowledge of site of lesion may provide clues for differential diagnosis of swallowing impairment if the clinician has knowledge of the origin of CN nuclei. CN nuclei involved in swallowing are primarily housed in the lower brain regions, with the exception of the nuclei for the olfactory (CN I) and optic (CN II) cranial nerves, both of which are contained with the cerebral cortex. The trigeminal motor and sensory nuclei (CN V) and the facial motor nucleus (CN VII) are both situated in the pons. Further down the neural axis, the brainstem houses the remainder of the important nuclei for swallowing. The NTS is the primary sensory nucleus for the facial (CN VII), glossopharyngeal (CN IX), and vagus (CN X) cranial nerves; all afferent information from the pharynx and larynx travel to the NTS via these cranial nerves. Additionally, the NTS receives secondary input from the trigeminal sensory nucleus of the pons. The NA is also housed in the brainstem and is the primary motor nucleus for the glossopharyngeal (CN IX), vagus (CN X), and spinal accessory (CN XI) nerves and has extensive interconnections with other motor nuclei, such as the hypoglossal (CN XII), facial (VII), and trigeminal motor (CN V) motor nuclei involved in pharyngeal swallowing.

Prior to the bolus entering the oral cavity, an individual sees the bolus, which activates CN sensory inputs from the occipital nerve (CN II). In addition, a person may smell the bolus, which activates similar receptors from the olfactory nerve (CN I). Input from these peripheral receptors travel via their respective CN to the primary visual and olfactory cortices before moving on to their respective association cortices for recognition and cognitive processing. At this early point in the preingestive process, and dependent on the stimulus, the individual may have activation of motor fibers of the chorda tympani branch of the facial nerve (CN VII) to initiate salivary flow from the submandibular gland and sublingual glands; activation of fibers of the glossopharyngeal nerve (CN IX) will assist in production of saliva from the parotid glands. Salivary production is critical for bolus preparation of more viscous textures. Additionally, dependent on the characteristics of the bolus, there may be very early activation of the motor fibers of the recurrent laryngeal branch of the vagus nerve (CN X), which initiates early onset of vocal adduction for airway protection, that occurs through contraction of the interarytenoid and cricoarytenoid muscles.

Bolus entry into the oral cavity requires paired inhibition and excitation of several muscle groups. Mouth opening generally requires inhibition of facial nerve (CN VII) fibers that contract orbicularis oris. However, for larger boli, there may be activation of other fibers of the facial nerve CN VII, which retract accessory facial muscles (such as risorius, zyomaticus, and quadratus labi superioris), thus allowing greater spread of the lips. Jaw opening is dependent on excitation of some fibers of the mandibular branch of the trigeminal nerve (CN V) resulting in active contraction of the jaw openers (anterior belly of digastric and mylohyoid); this movement is further facilitated by activation of the ansa cervicalis (C1, C2)[1] for contraction of geniohyoid.[2] Jaw opening is dependent on relaxation of the jaw closers (temporalis, masseters) and stabilization of the hyoid bone via contraction of the collective strap muscles through ansa cervicalis (C1, C2).

As the bolus enters the oral cavity, the base of tongue approximates the palate to contain the bolus orally. This is accomplished primarily via excitation of the pharyngeal plexus (CN IX, X), which results in contraction of the palatoglossus muscle. Additional fibers of the facial nerve (CN VII) may result in contraction of stylohyoid and posterior belly of digastric; the hypoglossal nerve (CN XII) also contributes to this movement via innervation and subsequent contraction of the styloglossus. This is an excellent example of redundancy in the neuromuscular system that facilitates airway protection even at this very early stage in the swallowing process.

Bolus acceptance requires excitation of the hypoglossal nerve (CN XII), to activate the intrinsic lingual muscles (verticalis, transverse, and longitundinal) to contour the tongue surface and the extrinsic muscles (genioglossus, hyoglossus, and styloglossus) to change the

---

[1]Discrepancies exist in the published literature on components of the ansa cervicalis. The reader is referred to Chhetri and Berke (1997).

[2]Discrepancies also exist regarding innervation of geniohyoid muscle. The reader is referred to Curtis, Braham, Karr, Holborow, and Worman (1988).

position of the tongue within the oral cavity. These muscles work collectively to groove the tongue with midline drop to collect the bolus. These same neuromuscular substrates consequently elevate the midline to transfer the bolus to the dental surfaces and manipulate the bolus for cohesive formation. Unlike some other biomechanical movement, bolus manipulation is heavily dependent on a single cranial nerve for neural control; all muscles that change the configuration of the lingual surface are innervated by the hypoglossal nerve (CN XII). Lingual position in the oral cavity may be secondarily facilitated by facial nerve (CN VII) innervation of the posterior belly of the digastric and stylohyoid to provide some compensatory function in the event of injury.

The motor tasks described above are completed under the guidance of sensory feedback from the maxillary branch of the trigeminal nerve (CN V) for the palate and teeth, the mandibular branch of the trigeminal (CN V) for the anterior two-thirds of the tongue, the facial nerve (VII) for the soft palate and adjacent pharyngeal wall, and the glossopharyngeal nerve (CN IX) for the posterior one-third of the tongue. This input facilitates immediate changes in lingual contour and position to contain and form a cohesive bolus. This sensory input pairs with taste input that is mediated through activation of sensory fibers of the facial nerve (CN VII) for the anterior two-thirds of the tongue and the glossopharyngeal nerve (CN IX) for the posterior one-third of the tongue and oral cavity. Cumulative oral sensory information transfers either directly from the facial and glossopharyngeal nerves or indirectly from the trigeminal sensory nucleus in the pons to the NTS of the dorsal medulla to contribute to motor planning for the pharyngeal swallow.

Throughout bolus preparation, the base of tongue is relatively more elevated than the tongue tip primarily through activation of the pharyngeal plexus (CN IX, X) that maintains tone in the palatoglossus muscle for glossopalatal approximation. Once the bolus is ready for transfer, the tongue base must drop to allow bolus transfer; this is accomplished passively via terminated activation of pharyngeal plexus for palatoglossal relaxation, paired with excitation of fibers of the hypoglossal nerve (CN XII) for active contraction of the genioglossus and hyoglossus, which pulls the base of tongue inferiorly. As the tongue base drops, the hypoglossal nerve (CN XII) also transmits the command to the collective intrinsic lingual muscles to pull the tip of the tongue to palate and then "squeeze" the bolus from the oral cavity.

Onset of pharyngeal swallow for deglutitive purposes requires three types of input into the NTS: cognitive cortical processing of the food to be ingested via descending corticobulbar pathways, sensory perception of bolus characteristics via trigeminal, facial and glossopharyngeal nerves, and perhaps some component of deep muscle receptor input linked to depression of tongue base for bolus transfer. This information converges on the NTS as a series of graded potentials, which summate until reaching an electrochemical threshold to trigger an action potential, which presents as the pharyngeal swallow. The dorsal nucleus then sends the motor command to the ventral nucleus or the NA for execution. Inconsistency in onset of pharyngeal swallow may represent variable contributions from these three sources of sensory input.

With onset of pharyngeal swallow, many CN and muscles activate in very rapid and overlapping succession to produce the complex movements required for ingestion. Anterior hyoid movement is considered to represent the leading complex of the pharyngeal swallow; velopharyngeal closure is another early event in the pharyngeal swallow. Activation of the pharyngeal plexus (CN IX, X) results in innervation of levator veli palatine to facilitate velopharyngeal closure. Anterior hyoid movement is accomplished via excitation of the trigeminal nerve (CN V) for contraction of the anterior belly of digastric and mylohyoid muscles and the ansa cervicalis (C1, C2) for contraction of the geniohyoid. With the importance of anterior hyoid movement to subsequent biomechanics, the redundancy in neural input is of significance. As the hyoid is pulled forward, there are concomitant forces pulling this bone up and back. The facial nerve (CN VII) activates the posterior belly of the digastric and the stylohyoid. Additionally, the pharyngeal plexus (CN IX, X) initiates activation of the middle pharyngeal constrictor which wraps from a posterior raphe and inserts into the cornu of the hyoid bone to biomechanically pull the hyoid back and up.

A delicate balance must exist between neuromuscular forces acting on the hyoid to allow for anterior movement required for deflection of the epiglottis and opening of the upper esophageal sphincter (UES). As a nonmuscular structure, the epiglottis requires external forces for deflection. As the hyoid moves forward, it effectively pulls the base of the epiglottis anteriorly, thus resulting in a functional deflection. Without this anterior movement, innervated by trigeminal (CN V) and ansa cervicalis (C1, C2), the epiglottis will simply elevate and thus fail to occlude the airway entrance, requiring other mechanisms to protect the airway. Excitation of fibers of ansa cervicalis (C1, C2) also will result in contraction of the anterior strap muscles, particularly thyrohyoid.[3] Both muscle groups result in supraglottic shortening, which consequently allows for compression of the quadrangular membrane over the anterior aspect of the airway entrance, thereby "corking" the laryngeal inlet. Vocal fold adduction via the vagus nerve (CN X) innervating the interarytenoid and cricoarytenoid muscles may have already occurred depending on bolus characteristics. Sensory mechanisms within the pharynx and larynx are critical for airway protection during the swallow and airway clearance immediately afterward. The pharyngeal plexus (CN IX, X) provides sensory innervation to the oropharynx and hypopharynx. The superior laryngeal nerve of the vagus (CN X) receives sensory input from the larynx and trachea, whereas the recurrent laryngeal nerve of the vagus accepts afferent information from the carina, or tracheal bifurcation. Importantly, sensory input from the superior laryngeal nerve transmits not only to the NTS as

---

[3]Thyrohyoid muscle innervation is also inconsistently reported in the literature. Refer to Curtis et al., 1988.

the primary sensory nuclei, but also transfers directly to the NA, the motor nucleus controlling swallowing, in order to facilitate reflexive cough within milliseconds of sensory receptor activation at the larynx. In summary, although the vagus nerve most directly influences the multilayered levels of airway protection, excitation of the trigeminal (CN V) and ansa cervalis (C1, C2) may facilitate closure in the case of impairment.

Bolus transfer through the pharynx is accomplished via contribution from the pharyngeal plexus, hypoglossal, and facial nerves. As the bolus is volitionally transferred into the oropharynx, the hypoglossal nerve innervates the styloglossus muscle to retract and elevate the tongue base. Additional contributions to this movement occur via excitation of the facial nerve (CN VII) for contraction of the stylohyoid and posterior belly of the digastric. The pharyngeal plexus (CN IX, X) innervates the glossopharyngeus muscle, part of the superior pharyngeal constrictor, which pulls the tongue base directly back to the posterior pharyngeal wall for positive pressure on the bolus. These same nerves and muscles contribute to pharyngeal shortening and are further facilitated in this movement by the glossopharyngeal (CN IX) activation of the stylopharyngeus, and pharyngeal plexus activation of the salpingopharyngeus and palatopharyngeus muscles. As the base of tongue to posterior pharyngeal wall movement provides the primary pressure on the descending bolus and the pharynx shortens to bring the UES to meet the oncoming bolus, the pharyngeal plexus innervates the superior, middle, and inferior constrictor muscles sequentially to clear the tail of the bolus from the pharynx.

The rostral branch of the superior laryngeal nerve of the vagus (CN X) maintains a state of excitation at rest which results in tonic contraction of the cricopharyngeus muscle. Bolus transport through the UES requires inhibition of this activation to allow the UES to be pulled open. The trigeminal nerve (CN V) activates the anterior belly of the digastric and mylohyoid, whereas the ansa cervicalis (C1, C2) innervates the geniohyoid to exert the external traction force to open the UES. As all pharyngeal structures are elevating, anterior hyoid movement is critical for opening. As the bolus passes through the UES, the pharyngeal plexus (CN IX, X) innervates the inferior pharyngeal constrictor to squeeze the tail of the bolus into the esophagus.

Postswallow pharyngeal residual is detected in normal swallowing via mucosal sensory receptors that initiate glossopharyngeal nerve fibers (CN IX). This information relays back to the NTS and subsequently results in initiation of a clearing swallow to manage pharyngeal residual.

Although central nervous system structures quite literally provide the brains for swallowing by developing and finely adapting the motor sequence necessary for bolus transfer, efficient function of the peripheral nervous system is required for carrying out that plan. The astute clinician caring for the stroke patient should be fluent in the language and concepts of neuroscience and learn to rely on this information for differential diagnosis.

3 Normal Swallowing Anatomy and Physiology

How does one define normal in the changing landscape of dysphagia research? In early clinical practice in this field, we adhered to a fairly rigorous definition of 'normal swallowing' with little recognition of the innate variance in the normal deglutitive process. However, it is important to recognize that as our knowledge base expands rapidly, definitions of normal will expand as well. We have greater information available to us that is described in subsequent sections, including changes in swallowing that occur as a function of the healthy aging process, as well as variations of swallowing in healthy adults due to other factors. Data regarding these factors, including consistency of bolus and type of swallowing (single versus sequential) are addressed. These differences from the perceived norm do not represent pathology, but rather the expected adaptation of a complex physiologic system to accommodate a variety of processes. Therefore, the clinician should be cautious not to base diagnosis on an inflexible definition of impairment and consequently overdiagnose.

The clinician also should be careful not to underdiagnose impairment. Although identification of aspiration risk is critical, this cannot be the only basis for determining impairment. One can have significant dysphagia without aspiration. Avoiding pulmonary compromise in the short term is an obvious and indisputable goal, but consideration must be given to long-term outcomes. Failing to recognize seemingly benign pathophysiology may ultimately result in the development of a more consequential impairment over the long term. Both short-term and long-term objectives for intervention should be addressed.

So again, how do we define normal? At a minimum, one could argue that "safe and efficient swallowing" is a workable definition of normal with "unsafe and inefficient swallowing" defining abnormal. But this leads to the inevitable questions of: How do you define safe and unsafe? How do you define efficient and inefficient? These definitions may be shaped by the overall health and history of the patient, their perception of disability, overall quality of life, risks associated with variance in swallowing, the type of diagnostic data collected, and the clinician's knowledge of normal. Additionally, our definition is limited or biased by the instrumentation we use for diagnosis. As availability of techniques expands, our understanding of swallowing will expand for greater diagnostic specificity. In the interim, the best one can do is to evaluate the documented range of behaviors in physiology and apply this to individual patients with all of their complexities.

An understanding of the fundamentals of swallowing is prerequisite for defining normal and abnormal swallowing. Following is a synopsis of our current understanding of normal swallowing physiology.

PHASES OF SWALLOWING

Swallowing is generally conceptualized as occurring in several distinct phases. Although these phases facilitate a common vocabulary and framework for discussion and definition, the clinician must realize that division by phase is an artificial construct. Swallowing is a continuous process with substantive interdependencies between features across the system. Isolating these features, without consideration of other influences, may lead the clinician to misdiagnose. As an example, patients with impaired cricopharyngeal opening may not have a primary abnormality of the upper esophageal sphincter (UES); rather, they may have substantial gastroesophageal reflux that impacts pharyngeal bolus transport. Thus, by limiting focus to the symptomatic phase, the true source of the pathology can be overlooked and, thus, treatment will be ineffective. However, for purposes of discussion, the delineation of phases certainly facilitates understanding. The three-phase model of oral, pharyngeal, and esophageal is more traditional; however, a more inclusive model which incorporates a preoral phase is used as a scaffolding to discuss normal and abnormal swallowing. Given the potential impairment of cognition and attention in stroke, the recognition of preparatory behaviors is considered essential.

Preoral Phase

Current models of dysphagia consider only the movement of the bolus through the aerodigestive tract. Using this traditional model, external influences such as attention, eating behavior, and feeding method, which may impact swallowing efficiency and safety, are not considered. A model of ingestion that considers both preswallowing and swallowing behavior has been proposed as a strong interaction between each has been suggested, particularly in neurogenic populations (Leopold & Kagel, 1997). Given the importance of supratentorial modulation of pharyngeal biomechanics, a failure in the preoral phase may have substantial consequences for pharyngeal swallowing efficiency. Consider the patient with right hemisphere damage who presents with reduced attention and impulsivity. As discussed, under certain conditions, airway protection may be initiated before the bolus enters the oral cavity. Thus, inattention may engender delayed airway protection. Additionally, the patient may not monitor rate of ingestion or amount delivered to the oral cavity; moreover, this patient may not be aware of deficits. Thus, these apparent cognitive deficits that affect preoral phase components can significantly impact swallowing events downstream. Furthermore, factors that may be manipulated in the preoral phase, such as cued versus non-cued swallow and sequential versus single swallow may modify swallowing.

Oral Phase

The oral phase begins once food or liquid enters the oral cavity. As the bolus is delivered into the oral cavity, the lips close anteriorly and the tongue contacts the velum to form a seal posteriorly to contain the bolus and prevent bolus loss. For boli of increased consistency, oral preparation is initiated to achieve an acceptable consistency for swallowing. This involves mixing the bolus with saliva during rotary and lateral jaw movement as well as rotary and lateral tongue movement. Preparation concludes when a bolus suitable for oral transfer is formed on the tongue.

Two events related to respiration frequently occur prior to onset of oral transfer and often with bolus loading: (1) apnea onset (Hiss, Strauss, Treole, Stuart, & Boutilier, 2004; Martin-Harris et al., 2005) and (2) approximation of the vocal folds and arytenoid cartilages (Ohmae, Logemann, Kaiser, Hanson, & Kahrilas, 1995; Shaker, Dodds, Dantas, Hogan, & Arndorfer, 1990). Although the specific onset of these events is highly variable, they are among the initial events to occur with swallowing.

Oral transfer generally is initiated by posterior lingual movement squeezing the bolus against the palate. Coordinated bolus transfer is critical for normal initiation and execution of pharyngeal events. The oral phase concludes when the bolus head reaches any point between the anterior faucial arch and the ramus of the mandible. Duration of the oral stage is dependent on determination of the starting point (bolus versus tongue movement, bolus head versus bolus tail) and identification of the endpoint (faucial pillar versus ramus of the mandible). However, duration of oral transfer is generally less than 1 second regardless of parameters measured.

During mastication numerous episodes of bolus preparation, that is, mastication, and transfer to the oropharynx, may occur prior to elicitation of the pharyngeal swallow (Dua, Ren, Bardan, Xie, & Shaker, 1997; Hiiemae & Palmer, 1999; Palmer, Rudin, Lara, & Crompton, 1992). Additionally, a liquid bolus may accumulate in the hypophaynx prior to onset of the pharyngeal swallow during sequential drinking (Chi-Fishman & Sonies, 2000; Daniels & Foundas, 2001). That is, during sequential swallowing via a cup or straw, lingual propulsion of the liquid may occur multiple times until a pharyngeal swallow is elicited. The accumulation of liquid in the pharynx during sequential swallowing may occur with the larynx lowered and epiglottis upright or with the larynx partially elevated and epiglottis inverted (Daniels & Foundas, 2001).

Pharyngeal Phase

Transition from the oral phase to the pharyngeal phase of swallowing occurs with elicitation of the pharyngeal swallow. Onset of the pharyngeal phase of swallowing is hallmarked by maximum hyolaryngeal excursion. Initiation of maximum excursion generally occurs when the bolus head is located between the anterior faucial arch and ramus of the mandible. Continued research is expanding our traditional notion of bolus location at swallow onset. As discussed earlier, as the bolus is processed during mastication, a portion of it is propelled into the valleculae until processing of the remaining material is completed at which point, the pharyngeal swallow is elicited (Dua et al., 1997; Hiiemae & Palmer, 1999; Palmer et al., 1992). Furthermore, during sequential swallowing of liquids either from a cup or straw, the bolus is frequently propelled to the hypopharynx prior to onset of the pharyngeal swallow (Chi-Fishman &

Sonies, 2000; Daniels et al., 2004; Daniels & Foundas, 2001). More recent research also is revealing considerable variability within and across individuals in bolus positioning of single liquid volumes at onset of the pharyngeal swallow (Martin-Harris, Brodsky, Michel, Lee, & Walters, 2007; Stephen, Taves, Smith, & Martin, 2005). It is not atypical to have the bolus inferior to the ramus of the mandible at onset of the pharyngeal swallow, particularly in healthy older adults. This more inferior location of the bolus at onset of the pharyngeal swallow is not associated with airway invasion in healthy adults.

The pharyngeal stage of swallowing involves the complex coordination of six components: (1) velopharyngeal closure, (2) laryngeal closure, (3) hyoid and laryngeal elevation, (4) UES opening, (5) base of tongue retraction, and (6) posterior pharyngeal wall contraction. The temporal coupling of these events in coordination with cessation of breathing is critical for a safe and efficient swallow (Figure 3–1).

Velopharyngeal closure involves retraction of the soft palate, medial movement of the pharyngeal wall, and anterior bulging of the adenoid pad. This closure provides a seal between the nasopharynx and oropharynx and contributes to the increase in pharyngeal pressure (Perlman, Schultz, & VanDaele, 1993).

Laryngeal valving involves multiple levels, from inferior to superior: true vocal folds, false vocal folds, arytenoids, aryepiglottic folds, and epiglottis. Although onset of glottic closure is one of the first events of swallowing (Ohmae et al., 1995; Shaker et al., 1990), complete true vocal fold (TVF) adduction along the entire length of the fold does not occur until after onset of laryngeal elevation (Ohmae et al., 1995). Entry of material into the pharynx during normal mastication or with pharyngeal water injection in an experimental paradigm is associated with brief partial TVF adduction, which is known as a pharyngoglottal closure reflex (Dua et al., 1997; Shaker et al., 2003). It is suggested that this reflex is preventive of preswallow aspiration.

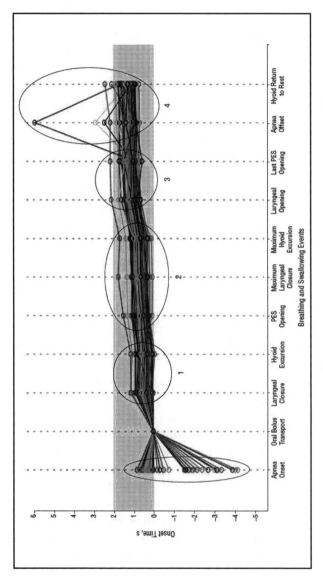

Figure 3–1. Temporal coordination of swallowing events and apnea. From "Breathing and Swallowing Dynamics Across the Adult Lifespan," by B. Martin-Harris, M. B. Brodsky, Y. Michel, C. L. Ford, B. Walters, and J. Heffner, 2005, *Archives of Otolaryngology-Head and Neck Surgery, 131,* p. 766. Copyright © 2005 by American Medical Association. All rights reserved. Reprinted with permission. PES = pharyngoesophageal segment.

Superior and anterior movement of the hyoid bone and the larynx is achieved through contraction of the suprahyoid muscles and the thyrohyoid muscle. Superior and anterior movement of the hyoid and larynx occurs due to the suprahyoid muscles (anterior belly of the digastric, mylohyoid, posterior belly of the digastric, stylohyoid, and geniohyoid). The superior movement of the hyolaryngeal complex facilitates supraglottic closure, and the anterior motion contributes to the opening of the UES (Jacob, Kahrilas, Logemann, Shah, & Ha, 1989).

Opening of the UES requires relaxation of cricopharyngeus muscle (a naturally tonic muscle) and sphincter opening from anterior movement of the hyolaryngeal complex. Bolus pressure contributes to obtaining the maximum sphincter diameter (Cook, 1993). When contracted, the cricopharyngeus muscle prevents passage of air into the stomach and prevents flow of esophageal contents from passing into the pharynx.

Base of tongue contact with the posterior pharyngeal wall is critical to create the dynamic pressure necessary to drive the bolus inferiorly through the pharynx (Cerenko, McConnel, & Jackson, 1989; McConnel, 1988). As the tongue propels the bolus into the pharynx and the tongue base makes contact with the posterior pharyngeal wall, contraction of the pharyngeal constrictors occurs superiorly to inferiorly. This descending sequence aids in clearing pharyngeal residue but minimally facilitates bolus propulsion (Kahrilas, Logemann, Lin, & Ergun, 1992). Base of tongue retraction involves continued posterior movement after passage of the bolus until the tongue base contacts the posterior pharyngeal wall. Bulging of the anterior pharyngeal constrictor contributes to muscular contact. Base of tongue contact with the posterior pharyngeal wall yields a buildup of pressure to drive the bolus through the pharynx. Pharyngeal contraction involves two processes: (1) pharyngeal shortening, which decreases the distance the bolus must travel and modifies pharyngeal recesses to prevent residualand and (2) pharyngeal constrictor contraction which progresses superiorly to inferiorly.

As with oral duration, there are varying reference points used to mark onset and offset of pharyngeal transfer. For onset, the points of measure include arrival of the bolus head at the ramus of the mandible (Robbins, Hamilton, Lof, & Kempster, 1992) or arrival of the bolus tail at the posterior tonsillar pillar (Shaw et al., 1995). For offset, measurement points may include passage of the bolus tail through the UES (Robbins et al., 1992) or UES closure (Shaw et al., 1995). Regardless of measure used, duration of movement of the bolus through the pharynx is approximately one second.

Breathing and swallowing are structurally linked via the oropharynx. Coordination of breathing and swallowing is exquisitely timed to prevent aspiration. Apnea, or cessation of respiration, occurs during swallowing. The onset of apnea is highly variable. As noted earlier, the onset of apnea frequently occurs prior to onset of oral transfer. If it does not occur prior to bolus transfer, it is suggested that apnea should occur at onset of transfer or immediately following (Hiss et al., 2004). Resumption of respiration is more specific occurring with lowering of the hyoid (Martin-Harris et al., 2005). Expiration preceding and following swallowing is the predominant respiratory phase pattern in healthy individuals (Hiss et al., 2004; Martin-Harris et al., 2005). Whereas inspiration after swallowing rarely occurs in healthy adults, inspiration prior to swallowing may occur in 10% to 20% of swallows (Martin-Harris et al., 2005; Perlman, He, Barkmeier, & Van Leer, 2005).

Esophageal Phase

The esophagus is bounded by the UES superiorly and the lower esophageal sphincter inferiorly. Both of these sphincters are actively contracted at rest but relax during swallowing, belching, and vomiting. This contracted resting state prevents retrograde flow of material into the upper aerodigestive tract. The upper one-third of the esophagus is composed of striated muscle and the lower two-thirds composed of smooth muscle. The esophageal phase of swallowing involves a sequential peristaltic wave that propels food and liquid into the stomach. Normal transit time varies between 8 to 20 seconds (Dodds, Hogan, Reid, Stewart, & Arndorfer, 1973).

Variability in Swallowing

Although specific events for normal swallowing are described above there is considerable variability in the system associated with intrinsic (e.g., aging) and extrinsic (e.g., bolus volume) factors. The influences of specific factors on normal swallowing are summarized in Table 3–1.

Table 3–1. The Influence of Intrinsic and Extrinsic Variables on Swallowing in Healthy Adults

Increased Age

- Increased oral transit time (Cook et al., 1994; Shaw et al., 1995)
- Increased stage transition duration (Logemann et al., 2000; Robbins et al., 1992; Tracy et al., 1989)
- Increased volume required to evoke a pharyngeal swallow (Shaker et al., 1994)
- Increased airway invasion (Daggett, Logemann, Rademaker, & Pauloski, 2006; Daniels et al., 2004)
- Increased pharyngeal residue (Cook et al., 1994)
- Decreased isometric tongue pressure (Robbins, Levine, Wood, Roecker, & Luschei, 1995)
- Decreased onset of submental contraction (Ding, Logemann, Larson, & Rademaker, 2003)
- Decreased extent of hyoid movement (Kern et al., 1999; Logemann et al., 2000)
- Decreased pharyngeal and laryngeal sensation (Aviv et al., 1994)
- Reduced pharyngeal contraction (Tracy et al., 1989)
- Delayed onset of UES relaxation (Shaw et al., 1995)

Table 3–1. *continued*

- Increased intrabolus pressure (Kern et al., 1999; Shaw et al., 1995)
- Increased duration of UES opening (Rademaker, Pauloski, Colangelo, & Logemann, 1998; Robbins et al., 1992)
- Decreased diameter of UES opening (Logemann et al., 2000; Shaw et al., 1995; Tracy et al., 1989)
- Increased duration of swallowing apnea (Hiss, Treole, & Stuart, 2001)
- Increased incidence of inhalation after swallowing (Martin-Harris et al., 2005)

Increased Volume

- Bolus held more posteriorly in the oral cavity (Tracy et al., 1989)
- Decreased oral transit time (Rademaker et al., 1998; Tracy et al., 1989)
- Decreased stage transition duration (Rademaker et al., 1998)
- Earlier onset of palatal elevation (Dantas et al., 1990)
- Increased duration of velopharyngeal closure (Rademaker et al., 1998)
- Earlier onset of anterior tongue base movement (Dantas et al., 1990)
- Earlier onset of laryngeal elevation (Dantas et al., 1990)
- Increased extent of hyoid movement (Dodds et al., 1988; Logemann et al., 2000)
- Increased duration of laryngeal closure (Logemann et al., 1992)
- Increased intrabolus pressure (Jacob et al., 1989; Kern et al., 1999)
- Earlier onset of UES opening (Cook et al., 1989; Dantas et al., 1990)
- Increased diameter of UES opening (Dantas et al., 1990)
- Increased duration of UES opening (Dantas et al., 1990; Rademaker et al., 1998; Tracy et al., 1989)
- Earlier onset of swallowing apnea (Hiss et al., 2004)
- Increased duration of swallowing apnea (Hiss et al., 2001)

Increased Consistency

- Increased oral transit time (Dantas et al., 1990)
- Increased stage transition duration (Robbins et al., 1992)
- Increased oral pressure (Pouderoux & Kahrilas, 1995; Shaker, Cook, Dodds, & Hogan, 1988)
- Increased amplitude and duration of contraction of the inferior orbicularis oris, submental, and infrahyoid muscles (Ding et al., 2003)

continues

Table 3–1. *continued*

- Increased duration of velar excursion (Robbins et al., 1992)
- Increased laryngeal elevation (Shaker et al., 1990)
- Increased duration pharyngeal contraction (Dantas et al., 1990)
- Increased duration of UES opening (Dantas et al., 1990)
- Later onset of swallowing apnea (Hiss et al., 2004)

Taste

- Increased tongue pressure (Pelletier & Dhanaraj, 2006)
- Earlier onset of submental and infrahyoid contraction (Ding et al., 2003)
- Increased submental amplitude (Ding et al., 2003)
- Increased pharyngeal pressure (Palmer, McCulloch, Jaffe, & Neel, 2005)
- Reduced swallowing speed (volume swallowed per second) (Chee, Arshad, Singh, Mistry, & Hamdy, 2005)
- Increased number of swallows to drink 50 ml (Chee et al., 2005)

Sequential Swallowing (as compared to single swallows)

- Decreased oral transit time (Chi-Fishman & Sonies, 2000)
- Increased stage transition duration (Chi-Fishman & Sonies, 2000)
- Decreased duration of UES opening (Chi-Fishman & Sonies, 2000)
- Repetitive activation and partial deactivation of surface electromyographic waveform patterns (Chi-Fishman & Sonies, 2000)
- Reduced amplitude and velocity of hyoid movement (Chi-Fishman & Sonies, 2002)
- Two patterns of HLC movement: lowering of the HLC with the epiglottis returning to upright between swallows; partial HLC elevation with continued epiglottic inversion between swallows (Daniels et al., 2004; Daniels & Foundas, 2001)

Cued Swallows (as compared to noncued)

- Bolus held more posteriorly in oral cavity (Daniels, Schroeder, DeGeorge, Corey, & Rosenbek, 2007)
- Decreased oral transit time (Daniels et al., 2007)
- Decreased stage transition duration (Daniels et al., 2007)

HLC = hyolaryngeal complex; UES = upper esophageal sphincter.

4 The Clinical Swallowing Examination

History and Patient Interview

As discussed in Chapter 1, the incidence of dysphagia in stroke is substantial. This paired with the fact that there is no clear association between site of lesion and dysphagia presentation makes assessment of all patients with acute stroke a mandate. The clinical swallowing examination (CSE) is the first step in evaluating all stroke patients. We hesitate to call this evaluation a "screening," as connotations emerge of a cursory, minimalist assessment. However, in practice, a thorough CSE is a type of screening. It is not diagnostic in nature (i.e., pathophysiology cannot be defined), but the information gleaned from the CSE will clearly contribute to the ultimate diagnosis of the patient when paired with more specific information. The instrumental examination provides detailed information about biomechanics and ultimately pathophysiology. Data from this detailed assessment are integrated with clinical observation and history and are used to develop a comprehensive and efficacious management approach.

PATIENT HISTORY

Medical history ideally is obtained from the patient's medical records prior to the CSE. Information obtained from the medical history may help guide the patient interview. If access to the patient's medical record is not available, the clinician should ascertain history information during the interview. For hospitalized patients, the medical chart review may be more detailed, particularly if the patient has had a protracted medical course. For inpatients, the clinician should begin with the history and physical report from the neurologist, whereas for outpatients, the clinician should begin with the note from the referring physician. Stroke onset, characteristics, and complications associated with stroke (if patient has been in the hospital for a period of time prior to consultation) should be noted. Subsequent notes that may relate to the underlying dysphagia process should be reviewed. Moreover, if the patient has a history of dysphagia, any available swallowing evaluation and treatment notes should be reviewed. Table 4-1 provides a focus for medical chart review. Numerous medications can negatively affect swallowing. Specific medications and their effects are too numerous to detail in this book. The interested reader may refer to Carl and Johnson (2006) or other pharmaceutical references for detailed information on this topic.

PATIENT AND FAMILY INTERVIEW

After review of the medical chart and prior to beginning the actual patient assessment, an interview with the patient or family should be obtained to determine specific complaints concerning swallowing. The depth of the interview is dependent on the acuteness of stroke, patients' responsiveness, and awareness of deficit. Patients seen in a rehabilitation or outpatient setting will generally warrant a lengthier interview than patients admitted with an acute stroke. For those stroke patients who are seen in outpatient settings but who have limited communication, it is advisable that they be accompanied by a caregiver who can provide information concerning swallowing.

During the initial swallowing evaluation, particularly for patients admitted to the acute care setting, the initial question may be "Are you having any problems with your swallowing?" If the patient indi-

Table 4–1. Medical Chart Review

- Diseases associated with dysphagia—with each note if dysphagia was identified
  - Prior history of stroke (note residual deficits)
  - Other neurologic diseases (e.g., Parkinson's disease, myasthenia gravis)
  - Head and neck cancer with radiation

- Surgeries associated with dysphagia—with each note if dysphagia was identified
  - Head and neck resection
  - Anterior cervical spine fusion
  - Carotid endarterectomy

- Pulmonary status
  - Current or prior sustained intubation or tracheostomy tube placement
  - Chronic pulmonary obstructive disease
  - Aspiration pneumonia

- Current nutritional intake
  - Nothing by mouth (NPO)—awaiting swallowing evaluation
  - Nasogastric tube (NGT)
  - Percutaneous endoscopic gastrostomy (PEG) tube
  - Intravenous fluids
  - Total parenteral nutrition (TPN)

- Medications that may affect swallowing
  - Functional status prior to hospitalization
  - Independent and active
  - Required assistance
  - Totally dependent
  - Bed bound

cates "No", the clinician should probe further with questions such as, "Do you cough or choke when eating or drinking?" If the answer remains "No", proceed with the rest of the CSE. It is important that the clinician not equate lack of acknowledgement of a swallowing deficit with no dysphagia, particularly in acute stroke patients. Silent aspiration has been identified in 67% of stroke patients who aspirated during the instrumental swallowing evaluation (Daniels et al., 1998). Furthermore, fewer than one-half of acute stroke patients are aware of dysphagia symptoms, for example, coughing, drooling (Parker et al., 2004). Even if acute stroke patients are diagnosed with dysphagia and are aware of symptoms, the majority of patients do not acknowledge having a "swallowing problem" (Parker et al., 2004).

If the stroke patient acknowledges dysphagia or is seeking consultation for a swallowing problem, the initial question may be "Tell me about your swallowing problem." If the patient has adequate communication skills, questions should initially be open-ended. By using open-ended questioning, the clinician will not be directing the patient's response. If communication is impaired or responses are vague, the clinician should ask more direct questions or questions requiring a yes/no response. Table 4–2 provides questions that may be asked during the patient or family interview.

If the clinician is seeing a patient with an acute stroke, but the patient has a history of prior strokes, questioning should attempt to determine a prior history of dysphagia. If the patient confirms previous dysphagia, the clinician will want to clarify if swallowing has changed. Additionally, for patients with a history of stroke and dysphagia it is important to determine if the patient has undergone previous evaluation and treatment for dysphagia. If the evaluation and treatment reports are not available at the initial interview, the clinician should attempt to discern from the patient the type of evaluation, findings from assessment, type of treatment, and progress made in treatment. If the patient previously was discharged from treatment, attempt to determine the reason why, for example, plateau in progress, or discharge from the medical facility. It is important to determine if the patient thinks swallowing has changed since discontinuation of prior treatment, particularly if there has been an extended length of time since treatment was terminated. The clini-

Table 4–2. Specific Questions Concerning Swallowing Ability

- When did your swallowing problem begin?
- Did it begin abruptly or gradually?
- Has your swallowing gotten better, worse, or remained the same?
- How often do you notice your swallowing problem?
  - Specific time of day?
  - Consistently? Intermittently?
- Does it hurt when you swallow?
  - Where?
  - Point to the exact spot where you feel pain
- Do you have problems swallowing a specific type or consistency of food?
  - What happens when you swallow this type of food/liquid?
- Do you cough or choke after swallowing?
- Does food get stuck?
  - Where?
  - Point to the exact spot where it gets stuck
- Do you avoid certain foods/liquids due to your swallowing problem?
  - What are these foods/liquids?
- Have you lost or gained weight since your swallowing problem began?
  - How much?
- Do you do anything that helps your swallowing?

cian may benefit by obtaining written consent from the patient to obtain the previous swallowing evaluation and treatment reports.

Upon completion of questioning, the clinician should have an idea of onset of symptoms, progression or resolution of deficits, characteristics of dysphagia, and food type associated with dysphagia.

The information obtained from the interview may identify specific areas on which to focus during the clinical and instrumental evaluations. For example, a patient's complaint of right-sided postswallow residual will alert the clinician to watch for this during the instrumental examination.

Improving quality of life is of equal importance as a goal of dysphagia management as is rehabilitating physiologic dysfunction. Thus, determining the impact of dysphagia on the patient's quality of life is important to obtain during the patient and family interview. The SWAL-QOL (McHorney et al., 2002) is a standardized 44-item questionnaire designed to measure a patient's perception of quality of life attributable to dysphagia. The questionnaire covers 10 categories (burden, eating duration, eating desire, symptom frequency, food selection, communication, mental health, social, fatigue, and sleep) and requires approximately 15 minutes to complete. Research has shown a modest relationship between the SWAL-QOL ratings (McHorney, Martin-Harris, Robbins, & Rosenbek, 2006) and bolus flow measures of oral and pharyngeal transit time and airway invasion. This suggests that the SWAL-QOL contributes unique information about dysphagia, which may be important both diagnostically and therapeutically. Administration of a questionnaire such as the SWAL-QOL prior to and during the course of therapy will allow the clinician to document the effect of improved swallowing on a person's quality of life. Documenting improved quality of life is as significant as documenting changes in swallowing biomechanics and may facilitate reimbursement from third-party payers.

5 The Clinical Swallowing Examination

Cognition and Communication Assessments

Evaluation of cognitive, speech, voice, language, and praxis status is important in stroke patients as function in these areas may have significant impact on the evaluation and treatment of swallowing disorders. The level to which a patient's cognition and communication are impaired depends on the location and extent of the stroke. A patient with right hemisphere damage (RHD) or a parietal or prefrontal stroke is more likely to present with cognitive impairment than a patient with an occipital stroke. Likewise, a patient with left hemisphere damage (LHD) is more likely to have aphasia than a person with RHD. A large vessel stroke is more likely to impair cognition and communication versus a single lacunar infarct. Hence, knowledge of the stroke location will provide the clinician with an idea of the levels to which cognition and communication may be impaired.

The depth of the evaluation is dependent on the cognitive-communication functioning of the patient; however, the impact of these processes on swallowing may require only a brief screening. Greater diagnostic exploration would be required to fully determine the magnitude of deficits and treatment strategies. At minimum, a screening of cognition and communication should be completed during the initial evaluation of all acute stroke inpatients. The level of cognitive and auditory comprehension deficits will impact the degree to which the remaining portion of the clinical swallowing examination (CSE) can be pursued, so screening of these functions should be completed first. Table 5–1 details cognitive and communication processes that are generally evaluated as part of the CSE in stroke patients.

Table 5–1. Evaluation of Cognition and Communication

Cognitive and Communication Processes	How to Evaluate
Cognition	
Attention	—Digit span—Repeating digits of increasing length
	—Vigilance-Patient signals (hand raise, finger tap) every time a target letter (e.g., "s") is verbalized in a series of randomly presented letters. The target letter is presented with greater than random frequency.
Sensory Neglect	
Visual	With the patient looking straight ahead, present visual stimulus (e.g., finger movement) to each visual field. The patient may report the side of stimulation either verbally or nonverbally.
Tactile	With the patient's eyes closed, touch the patient lightly with finger tip or cotton-tipped applicator.
Auditory	With the patient's eyes closed, snap fingers by each ear.
Simultaneous	Bilateral stimulation (visual, tactile, auditory) to both sides of the body is interspersed with unilateral stimuli.
Spatial Neglect	
Cancellation	Stimuli are randomly positioned on a page. The patient is asked to cross out all of the stimuli. Stimuli may consist of lines, a specific letter interspersed with other letters.
Line Bisection	A single line is drawn on unlined paper and the patient is asked to divide a line into two equal halves. Lines should vary in length.
Drawing— spontaneous, copy	On unlined paper, patients are asked to draw (and then copy) figures such as a clock, man, flower, and/or house.
Awareness of Deficits	Ask patient about reason for hospitalization, deficits, etc.
Memory	—Orientation—person, place, time
	—Short-term memory—forward digit repetition of increasing length. Digit backward challenges cognitive processes in addition to memory.

Table 5–1. *continued*

Cognitive and Communication Processes	How to Evaluate
Memory *continued*	—Remote memory—recall of personal information such as family information and occupation, historical facts such as current president, presidents in life time.
	—New learning—patient learns a set of 3–4 words and recalls them after delays of 1, 5, and 10 minutes.

Communication

Language	
Auditory Comprehension	—Yes/no questions—related to self, "Do you live in New Orleans?" and unrelated questions "Do you wear shoes on your hands?"
	—Patient follows single step and multiple step commands.
Verbal Expression	—Confrontation naming—high frequency (pencil), low frequency (eraser)
	—Responsive naming—"What do you wear on your feet?"
	—Repetition of words and sentences
	—Conversational speech
Speech	—Conversational speech
	—Repetition of single and multisyllabic words and nonwords; challenge patient to increase speed if possible
Voice	—Conversational speech
	—Maximum phonation time-patient takes a deep breath and says "ah" for long as possible. Clinician measures duration with a stopwatch.

Other

Buccofacial apraxia	Patient performs various meaningful respiratory and nonrespiratory gestures. Respiratory—"Show how you would blow out a candle," Nonrespiratory—"Show how you would lick milk off your top lip"
Limb apraxia	Patient performs gestures with unaffected upper extremity. Transitive—"Show how you use a key to unlock a door" Intransitive—"Show how you wave goodbye"

THE COGNITIVE ASSESSMENT

Executing the Cognitive Assessment

Several aspects of cognition may impact swallowing and thus require at a minimum a brief screening. These areas of cognition include:

- Level of Consciousness
- Attention
  - Focus/Concentration
  - Neglect
    - Sensory Neglect (Inattention)
    - Motor Neglect (Intention)
    - Spatial Neglect
    - Awareness of Deficits
- Memory

There are five principal levels of consciousness: alert, lethargy, obtunded, stupor/semicoma, and coma (Strub & Black, 2000). Each level is described in Table 5–2. The alert patient is awake and interactive when the clinician enters the room. If asleep, the alert patient readily arouses with verbal or light tactile stimulation and easily maintains interaction with the clinician. If the patient is asleep and does not easily awaken, the volume of verbal stimulation and the vigor of tactile stimulation should be increased. If the patient demonstrates lethargy or a lower level of consciousness, it is important to determine the patient's baseline by conferring with medical staff. It may be that the patient slept poorly the previous night or has been sedated. If possible, determine the optimum time of alertness and proceed with the CSE at that time.

After establishing level of consciousness and determining that the patient is alert enough to pursue further evaluation, attention should be addressed. In addition to assessing basic focus to task and

Table 5–2. Levels of Consciousness

Level of Consciousness	Response
Alert	The patient is awake, fully aware of stimuli, and interactive. If totally paralyzed, interaction can be established with eye contact and eye movement.
Lethargy	The patient requires constant stimulation to maintain wakefulness. Attention is reduced even if eyes are open. Impaired cognitive performance should be interpreted with caution.
Obtunded	This is a transitional state between lethargy and stupor. The patient is difficult to arouse and cannot maintain alertness even with constant stimulation. The patient is confused when aroused.
Stupor/Semicoma	The patient responds only to persistent and vigorous stimulation. When aroused, the patient responds with groaning or mumbling.
Coma	The patient is completely unarousable.

vigilance, the clinician should evaluate the stroke patient for neglect. Assessment of basic attentional processes can be done through general observation during testing and identifying distractibility or difficulty focusing on the clinician.

Neglect is defined as failure to respond or orient to stimuli presented to the contralesional side in the presence of intact elemental sensory and motor functioning (Heilman, Watson, & Valenstein, 2003). Neglect may be evident by sensory inattention, motor neglect (intentional disorders), spatial neglect, and/or unawareness of deficits. Sensory inattention and unawareness of deficits may have a greater impact on swallowing as compared to other aspects of neglect. The clinician, therefore, may focus primarily on these aspects of neglect during the CSE and rely on further testing during expanded cognitive evaluation or results of the neurologic evaluation to determine the full range of neglect.

Inattention refers to unawareness of sensory stimuli presented to the contralesional side and generally is tested in three modalities: visual, auditory, and tactile. The patient verbalizes (or points if verbal language is impaired) the location and side stimulated. For example, standing behind the patient, the clinician presents auditory stimuli (finger snapping) by the patient's left ear. The patient would in turn raise his left hand. If the patient accurately responds to unilateral sensory stimulation, bilateral simultaneous stimulation in each modality can be used to further challenge the patient. Patients with extinction to simultaneous stimulation will fail to respond to the contralesional stimuli.

Motor neglect refers to failure to initiate movement in the presence of awareness of a stimuli and intact strength. Intentional disorders may present as akinesia, motor extinction, hypokinesia, and motor impersistence. Evaluation of motor neglect is generally completed by the neurologist, but the interested clinician may refer to Heilman et al. (2003) for details concerning examination of motor intentional disorders.

Spatial neglect refers to omission of contralesional hemispace when performing tasks. Patients with spatial neglect may fail to draw portions of a picture that are in the contralesional hemisphere or when asked to bisect a line into two equal halves, they may quarter it. Spatial neglect may be evaluated with numerous tasks such as cancellation, line bisection, and drawing—both spontaneously and to copy. During cancellation tasks, patients with spatial neglect will fail to cross out stimuli on the contralesional side of the paper. With line bisection, patients with neglect will place their mark to the ipsilesional side of the line. Longer lines will yield a more pronounced deviation from center. During drawing, a patient with neglect may omit half of the figure on the contralesional side.

Determination of awareness of deficits can be assessed by asking patients why they are in the hospital or for outpatients, what deficits they are experiencing since the stroke. Evidence of anisodiophoria or anosognosia should be noted. Anisodiophoria refers to the patient who is aware of deficits but unconcerned by them. Anosognosia refers to the patient who is unaware of deficits or denies them.

As with attention, memory may be assessed informally with brief tasks. Short-term recall, remote memory, and new learning each should be examined as all can have a significant impact on the evaluation and management of swallowing disorders.

Interpreting the Cognitive Assessment

Level of consciousness will dictate if the rest of the cognitive assessment as well as the remainder of the CSE can be pursued. If patients cannot maintain alertness for a sustained period without rearousal, for example, 5 minutes, postponement of the swallowing evaluation should be considered.

Deficits in cognition not only have significance for the instrumental evaluation and treatment but also for eating and nutritional intake. If the patient cannot attend to task, completing rehabilitation protocols may prove challenging as the clinician must constantly redirect the patient to task. Likewise, if a chin tuck posture is found to reduce airway invasion, but the patient cannot remember to employ this compensatory strategy, it is of little benefit. Many management approaches, such as super supraglottic swallow have multiple and temporally specific levels of instruction that the patient must recall to correctly implement; therefore, intact memory is critical to swallowing treatment. Visual inattention impacts eating and swallowing in that the patient may not be aware of food in contralesional visual field, thus eating only part of the meal and thereby decreasing nutritional intake. Tactile inattention may result in a patient with food remaining in the contralesional lateral sulcus even though sensation is intact.

Although it seems intuitive to the clinician working with stroke patients that cognitive impairments may impact eating and swallowing, little research in this area has been conducted. Results from a recent study suggest that stroke patients who have poor awareness of their dysphagic symptoms do not modify swallowing behavior, whereas patients who are aware of their dysphagia modify rate and volume of ingestion (Parker et al., 2004). In this study, it also was noted that patients with poor awareness developed more medical complications at three months postonset as compared to the group with good awareness of dysphagia symptoms. Another current study found spatial neglect to be associated with initial nonoral intake in acute stroke patients (Schroeder, Daniels, McClain, Corey, & Foundas, 2006). It may be that patients with RHD or LHD present with similar swallowing pathophysiology, but patients with cognitive deficits, for example, neglect, inattention, or anosognosia pose a greater risk of aspiration. This may lead the clinician to suggest restricted intake or eventually may lead to increased morbidity and mortality. Moreover, these patients may be more difficult to rehabilitate as a result of their cognitive deficits. Further research is warranted to determine the relationship between cognitive dysfunction, dysphagia, and recovery of swallowing function.

THE COMMUNICATION ASSESSMENT

Executing the Communication Assessment

Language, speech, and voice may be assessed in a general fashion. Evaluation procedures are discussed in Table 5–1. Language should be assessed for the presence of aphasia. Speech and voice should be assessed for the presence of dysarthria, apraxia of speech, and dysphonia. Articulation, vocal quality, pitch, resonance, intensity, prosody, and overall intelligibility should be detailed. The type of dysarthria, for example, spastic, flaccid, should be identified. The interested reader is referred to Duffy (2005) concerning the differential diagnosis of dysarthria. Vocal quality should be reported in terms of hoarse, strained, wet, or hypophonic.

Preoral behavior such as self-feeding may affect swallowing, particularly in stroke patients (see Chapter 3 for review), but this has not been empirically studied. It is known, however, that limb apraxia adversely affects activities of daily living (Hanna-Pladdy, Heilman, & Foundas, 2003). Furthermore, severity of limb apraxia has been associated with self-feeding difficulties in stroke patients (Foundas et al., 1995). Thus, assessment of limb apraxia as well as buccofacial apraxia in the stroke population may be important. Transitive gestures, which are gestures that involve tool use, and intransitive (symbolic) gestures generally are assessed. For transitive gestures, patients pretend as if they are holding and using the tool as opposed to actually demonstrating use of a specific tool. Comprehension and motor strength must be intact to make an accurate diagnosis of buccofacial or limb apraxia.

Interpreting the Communication Assessment

Language ability will impact interpretation of the cognitive assessment and thus responses should be analyzed according to language functioning. Reduced auditory comprehension will impact the conduction of the swallowing assessment and management. A patient with reduced comprehension may not understand instructions such as swallowing on cue, coughing, or the instructions to a therapeutic strategy. Visual cues and imitation may facilitate comprehension necessary for completion of the CSE and instrumental examination, but they may prove of limited assistance in the actual rehabilitation of dysphagia.

The upper aerodigestive tract is common to speech, voice, and swallowing. Damage to specific cranial nerves may affect one, two, or all three functions. Abnormality in speech and voice has frequently been related to risk of aspiration in acute stroke patients (Daniels et al., 1998; McCullough et al., 2005). Although not every patient with a motor speech or voice disorder has dysphagia, the presence of these should alert the clinician to the increased potential for dysphagia in the acute stroke patient.

6 The Clinical Swallowing Examination

Evaluation of the Oral Mechanism

Before beginning the evaluation of the oral mechanism, it is recommended that the clinician briefly observe the patient at rest to obtain a global idea of the patient's status. The clinician should note the patient's appearance, alertness, posture, positioning, and respiratory rate. For example, the clinician may note if the patient is disheveled or neat in appearance, drowsy or alert, sitting upright or leaning to a hemiparetic side, or using rapid mouth breathing or slow nasal breathing. Although it is a widely held notion that aspiration risk is increased if the respiratory rate is over 20 breaths per minute, this has not been empirically confirmed.

Executing the Evaluation of Structural Integrity

The appearance of the oral mucosa should be evaluated in terms of salivation and color. The mucosa should be moist without evidence of excess saliva or drooling. The color of the oral mucosa should be pink. Any structural abnormality such as sores or lesions in the oral cavity should be identified, and the presence and awareness of food should be noted.

Dentition should be inspected for number and appearance of teeth as well as evidence of dental prostheses. The clinician should note missing teeth and provide a general report of the quality of remaining teeth, such as decay, cracked, and so forth. The presence and fit of dentures should be noted. For inpatients in particular, dentures may be available but not inserted.

Interpreting the Evaluation of Structural Integrity

Pooling of saliva in the oral cavity generally does not indicate hypersalivation in stroke patients, rather it may indicate dysphagia. For example, patients with a lateral medullary stroke frequently have severe dysphagia with inability to swallow saliva. This in turn may cause collection of saliva in the oral cavity. The clinical picture of an acute stroke patient expectorating saliva into a cup is frequently evident in individuals with for lateral medullary stroke. The presence of drooling should alert the clinician to facial nerve weakness. If hydration is not optimal, the mucosa may appear dry with cracks and flaking along the tongue surface. As discussed in the cognitive evaluation, the presence of residual food may be due to sensory deficit or inattention.

Poor dental care in combination with decreased mobility, sensation, and awareness of dysphagia, may increase the risk of pneumonia in stroke patients. Dental decay and dependence for oral care are significant contributors to the development of aspiration pneumonia (Langmore et al., 1998).

THE CRANIAL NERVE EXAMINATION: INFERRING PHYSIOLOGY

Basic neuroscience is considered a standard component of professional training programs in speech-language pathology, but merging that information into dysphagia management practice eludes many clinicians when faced with the demands of a full clinical load. The astute clinician will integrate a thorough cranial nerve examination into their clinical swallowing examination (CSE) and use this information to infer aspects of potential pathophysiology. Asking the patient to execute various motor and sensory tasks as clinical indicators of cranial nerve function provides valuable information about the functional status of the task assessed. More importantly, however, a thorough cranial nerve assessment allows the clinician to "see" what they "cannot see"; it allows the clinician inferred insights into unobservable pharyngeal physiology.

Executing the Cranial Nerve Examination

The earlier review of basic neurophysiologic substrates discussed in Chapter 2 provides the foundation for the clinical assessment. Execution of a cranial nerve examination in a neurologically impaired patient optimally will consist of a well-organized protocol of specifically tested information that allows the clinician access to maximal information with minimal invasiveness and discomfort to the patient. To accomplish this it is often more logical to organize the examination not by cranial nerve, but rather by starting at the front of the swallowing system and working to the back of the system. The clinician must be methodical.

- *Face:* Assessment of facial sensation and symmetry with careful observation of differentiation in upper and lower facial movement. Attention to facial grooving/folds (nasolabial fold, forehead, and circumorbital and circumlabial wrinkling) for indication of asymmetry that would suggest unilateral weakness.
- *Lips:* Labial symmetry at rest; range of motion, symmetry, and resistance during functional activity.
- *Tongue:* Observation of lingual structure at rest with careful attention to subtle fasciculations and muscle

wasting. Lingual range of motion and symmetry; strength to resistance. Taste and touch perception on lingual surface.

▩ *Palate:* Assessment of velopharyngeal sensation via touch and symmetry of movement on phonation of non-nasal phonemes. Observation of velar elevation and movement of pharyngeal walls in response to gag elicitation.

▩ *Pharynx:* Little observation can be made of the pharynx outside of pharyngeal wall contraction during gag. Palpation of the thyroid cartilage will provide the clinician with a subjective marker of laryngeal excursion during swallowing; however, it must be recognized that presence, not adequacy, of hyolaryngeal ascent is provided by palpation. The adequacy of hyolaryngeal ascent can only be ascertained through observation of epiglottic deflection and upper esophageal sphincter (UES) opening.

▩ *Larynx:* As above, direct evaluation of laryngeal function is not possible from clinical assessment; however, evaluation of phonatory ability can provide clues as to the integrity of laryngeal structure and function. Vocal quality, glottal coup, and cough should be assessed.

▩ *Speech:* Although speech and swallowing share some common structures and neurophysiologic substrates, there is not a robust association between these two tasks. Evaluation of speech sound production for isolated phonemes (particularly /g, k/) and connected speech will provide information about overall strength and coordination of muscles as they are recruited for voluntary tasks. Findings may carry over to swallowing tasks in the case of lower motor neuron (LMN) impairment; however, the clinician will need to recognize that upper motor neuron (UMN) pathway activations for swallowing vary from those for speech and thus may reflect differentially on functional outcomes.

▩ *Dry swallow:* Initiation of voluntary swallow and reflexive swallow for secretion management.

Interpreting the Cranial Nerve Examination

Interpretation of cranial nerve examination findings are outlined in Table 6-1, which provides a summation of cranial nerves primarily involved in swallowing biomechanics.

Included are instructions for direct assessment of motor and sensory components, the innervation patterns of those nerves, and a summary of *potential* biomechanical implications of involvement of those muscles. The astute clinician will make every effort to link clinical observations of cranial nerve impairment to suspected pharyngeal pathophysiology. By doing this, the clinical swallowing examination is extended from observed behavior to intelligently inferred behavior and thus may increase sensitivity for detecting pharyngeal swallowing impairment.

Findings of the cranial nerve examination need to be seen in light of the patient's overall status. A robust patient with adequate cognition and reasonable health may provide clear and unambiguous information. However, acutely ill patients and those with substantive neurologic impairment frequently exhibit difficulty in executing the required tasks. It is important to keep in mind that just because patients do not perform the tasks, does not mean that neurologically they cannot. Lack of execution does not always implicate a neurologic deficit. If eliciting a response proves difficult, attempts should be made to observe the behavior in spontaneous activity (i.e., volitional cough versus reflexive cough, tongue lateralization versus protrusion versus licking dry lips). Evaluation of the patient at another time, particularly those in the acute poststroke phase, may yield dramatically different results if their overall status improves.

There are several primary factors to consider in the interpretation of cranial nerve assessment.

■ Direct motor and sensory innervation patterns will allow the clinician to bridge the gap between observed behaviors and inferred physiology.

Table 6–1. Clinical Testing of Cranial Nerve Function with

Cranial Nerve	Tested by:	Motor Innervation:

V Trigeminal	Motor:
	  Jaw open to resistance
	  Jaw lateralization, bite
	Sensory:
	  Sensory to face, hard
	  palate, anterior tongue
		Temporalis
		Masseters
		Medial & lateral pterygoids
		Anterior belly of digastric
		Mylohyoid
		Tensor veli palatini

VII Facial	Motor:
	  Close eyes, wrinkle brow
	  Smile, kiss, whistle
	  Flatten cheeks, Lateralize
	  lips
	Sensory:
	  Taste to anterior 2/3 tongue
	  Sensory to soft palate and
	  Adjacent pharyngeal wall
		Posterior belly of digastric
		Stylohyoid
		Submandibular & sublingual
		glands
		Muscles of face & lips
		(orbicularis oris)

IX Glosso-
pharyngeal
	Motor:
	  Gag reflex*
	Sensory:
	  Gag reflex
	  Estimation of onset of
	  swallow**
	
	  *high risk of false positive
	**very difficult to assess clinically
		Stylopharyngeus
		Taste and sensation to
		posterior
		1/3 tongue and oral cavity,
		faucial arches

X Vagus	Motor:
	  Vocal quality
	  Volitional cough, glottal
	  coup
	Sensory:
	  Reflexive cough
	  Inhalation cough challenge
		Cricothyroid
		Intrinsic/extrinsic laryngeal
		muscles (interarytenoid,
		lateral cricoarytenoid)
		Sensory input to lower
		pharynx, larynx
		Cricopharyngeus

IX & X Pharyngeal Plexus	See IX, X	Superior, middle, and inferior pharyngeal constrictor Palatoglossus Palatopharyngeus Salpingopharyngeus Levator veli palatini

Potential Implications:

- Bolus breakdown and preparation of solids
- Reduced anterior hyoid movement with consequent
  - Decreased epiglottic deflection
    - → intraswallow aspiration 2° impaired supraglottic closure
  - Decreased opening of the upper esophageal sphincter
    - → with piriform sinus residual and postswallow aspiration
- Decreased bolus recognition/awareness

- Reduced elevation of hyoid
  - Decreased pharyngeal shortening and supraglottic compression,
    - → risk of intraswallow aspiration
- Reduced superior, posterior displacement of tongue, hyoid, larynx
  - May have 2° implications for oral containment of the bolus
    - → Premature spillage and preswallow pooling
  - Base of tongue to posterior pharyngeal wall approximation
    - → Postswallow vallecular residual
- Decreased salivation

- Reduced pharyngeal motility and reduced pharyngeal shortening
  - Postswallow diffuse residual
- 2° Reduced supraglottic compression,
  - risk of intraswallow aspiration
- Decreased base of tongue to posterior pharyngeal wall approximation
  - Postswallow vallecular residual
- Decreased bolus recognition/awareness

- Diminished capacity for laryngeal adduction
  - Intraswallow aspiration
- Decreased effectiveness of cough on aspiration (motor)
- Silent aspiration (sensory)
- Impairment opening of the upper esophageal sphincter
  - Postswallow pyriform residual
  - Postswallow aspiration

- Poor preswallow bolus containment
  - Premature spillage and preswallow pooling
  - Preswallow aspiration
- Decreased pharyngeal shortening and supraglottic compression,
  - Risk of intraswallow aspiration

continues

Table 6–1. *continued*

Cranial Nerve	Tested by:	Motor Innervation:
XII Hypoglossal	Motor only: Lingual movement— superior, lateral Protrusion, retraction	Intrinsic Extrinsic muscles of tongue Genioglossus, styloglossus Hyoglossus Strap muscles & geniohyoid when paired with C1-C2 (ansa cervicalis)

■ An assessment of laterality of presentation of pathologic findings will provide insights into site of lesion and potential neuromuscular presentation as well as recovery potential. As the cranial nerves involved in swallowing are bilaterally, but asymmetrically represented, (with the exception of the lower face), strong asymmetry of clinical presentation beyond the acute phase would tend to suggest ipsilesional LMN involvement as the bilateral representation softens clinical presentation over time. Lateralizing presentation in the early acute phase can be difficult to specify as this could reflect either ipsilesional LMN damage or contralesional UMN damage that has not yet softened due to bilateral inputs.

■ An understanding of redundancy in the physiologic system will allow for a more realistic reflection of inferred pathophysiology. There are only rare situations in swallowing physiology where a single nerve that feeds a single muscle group accomplishes a task. More often than not, there is redundancy in the system. As an example, apparent damage to the trigeminal nerve may have significant adverse consequences on anterior hyoid

Potential Implications:

- Poor bolus manipulation, preparation and transfer
  → Lack of cohesive bolus
  → Postswallow oral residual (buccal and sublingual)
- Decreased base of tongue to posterior pharyngeal wall approximation
  → Postswallow vallecular residual

movement as the anterior belly of digastric and the mylohyoid muscles are innervated by this nerve. However, if the hypoglossal nerve remains intact and thus, the geniohyoid is likely unimpaired, the clinical inference of impaired anterior hyoid movement may be tempered, leading the astute clinician to suspect impairment of lesser severity.

By taking these factors into account, a clinical picture will emerge that allows the clinician substantial insights into swallowing behavior.

Specific Comments on the Gag Reflex

The gag response historically has been utilized as a standard test of pharyngeal sensation to aid in prediction of a patient's ability to swallow without risk of airway compromise (Linden & Siebens, 1983). A recent report has indicated that assessment of the gag response in clinical evaluation provides high sensitivity (but low specificity) when compared to bedside evaluation alone in identifying aspiration in acute stroke patients (Ramsey, Smithard, Donaldson, & Kalra,

2005). However, other authors report that the presence or absence of gag response does not predict the swallowing ability or airway protection (Davies, Kidd, Stone, & MacMahon, 1995; Leder, 1996, 1997). Variability in responsiveness to gag in individuals without swallowing impairment is common (Schulze-Delrieu & Miller, 1997) with as many as 37% out of a cohort of 140 healthy adults, young and old, not demonstrating a gag response (Davies et al., 1995). Aviv (1997) points out that assessment of the gag response measures integrity of sensory fibers of the glossopharyngeal nerve; this is valuable information. However, it is the superior laryngeal branch of the vagus nerve that provides sensation to the hypopharynx and larynx and thus is critical for 'last chance' airway protection. Due to conflicting reports on association with pharyngeal biomechanics and airway protection, the clinician is left with a conclusion that presence of a gag response indicates integrity of glossopharyngeal sensory fibers; absence of a gag response indicates very little reliable information in isolation but may help to complete the clinical picture when taken in context of other derived information.

CASE EXAMPLE

As an example, a clinician receives a referral on an elderly patient, 4 weeks postonset, who was involved in a motor vehicle accident and has sustained traumatic insult to the base of skull region. In the emergency department, he experiences acute onset of confusion and dysarthria and is diagnosed with an acute stroke. On the clinical examination, the patient presents with significant dense, right upper and lower facial weakness, the smile is asymmetric with weakness on the right, and the patient is unable to tightly purse the lips. The tongue deviates to the right on protrusion. There is bilateral protrusion of the masseters on biting; however, this is less pronounced on the right and the jaw deviates mildly to the right when opening against resistance. The gag response is present; volitional cough is strong with a clear and loud vocal quality. Based on the history and the clinical presentation, the clinician is in a position to query potential physiologic impairments and identify both positive and negative predictors that support the decision making process. Clinical reasoning for this patient is outlined in Table 6–2.

The ability to make clinical deductions that pair findings of cranial nerve examination with observations of oral ingestion, as described in Chapter 7, will provide the clinician with a more thorough diagnostic picture. This skill is one that distinguishes a very strong diagnostician.

Table 6–2. Clinical Problem-Solving from Cranial Nerve to Physiologic Probabilities in a Patient with Closed Head Injury and Acute Onset Stroke

CN	Query	Positive Predictors	Negative Predictors
Possible residual effects of UMN lesion of left V or mild LMN of right V	Impairment of mastication (massetters, temporalis)		Not reported from clinical presentation
	Reduced anterior hyoid movement (anterior belly of the digastric, mylohoid)	There was questionable aspiration on solids in clinical assessment which may suggest postswallow aspiration of piriform sinus residual that would be consistent with decreased anterior hyoid movement.	Mild impairment overall; aspiration of liquids which would be consistent with poor epiglottic deflection from decreased anterior hyoid movement is not observed on clinical examination.
Right LMN of VII	Reduced elevation (not anterior) of hyoid secondary involvement of posterior belly of digastric and stylohyoid resulting in decreased pharyngeal shortening and reduced supraglottic compression. May lead to risk of intraswallow aspiration.		Pharyngeal constrictors may more directly facilitate pharyngeal shortening, and there is no evidence of pharyngeal plexus impairment.

CN	Query	Positive Predictors	Negative Predictors
Right LMN of VII (*continued*)	May have secondary implications for oral containment of the bolus, premature spillage, and preswallow pooling.	Potential impairment of posterior belly of diagastric and stylohyoid may be exacerbated by damage to hypoglossal that innervates styloglossus. This may adversely affect elevation of posterior tongue.	Palatoglossus muscle is primarily responsible for glossopalatal approximation and there is no evidence of pharyngeal plexus impairment which would suggest impairment of this muscle.
	Base of tongue to posterior pharyngeal wall approximation with postswallow vallecular residual.	Posterior belly of digastric and stylohyoid may assist with approximation of the tongue to the posterior pharyngeal wall.	This movement is more significantly influenced by fibers of the superior pharyngeal constrictor, of which there is no indication of impairment.
	Decreased salivation: difficulty with bolus preparation	Most salivary flow from CN VII.	Some salivary flow via CN IX. No clinical reports of dry mucosa.
Right LMN of XII	Poor bolus manipulation, preparation, and transfer resulting in lack of cohesive bolus; postswallow oral residual (buccal sublingual).	No redundancy in innervation or muscle function for bolus manipulation; fits clinical description. Aspiration of solids that is observed clinically may be from oral residual.	Unilateral involvement.

continues

Table 6–2. *continued*

CN	Query	Positive Predictors	Negative Predictors
Right LMN of XII (*continued*)	Decreased glossopalatal approximation and decreased base of tongue to posterior pharyngeal wall with postswallow vallecular residual (styloglossus).	When paired with facial involvement (as above), this increases likelihood.	No evidence of difficulty with pharyngeal plexus, which would impair contribution of palatoglossus to glossopalatal approximation and pharyngeal plexus to superior constrictor.
	Contribution to delayed pharyngeal swallow secondary to inefficient base of tongue transfer of the bolus.	Associated cognitive impairment may also inhibit contribution to onset of swallow.	No strong evidence of impaired sensation otherwise in oral cavity CN V and pharyngeal cavity CN IX.

CN = cranial nerve, UMN = upper motor neuron, LMN = lower motor neuron.

7 The Clinical Swallowing Examination

Assessment of Oral Intake

As described earlier, completion of a thorough cranial nerve examination will allow the clinician to problem-solve their way to educated deductions regarding potential impaired features of swallowing. Direct observation of oral intake can provide specific and direct information about observed oral phase swallowing impairments and, through careful observation and *realistic* interpretation, can offer suggestions regarding pathophysiologic features of swallowing in other phases. Integration of cranial nerve function with observed behavior of ingestion should lead the astute clinician to a clinical assessment with greater sensitivity and specificity for pharyngeal swallowing impairment.

EXECUTING THE ASSESSMENT OF ORAL INTAKE

Several factors need to be considered in completing the direct swallowing assessment. First, there may be situations where ingestion is not immediately appropriate. Receipt of a referral for swallowing assessment does not necessarily stipulate that the patient must be fed. The overall assessment of cognition, language, and cranial nerve function may suggest that any type of oral intake is premature. An obtunded patient may not be dysphagic but would not be a candidate for oral ingestion until consciousness has improved. Likewise, a patient with concomitant respiratory disease who struggles to maintain baseline ventilation also may not be appropriate for initiation of oral intake until respiratory stability is ensured. In the shorter term, a patient who is receiving nothing by mouth (NPO) and with neglected oral care who presents with unhealthy oral mucosa and an environment ripe for the proliferation of bacteria would first warrant a recommendation for nursing care prior to direct assessment of oral intake in order to inhibit the potential aspiration of colonized oral bacteria. The assessment of oral intake should be completed as the patient would normally eat, or a close approximation to this. The patient should be upright at 90 degrees if possible and should be wearing dentures if this is the norm.

As with the cranial nerve assessment, an organized protocol for evaluation of oral ingestion will ensure efficient and comprehensive observation of a variety of behaviors. No data exist to support that one protocol is more appropriate than another, although certainly clinical biases exist. Although standard protocols can ensure that the inexperienced clinician assesses all required information, the skilled therapist will likely elect to tailor an existing protocol to the needs of the presenting patient. For the patient who is NPO going into the examination, the clinician may opt for a careful and measured approach of moving through each consistency level. A patient who is currently ingesting a regular diet will require an approach that perhaps challenges more difficult consistencies or which targets specific food that are known to the patient to be problematic, but only "screens" less problematic textures. One suggested approach to completion of the comprehensive clinical assessment includes:

1. *Presentation of ice chips/crushed ice:* For the patient with significant cognitive or attentional deficits, it may be of benefit to initiate the examination with crushed ice by instructing the patient to chew and swallow promptly. This strong sensory stimulus may assist in directing the patient's attention to the task and lays a foundation for subsequent trials. If a patient fails to respond to this strong stimulus, the clinician may need to reconsider the timing of the assessment and may choose not to

proceed with other textures. As a clinical note, in a patient who is NPO, it will be most useful to advise the patient to actively chew and swallow rather than acquiesce to the temptation of holding the stimulus in the oral cavity while it melts.

2. *Thin liquids:* After the patient is attentive and cued to the task, the examination may be best continued with evaluation of liquids. In the case of the patient with significant pharyngeal dysmotility and subsequent residual, initiating the examination with heavier textures may consequently "soil" the pharynx such that unbiased evaluation of physiology with liquids is consequently not possible. Although liquids are most frequently aspirated in patients with neurogenic dysphagia (Clave et al., 2006; Linden & Siebens, 1983) simply allowing the patient ample time to recover from any discomforting coughing episodes before moving to subsequent trials will ensure that appropriate information is received.

3. *Thickened liquids:* If thin liquids are not well tolerated, the clinician may then elect to proceed to an assessment of thickened liquids to evaluate differential effects of viscosity. As outlined in Chapter 3, Table 3–1, viscosity has been shown to influence both spatial and temporal characteristics of swallowing biomechanics; thus, all assessment protocols should include evaluation of varying consistencies.

4. *Puree:* Puree consistency may consist of textures similar to applesauce, or other pureed fruit or vegetable, or may extend to a more viscous puree such as pudding or mashed potatoes.

5. *Mashable moist solid:* There are likely as many described food consistency levels as there are facilities in which dysphagic patients reside. A mashable moist solid would represent a texture that easily deforms or mashes with a fork or spoon but is able to be picked up with the fingers. This might be represented by a well-cooked carrot or other vegetable or a ripe banana. Assessment of this consistency level will provide greater information about bolus formation and control.

6. *Firm solid:* This food level will challenge the patient for mastication, bolus formation, and control and may also assist in identification of patients with specific impairment of the cricopharyngeus as transfer through the upper esophageal sphincter (UES) requires substantial deformation of the bolus.

For each bolus consistency, it is important to assess a number of trials. Based on research by Lazarus and colleagues (1993), 2 to 3 trials of each evaluated consistency optimally are suggested to ensure that a reliable clinical picture is obtained. Certainly, clinical reason will dictate the actual number of trials and the range of texture for a given patient. Circumventing multiple trials and textures would be appropriate in a patient with obvious dysphagic symptoms who clearly is distressed with oral intake. However, the clinician will need to be aware that a single bolus of any texture may be misleading with the potential for overestimation or underestimation of risk.

Additionally, within reason of time and patient tolerance, evaluation of each texture within the following progressive conditions is recommended.

1. *Controlled ingestion:* Single sips or bites that are dictated in size and generally provided by the examiner. Bolus size may be precisely measured in increasing increments (5 ml, 10 ml, etc.), or may be presented as more functional measures (a tablespoon, a hand-over-hand cup sip, etc.).

2. *Monitored ingestion:* Bolus size and rate of intake that are at the discretion of the patient but are monitored carefully by the clinician to ensure safety. The patient is encouraged to self-feed such that self-monitoring behavior can be observed. Very little is understood about the phenomenon of 'apraxia of swallowing' (Daniels, 2000; Daniels, Brailey, & Foundas, 1999); however, if this exists as a component of dysphagic presentation, the ability of the patient to self-feed may significantly influence performance.

3. *Independent ingestion:* Intake rate and bolus size that are fully at the discretion of the patient and not restricted, but are observed by the clinician. Independent feeding behaviors may place the patient at significant risk, and thus, the clinician will want to allow opportunities for observation of these behaviors.

4. *For liquids only:* Rapid ingestion of liquids (i.e., sequential swallowing). As discussed in Chapter 3, Table 3–1, continuous swallows create a significantly different biomechanical swallow than single sips (Chi-Fishman & Sonies, 2000, 2002; Daniels et al., 2004; Daniels & Foundas, 2001; Dozier, Brodsky, Michel, Walters, & Martin-Harris, 2006). Thus, assessment of this type of ingestive behavior will challenge the flexibility of the neuromuscular system. In the subsequent section of this chapter, details are provided for the execution of a specific water swallow test for which normative data are available in the literature.

5. Following the formal swallowing evaluation, if the decision is made to initiate or continue oral intake without benefit of instrumental assessment, observation of a full meal by the assessing clinician would be appropriate. This final assessment would allow the clinician great insights into the effects of behavior, fatigue, and increased quantity on clinical swallowing presentation.

INTERPRETING THE ASSESSMENT OF ORAL INTAKE

Observation of oral intake can provide substantial information about the efficiency of the oral phase and can allow the clinician, when supported by other data, to infer characteristics of pharyngeal physiology. The assessment of multiple consistencies is important to maximize the probability of identifying impairment. It is well documented that pharyngeal swallowing adapts to different bolus consistencies, or in the case of neurogenic impairment, may fail to adapt. Pathophysiologic features of swallowing thus will be differentially highlighted based on the consistency being assessed. As an example, decreased neurosensory input that underlies the abnormality of delayed swallowing will be present regardless of bolus consistency; however, the diagnostic feature of delayed swallow, or prolonged duration of stage transition, will be more readily detected on liquid or smaller boluses that inherently provide decreased sensory stimulation. Likewise, the weakness that may underlie poor pharyngeal motility will be present regardless of bolus consistency; however, heavier and more viscous consistencies will exacerbate the development of symptoms secondary to that pathophysiologic feature. Although this may seem a somewhat pedantic distinction, it is important that the clinician understand that they are evaluating swallowing physiology through the use of different consistencies, rather than evaluating ingestion of different textures.

From the initial bolus presentation, the clinician can glean information about preoral parameters of swallowing, including awareness of the bolus, attention to task, and problem-solving abilities. Does the patient actively accept the bolus, is the bolus placed in the patient's oral cavity, or does the patient actively refuse the bolus? Regardless of pharyngeal physiology, answers to these questions may supercede all else and ultimately dictate the treatment plan. As the bolus enters the oral cavity, does the mandible actively open and close to accept the cup, spoon, straw, or bolus itself? Is there adequate lip seal to inhibit anterior leakage of liquids and clear a spoon of a more viscous bolus? It will be important to determine if poor abilities at bolus acceptance are reflective of neuromuscular impairment or of impaired cognition and attention and are failing to drive the patient to volitionally participate in the feeding process. Prior assessment of cranial nerve and cognitive function may aid in this differential diagnosis.

Once the bolus is contained within the oral cavity, observation of behaviors becomes more inferential. Requesting that a patient masticate a solid bolus and then allow visualization of the bolus prior to transfer will provide information about bolus preparation and cohesion. Observations of a poorly cohesive bolus would suggest weakened or inefficient neuromuscular function of the intrinsic lingual muscles. This finding should correlate well with evidence of hypoglossal damage on cranial nerve examination either through assessment of strength or ease of movement and might be supported by decreased diadochokinetic speech rates. A solid bolus that has not been broken down would suggest either impairment of the masticatory process or an inability of the lingual muscles to position the bolus between the teeth. A pre-existing understanding of cranial nerve function will aid the clinician in making this distinction. Evidence of trigeminal involvement would lead to a clinical speculation of impaired masticatory ability, whereas evidence of hypoglossal nerve involvement supports a speculated diagnosis of impaired bolus positioning. Once the clinician has observed bolus preparation, the patient is allowed to continue with the ingestive process. Reflexive cough or vocal quality changes during the preparatory process *may* suggest inadequate glossopalatal approximation (palatoglossus and styloglossus muscles) that allows for premature spillage of the bolus and the potential for preswallow airway compromise. In order to gather supporting evidence for this pathophysiologic feature, the clinician can ask the patient to hold a fairly large liquid bolus in the oral cavity before either swallowing it, or expectorating it if intraswallow aspiration is a substantial concern. An inability to perform this task would support that glossopalatal approximation is insufficient. Postswallow observation of the oral cavity will provide further information about orolingual control of the intrinsic lingual muscles, as well as the extrinsic lingual muscles if the patient has been unable to transfer a bolus from the oral cavity. Observations of sublingual and buccal pocketing should be undertaken; allowing a delay before asking the patient to clear with a lingual sweep or finger sweep will provide information about oral sensory perception. Assessment of oral phase pathophysiology often is more apparent on solid or more viscous textures that challenge the neuromuscular system to a greater degree.

Clinical inferences about timing of onset of pharyngeal swallow after transfer of the bolus from the oral cavity are difficult. Although thyroid palpation may be assistive in identifying onset of pharyngeal swallowing, after the bolus enters the oral cavity and the lips are closed, even the most skilled clinician would be unable to know the location of the bolus within the aerodigestive tract in relation to onset of swallowing. Preswallow coughing or vocal changes may reflect the sensory impairment of delayed onset of the pharyngeal swallow, but these also may reflect premature spillage from poor bolus control. A careful assessment of oral sensation during the cranial nerve examination may be helpful in differential diagnosis. Additionally, delayed swallow may be more apparent on liquid consistencies as they provide less input to trigger sensory receptors, thus exacerbating the presentation of delay. Although not empirically validated, having the patient perform a "3-second prep" compensatory technique, as described by Huckabee and Pelletier (1999), may help in differential diagnosis as well. Patients with oral phase impairment may demonstrate signs of airway compromise before being instructed to swallow, whereas patients with a pure sensory deficit more likely may present this clinical presentation after the instruction to swallow. Additionally, as described in subsequent sections of this chapter, cervical auscultation is advocated by some as a means to identify delay in swallowing onset.

As the bolus moves farther into the lower aerodigestive tract, fewer reliable indicators of swallowing physiology are available, and the clinician has to rely heavily on nonspecific symptoms and quite often qualitative judgments to suggest pharyngeal impairment. During swallowing, the clinician can observe the patient for struggling behavior that might suggest discoordination of pharyngeal motility. Palpation of the thyroid cartilage often is used by clinicians to identify onset of the pharyngeal swallow; however, clinicians must be very cautious not to infer adequacy of excursion based on palpation. The measure of adequacy of hyolaryngeal excursion is subsequent epiglottic deflection and UES opening; these behaviors cannot be observed clinically. Thus, any estimation of hyolaryngeal excursion outside of "presence" or "absence" of movement is speculative at best.

Pharyngeal phase impairment may be detected nonspecifically by presentation of symptoms after swallowing. Pharyngeal residual may present as a subtle change in vocal resonance or audible movement within the pharynx that can be differentiated from vocal dysphonia, particularly if these symptoms appear to increase with increasing consistency or quantity of ingested material. Asking the patient to attempt expectoration of pharyngeal residual into a cup will aid in identification of residual and will provide valuable information about the patient's ability to expectorate as a compensatory airway protection mechanism. A spontaneous multiple swallow pattern also may suggest pharyngeal impairment in the presence of reserved sensation. Clinically, this appears more frequently to be observed in patients with specific UES abnormalities; however, there are no data to support this observation. Multiple swallows also may reflect oral residual that falls into the pharynx postswallow. The identification of pharyngeal residual as a probable symptom is nonspecific; the clinician will be unable to determine if the residual is due to impaired base of tongue to posterior pharyngeal wall approximation, impaired UES opening, or overall weakened or otherwise impaired pharyngeal motility. Knowledge of cranial nerve findings unfortunately is less helpful in differential diagnosis in the pharynx. Clear evidence of trigeminal involvement in the absence of observed deficits of glossopharyngeal and vagus nerves may lead the clinician to suspect that hyolaryngeal excursion is impaired; thus, pharyngeal symptom presentation may reflect impaired epiglottic deflection with postswallow vallecular residual and impaired UES opening with piriform sinus residual. Additional facial nerve damage would increase suspicion of vallecular residual secondary to decreased base of tongue to posterior wall approximation. Evidence of cranial nerve damage involving glossopharyngeal and vagus nerves, if trigeminal and facial are intact, would suggest a more likely scenario of overall impaired pharyngeal motility or specific abnormalities of the crico-pharyngeus muscle.

Certainly cough is a visible and audible indicator of aspiration, although once again it is nonspecific to physiology. Timing of the cough response can provide some additional clues with preswallow coughing suggesting oral phase abnormalities or delayed initiation of the pharyngeal swallow, and intraswallow or postswallow cough-ing suggestive of pharyngeal phase involvement or the possibility of postswallow aspiration of oral residual. Subtle throat clear or phona-tory efforts or wet dysphonia may be detected by careful observa-tion if the cough response is impaired. Detection may be augmented by cervical auscultation. The skilled clinician will want to discriminate between laryngeal dysphonia from vocal fold pathology and wet dysphonia suggestive of penetration or aspiration.

Specific data regarding interpretation of clinical findings are summarized in Chapter 8. The published data focus heavily on the balance between sensitivity and specificity in identification primarily of aspiration. Little data exist regarding the sensitivity and specificity of identifying other pathophysiologic features of swallowing. It is important that the clinician not overinterpret the information they can attain through clinical assessment. Accurate diagnosis is not pos-sible through observation of oral intake. However, by integrating this information with other components of a thorough clinical assess-ment, the clinician can blend a balance of art and science to increase appropriateness of referrals for instrumental assessment.

8 The Clinical Swallowing Examination

Predicting Dysphagia and Aspiration

THE WATER SWALLOW TEST

As part of the clinical swallowing examination (CSE), many water swallow tests have been developed primarily to screen for aspiration, although the timed water swallow test (Hughes & Wiles, 1996) also assesses swallowing efficiency. Water swallow tests may incorporate calibrated single swallows and/or ingestion of a large volume. For example, Daniels et al. (1998) suggest using water volumes of 5, 10, and 20 ml to assess for risk of aspiration in acute stroke patients. Kidd, Lawson, Nesbitt, and MacMahon (1993) suggest evaluating swallowing with a 50 ml volume by having the patient ingest it in 5 ml portions. Others suggest providing the patient with an entire volume of 3 ounces (90 ml) (DePippo, Holas, & Reding, 1992) or 100 to 150 ml (Hughes & Wiles, 1996).

Executing the Water Swallow Test

For the typical 3-oz water swallow test, patients are given the pre-scribed volume of water in a cup and instructed to drink without stopping. Clinically positive aspiration is classified as coughing or the presence of wet hoarseness for up to 1 minute after ingestion of the liquid (DePippo et al., 1992).

In addition to noting coughing or voice change after swallow-ing, the average volume per swallow, average time per swallow, and swallowing capacity are determined in the timed water swallow test (Hughes & Wiles, 1996). To complete the timed water swallow test, patients are given a prescribed volume and instructed to drink as rapidly and comfortably as possible. Duration of the task is measured with a stopwatch; onset is initiated when the water reaches the lips and offset is identified by return of the larynx to rest after completion of the sequential swallowing task. The number of swallows is determined by visual observation of thyroid cartilage elevation and lowering. Any residual left in the cup is subtracted from the initial amount of water provided to determine total volume swallowed.

Interpreting the Water Swallow Test

Results are conflicting concerning the ability of the 3-oz water swallow test to accurately identify patients with aspiration. One study found that it identified 80% of patients who aspirated on the videofluoroscopic swallow study (VFSS) (DePippo et al., 1992), whereas another found that it identified only 35% of patients with evidence of aspiration on the VFSS (Garon, Engle, & Ormiston, 1995). This last finding noted that 65% of the patients who aspirated on VFSS passed the 3-oz water swallow test. Differences in findings may relate to the study population as well as diagnostic measures. DePippo et al. evaluated patients who were 5-weeks poststroke and used cough *or* a wet-hoarse vocal quality to indicate failing the 3-oz water swallow test. Garon et al. evaluated a heterogeneous population including patients with stroke, dementia, and so forth, and used cough or throat clearing to define failing the clinical test.

By adding a time component to the 3-oz water swallow test, the clinician can determine the stroke patient's swallowing efficiency in addition to testing for the presence or absence of aspiration. Normative data for the timed water swallow test for specific age groups are shown in Table 8–1. Volumes in which these norms were obtained are 150 ml for individuals under age 75 years and 100 ml for individuals over the age of 75 years.

Table 8–1. Normative Data for the Timed Water Swallow Test

		Water Swallow Test					
		V/S		T/S		V/T	
	Age	*V/S*	*Range*	*T/S*	*Range*	*V/T*	*S/D*
Male	19–34	37.5	25–50	1.2	1.0–1.3	31.9	9.5
	35–55	30	21.4–37.5	1.2	1.0–1.4	24.8	7.8
	56–73	23.2	20.8–30	1.3	1.2–1.4	18.7	5.2
	74+	20	15.7–25	1.5	1.3–1.8	14.6	5.9
Female	19–34	18.8	15–30	1.1	1.0–1.3	18.7	6.0
	35–55	16.7	13.6–21.4	1.3	1.1–1.7	13.6	4.8
	56–73	16.7	13.6–21.4	1.5	1.1–2.1	12.3	4.9
	74+	10.6	9.1–13	1.5	1.4–1.8	7.5	3.3

= Number; V/S = total volume/# of swallows; T/S = time in second/# of swallows; V/T = total volume of fluid/time taken to ingest.

Source: From "Clinical Measurement of Swallowing in Health and in Neurogenic Dysphagia," by T. A. Hughes and C. M. Wiles, 1996, *Quarterly Journal of Medicine, 89,* p. 111. Copyright © 1996 by Oxford University Press. Adapted with permission.

Limitations of the Water Swallow Test

The primary focus of the water swallow test is to identify aspiration. As a patient's overt response to aspiration (cough, voice change) is necessary to identify aspiration on the CSE, silent aspiration may be missed. Splaingard, Hutchins, Sulton, and Chaudhuri (1988) were among the first to report the high incidence of silent aspiration (42%) in neurologically impaired patients that went undetected during the CSE.

Self-regulation of ingestion of large volumes during the water swallow test should also cause the clinician concern, especially in acute stroke patients or patients with cognitive deficits. Parker et al. (2004) noted that all dysphagic stroke patients with poor awareness of their swallowing problem drank the entire volume provided, with some patients requiring the clinician to stop them from drinking due to significant coughing. Conversely, most stroke patients with awareness of dysphagia did not complete the entire volume offered. The clinician would be wise to initiate the water swallow test with small volumes and progress accordingly, particularly in acute stroke patients. Compromised medical status or signs of aspiration on smaller trial volumes should alert the clinician not to administer a 3-oz volume (McCullough et al., 2005).

Although the timed swallow test may provide the clinician more information about swallowing in addition to documentation of aspiration, details concerning swallowing physiology cannot be determined. In using this test, the clinician has no knowledge of critical information such as laryngeal excursion; thus, evaluation of important components of swallowing is missed. Without this information, the appropriate selection of specific management techniques would be lost.

THE CSE WITH A FOCUS ON CLINICAL FEATURES PREDICTING DYSPHAGIA AND ASPIRATION

Clinical features associated with aspiration and dysphagia are presented in Table 8–2. Assessing and interpreting responses for each feature is fairly standard to clinical practice, and evaluation techniques for most are discussed in detail in earlier sections of this chapter. Although many of the research articles provide no specific detail concerning administration of test items from the CSE (Horner, Massey, Riski, Lathrop, & Chase, 1988), others provide detailed instruction on administration of items and interpretation of a patient's response (Logemann, Veis, & Colangelo, 1999). Therefore, it is recommended that the interested clinician thoroughly review specific references to obtain detailed information concerning features for which they are interested.

Clinical features predicting risk of aspiration or dysphagia generally are based on subjective scoring; however, volitional cough characteristics may be quantified allowing for objective confirmation of abnormality (Smith Hammond et al., 2001). To quantify cough characteristics, a mask is placed over the patient's nose and mouth. A recording of airflow is obtained with a pneumotachograph and a microphone attached to the mask, which allows recording of sound pressure level during the cough. The patient is instructed to produce a strong cough with recording obtained over a series of three to five trials. Numerous measures such as inspiration phase, peak flow, and sound pressure level have been identified as related to aspiration, but expulsive phase rise time appears to have the strongest relationship to aspiration. If the clinician has access to the necessary equipment, measurement of volitional cough may facilitate accuracy of identifying stroke patients with a risk of aspiration.

When discussing how well a feature predicts aspiration (or dysphagia), the terms **sensitivity** and **specificity** generally are used. Sensitivity refers to the ability of a sign to determine the presence of a disease given that the disease is truly present. Specificity refers to the ability of a sign to determine the absence of a disease given that the disease is truly absent. For example, consider that dysphonia is the sign and aspiration is the disease. If dysphonia has high sensitivity in predicting aspiration, most patients who aspirate will present with dysphonia. High sensitivity yields a low false-negative result; that is, the clinician would be confident that most patients who aspirate would be identified. Conversely, if dysphonia has low sensitivity in predicting aspiration, patients will not present with dysphonia yet they will actually be aspirating. Low sensitivity yields a high false-positive result, and the clinician must be concerned that a large percentage of patients with aspiration would not be identified. On the other hand, high specificity occurs if patients present with neither dysphonia nor aspiration. As with high sensitivity, this would yield a low false-negative result indicating that the clinician was not overidentifying aspiration. Low specificity occurs when patients have dysphonia but no aspiration. Low specificity would result in a high false-positive with the clinician identifying a large percentage of patients as aspirators due to the presence of dysphonia, yet patients would actually not be aspirating.

Table 8–2. Summary of Clinical Features Associated with Aspiration

Study	Population	CSE Focus	Instrumental Protocol
Linden & Sibens (1983)[a]	15 neurologic patients referred for swallowing evaluation	Structural assessment Voice Gag reflex Pharyngeal sensation Trial swallows	VFSS: thin and thick liquid, semisolid, solid
Horner et al. (1988)[a]	47 stroke patients referred for swallowing evaluation	Oral motor-sensory assessment	VFSS: not detailed
Horner, Massey, & Brazer (1990)[a]	70 bilateral stroke patients who had VFSS	Chart review of specific features	VFSS: ½ teaspoon, 1 teaspoon, 1 tablespoon, multiple sips from straw of liquid, ½ teaspoon pudding, cookie
Horner, Brazer, & Massey (1993)[a]	38 bilateral stroke patients who underwent a CSE and VFSS	Oral motor-sensory assessment	VFSS: not detailed
Alberts et al. (1992)[b]	44 consecutive rehab stroke patients with risk of dysphagia	3 oz water	VFSS: 5 ml thin, thick liquid; 20, 30 ml thin liquid; 5 ml pudding; ¼ cookie

Outcome Measures	Features	Sensitivity/ Specificity
Aspiration	Wet hoarseness	91/50
	Abnormal gag	91/50
Aspiration	Unilateral cranial nerve signs	29/61
	Bilateral cranial nerve signs	71/61
	Abnormal vocal quality	91/32
	Reduced sensation	22/48
	Abnormal cough	68/38
	Abnormal gag	60/48
Aspiration	Unilateral neurologic signs	18/69
	Bilateral neurologic signs	82/31
	Abnormal gag reflex	67/73
	Abnormal volitional cough	84/56
	Dysphonia	97/29
Aspiration	Unilateral neurologic signs	37/64
	Bilateral neurologic signs	63/36
	Abnormal gag reflex	74/64
	Abnormal volitional cough	89/64
	Dysphonia	93/09
Aspiration	Cough or wet-hoarseness during or 1 minute after 3-oz test	80/54

continues

Table 8–2. *continued*

Study	Population	CSE Focus	Instrumental Protocol
Linden, Kuhlemeier, & Palmer (1993)	249 patients, primarily neurologically impaired but no details provided	Assessment of respiratory, oral, and laryngeal function	VFSS: not specified
Kidd et al. (1993)	60 consecutively admitted acute stroke patients	Pharyngeal sensation Trial swallow: 50 ml provided in 5 ml portions	VFSS: 2, 5, 10 ml liquid, custard, jelly, mince, biscuit
Garon et al. (1995)[b]	100 consecutive patients with risk of dysphagia; various diagnosis	3-oz water	VFSS: four swallows each of 5 ml thin, thick liquid; 5 ml pudding
Daniels et al. (1998)	55 consecutively admitted acute stroke patients	Voice Speech Volitional cough Gag reflex Trial swallows of 5, 10, 20 ml liquid, 2.5 ml semisolid, ½ cookie	VFSS: two swallows each of liquid (volumes 3, 5, 10, 20 ml); 2.5 ml pudding
Daniels et al. (1997)	59 consecutively admitted acute stroke patients	Voice Speech Volitional cough Gag reflex Trial water swallows of 5, 10, 20 ml	VFSS: two swallows each of liquid (volumes 3,5, 10, 20 ml); 5 ml pudding; ½ cookie; sequential swallowing

Outcome Measures	Features	Sensitivity/Specificity
Aspiration	Reclining/lying posture Dsyphonia Wet phonation Abnormal laryngeal elevation Reduced swallowing of secretions Wet spontaneous cough Abnormal palatal gag Harsh phonation Breathy phonation	Values not provided for each feature but overall value for any one feature: Sensitivity—64 Specificity—67
Aspiration	Abnormal pharyngeal sensation	100/60
	Cough or voice change	80/86
Any single incidence of aspiration	Cough or throat clear during or for 1 minute after 3-oz test	35/89
Risk of aspiration: any single incidence of laryngeal penetration with postswallow residual or actual aspiration	Dysphonia Dysarthria Abnormal volitional cough Abnormal gag reflex Cough after trial swallow Voice change (any type) after trial swallow	76/68 76/53 48/94 62/82 57/85 38/85
Risk of aspiration: any single incidence of laryngeal penetration with postswallow residual or actual aspiration	Dysphonia Dysarthria Abnormal volitional cough Abnormal gag reflex Cough after trial swallow Voice change (any type) after trial swallow Any 2 of the 6 features	73/76 77/61 39/85 54/67 62/79 31/88 92/67

continues

Table 8–2. *continued*

Study	Population	CSE Focus	Instrumental Protocol
Logemann et al. (1999)	200 consecutive patients referred for dysphagia evaluation; various diagnosis	History: 4 items Behavior: 6 items Gross motor: 2 items Oral motor: 9 items Trial swallow: 7 items: 1 ml thin liquid, 1 ml pudding, ¼ cookie	VFSS: details not provided
McCullough, Wertz, & Rosenbek (2001)	60 patients consecutively admitted within 6 weeks of stroke	History: 15 items Oral motor: 18 items Voice: 6 items: speech/"ah" Trial swallows: 10 items: 5 ml thin and thick liquid; 5 ml puree, ¼ cookie, 3 oz water	VFSS: two swallow each of 5, 10 ml thin liquid; 5–10 ml thick liquid; 5 ml puree, ¼ cookie

Outcome Measures	Features	Sensitivity/ Specificity
Aspiration	Throat clear/cough on trial swallow	78/58
	Presence of 2 of 3: cough/throat clear on trial swallow, reduced laryngeal elevation on trial swallow, recurrent pneumonia	69/73
Oral stage problem	Dysarthria	64/75
Delayed pharyngeal swallow	Unsafe on more than 8 of the 28 test items	69/71
	Presence of 2 of 3: unsafe on more than 8 of the 28 test items, pharyngeal delay on trial swallow, facial weakness	71/73
Pharyngeal stage problem	Reduced laryngeal elevation	72/67
Any single incidence of aspiration	Pneumonia history	32/92
	Poor nutrition	50/76
	Presence of tube feeding	36/95
	Dysarthria	77/55
	Poor intelligibility	73/58
	Poor secretion management	50/84
	Wet voice (speech)	50/78
	Abnormal resonance	46/81
	Dysphonia (ah)	100/27
	Cough after trial swallow	68/82
	Judgment of airway invasion	77/63
	Reduced laryngeal elevation	41/84
	Cough on 3-oz water swallow	86/50
	Clinician rating of dysphagia	91/47

continues

Table 8–2. *continued*

Study	Population	CSE Focus	Instrumental Protocol
Mann & Hankey (2001)[c]	128 consecutive stroke patients	Demographic items and the Mann Assessment of Swallowing Ability	VFSS: 5, 10 ml thin liquid, thick liquid, and pudding, 20 ml thin liquid
Leder & Espinosa (2002)	53 consecutive stroke patients referred for swallowing evaluation	Voice Speech Volitional cough Gag reflex Trial water swallows via straw	Videoendoscopy: 5 ml puree, liquid, solid
McCullough et al. (2005)	165 consecutive acute stroke patients	History: 23 items Oral motor: 20 items Voice/Speech praxis: 9 items Trial swallows: 23 items: 5–10 ml thin liquid thick liquid, puree, ¼ cookie, 3 oz water	VFSS: two swallow each of 5 ml thin and thick liquid, 5 ml puree, ¼ cookie, 3 oz thin liquid

[a]Sensitivity and specificity calculated from data; [b]Sensitivity and specificity recalculated from data; [c]Data not available to calculate sensitivity and specificity. *Regression identified these

Outcome Measures	Features	Sensitivity/ Specificity
Dysphagia (defined as a disordered bolus flow)—rated as normal, moderate, severe, complete	Impaired pharyngeal response Male gender Barthel score <60 Incomplete oral clearance Palatal weakness or asymmetry Age >70	All items listed in features significant based on logistic regression
Aspiration: rated as normal, mild, moderate, severe, complete	Delayed oral transit Incomplete oral clearance	
Risk of aspiration: any single incidence of aspiration or significant spillage or residue of a bolus into the valleculae, pyriform sinus, or laryngeal vestibule	Presence of any 2 of 6: dysphonia, dysarthria, abnormal volitional cough, abnormal gag reflex, cough after trial swallow, voice change after trial swallow	86/30
Any single incidence of aspiration	Weak jaw bilaterally*	15/99
	Aspiration 3-oz swallow*	48/95
	Aspiration 10 ml thin liquid	38/96
	Aspiration thick liquid	21/98
	Aspiration 5 ml thin liquid	44/94
	Breathy voice	16/98
	Pneumonia	9/98
	Weak jaw unilaterally	26/96
	Aspiration puree	9/99
	Wet/gurgly voice	22/96
	Poor oral hygiene	14/97
	Aspiration solid	14/97
	Dysphonia*	54/86
	Strained voice	30/92
	Drooling	23/94
	Abnormal velum structure	24/93
	Nonoral feeding	49/84

measures as best for detecting aspiration. VFSS = videofluoroscopic swallowing study.

Interpreting the CSE with a Focus on Clinical Features to Predict Dysphagia and Aspiration

Sensitivity and specificity are both important and ideally a feature would be equally high in both. A clinical feature used to determine aspiration or dysphagia should have a score of at least 70% to be minimally sensitive and specific, scores closer to 100% of course are better. When deciding whether to choose measures with high sensitivity or high specificity, clinicians must consider their relative risk tolerance and the environment in which they work. For example, suppose there are two clinicians from two very different facilities who are using specific features from the CSE to determine which patients are at risk for aspiration, thus warranting an instrumental examination. One clinician works in a setting with a large percentage of acute and complicated stroke patients and has ready access to VFSS. This clinician may choose to select features with high sensitivity to identify the majority of patients with aspiration and reduce chances of missing patients with risk of aspiration. In doing this, the clinician must understand that the potential for over-recommendation of the VFSS if specificity is low. This may lead to unnecessary expense and radiation exposure as well as the potential for unwarranted diet restriction if there is delay in obtaining the VFSS. The other clinician works in a nursing home where patients are without acute illness and access to VFSS is limited. This clinician may want to focus on features with high specificity with the caveat that some patients with dysphagia or aspiration will not receive an instrumental assessment if sensitivity is low. Although decreasing the expense and burden of travel for VFSS, the potential for increased morbidity and mortality may increase if patients with aspiration are not identified. Again, a balance between both sensitivity and specificity cannot be overly stressed and may be best accomplished by using a cluster of features as compared to a single clinical feature as discussed by Daniels, McAdam, Brailey, and Foundas (1997) and Logemann et al. (1999) and reviewed in Table 8-2.

Limitations of the CSE with a Focus on Clinical Features to Predict Dysphagia and Aspiration

By focusing only on specific features to predict aspiration, the clinician may ignore extremely important data collected as part of the global CSE. A focus only on aspiration will miss patients with dysphagia but no airway invasion. A complete CSE will allow the astute clinician to make judgments swallowing on ability, diet, and potential for treatment. With a focus only on a few clinical features, the clinician can only address the potential for aspiration and not other aspects critical to swallowing and recovery of function. Many stroke patients can have clinically significant dysphagia without aspiration. As noted previously, only two studies have identified clinical features that relate to dysphagia. Although important, both studies report only moderate sensitivity and specificity in identifying dysphagia as confirmed by the VFSS. Moreover, both studies classified dysphagia in terms of bolus flow. Future research studies are needed that are highly sensitive and specific in determining stroke patients at risk for dysphagia, not just aspiration.

Whether using the CSE as a global evaluation of swallowing or extracting specific features to identify aspiration, fewer than 50% of items from the examination have adequate inter- and intrajudge reliability (McCullough et al., 2000). That is, whereas one clinician may identify a patient with dysfunction in one area (i.e., volitional cough) another clinician may assess no dysfunction. In addition, the same judge may have completely different findings between two evaluations completed on the same person. Reliability is critical for an examination to be meaningful. Clinical measures of oral motor functions and voice have proven more reliable than measures of history information or trial swallows (McCullough et al., 2000). It is strongly recommended that clinicians in the same facility determine a definition of normal and abnormal on the clinical measures used to evaluate swallowing and then work together to establish reliability within and across the department.

THE MANN ASSESSMENT OF SWALLOWING ABILITY

If the clinician is uncomfortable integrating findings from a comprehensive CSE, The Mann Assessment of Swallowing Ability (MASA) may be used (Mann, 2002). The MASA is the only standardized clinical swallowing tool that has undergone rigorous psychometric testing. The MASA was designed by the author to be an independent measure of dysphagia and aspiration. It is suggested that results from the MASA should help the clinician identify the pathophysiology of the swallowing problem, facilitate development of a treatment plan, and determine the need for further instrumental assessment.

Executing the Mann Assessment of Swallowing Ability

The MASA is composed of 24 test items in four categories: general patient examination, oral preparation, oral phase, and pharyngeal phase. Each component is evaluated in terms of normal or level of impairment: mild, moderate, severe, or inability to test. The test requires approximately 15 to 20 minutes to administer. If the patient cannot complete the first item, administration of the test should be postponed until a later date. It is suggested that swallowing assessment begin with saliva and advance to 5 and 20 ml of water and thickened liquid as appropriate (Mann et al., 2000), although other consistencies may be provided.

Interpreting the Mann Assessment of Swallowing Ability

After completing the MASA, scores are tallied and composite dysphagia and aspiration scores are calculated. The maximum score is

200 indicating no swallowing deficit. Based on scores the clinician determines the severity of dysphagia and aspiration as well as the likelihood of occurrence of each:

- *Unlikely*—minimal or no evidence of a disorder
- *Possible*—limited probability of a disorder requiring continued monitoring
- *Probable*—greater risk of a disorder requiring intervention or further evaluation
- *Definite*—high likelihood for a disorder requiring immediate intervention or instrumental assessment.

Diet recommendations are determined by identifying the intake mode that best fits the clinical impairment profile.

Limitation of the Mann Assessment of Swallowing Ability

The MASA provides a relatively good summary of items important in swallowing; however, it is relatively brief without accounting for further exploration of cognitive, cranial nerve, or swallowing impairment. As with all CSE, pathophysiology can only be inferred; thus, instrumental assessment is required to develop specific management plans.

9 Adjuncts to the Clinical Swallowing Examination

Instrumentation may be added to the clinical swallowing examination (CSE) to increase objectivity and accuracy of findings. This instrumentation may include pulse oximetry and cervical auscultation. In addition, the cough reflex test has been proposed to facilitate identification of patients at risk for development of aspiration pneumonia. Methods for implementing each CSE adjunct as well as current limitations are reviewed.

PULSE OXIMETRY

Executing Pulse Oximetry

It has been suggested that the inclusion of pulse oximetry during evaluation of trial swallows on the CSE will increase accuracy of identification of aspiration. The notion behind pulse oximetry is that aspiration results in reduced oxygen saturation of arterial blood. The device is attached to the earlobe or finger and oxygen saturation is monitored during oral intake. Pulse oximetry should decrease from baseline by a specific amount if aspiration occurs. The optimal way to evaluate the accuracy of pulse oximetry in an experimental paradigm is to complete simultaneous pulse oximetry and instrumental evaluations. The reviewer coding aspiration on the instrumental examination should be blinded to the pulse oximetry results and vice versa.

Interpreting Pulse Oximetry

Numerous studies have been conducted concerning the reliability of pulse oximetry to identify aspiration in stroke patients; however, contradictory findings are prominent. Some studies suggest that pulse oximetry is accurate in identifying aspiration (e.g., Collins & Bakheit, 1997; Zaidi et al., 1995), whereas others show no association between the occurrence of aspiration identified during the instrumental examination and a decrease in oxygen saturation identified with pulse oximetry (Colodny, 2000; Leder, 2000).

Desaturation criteria may account for some of the different findings. Many studies used greater than 2% change in saturation as criterion for aspiration, whereas others used greater than 4% criterion. It is reported that 59% of healthy adults desaturate greater than 2% during swallowing, and 15% desaturate greater than 4% during swallowing (Hirst, Ford, Gibson, & Wilson, 2002). Moreover, many studies did not complete simultaneous pulse oximetry and instrumental swallowing evaluation, which may contribute to differences in findings. Thus, there remains no consensus as to whether the implementation of pulse oximetry as part of the CSE can increase accuracy in identifying aspiration.

Pulse oximetry, however, may provide other benefits to the CSE. As it is not uncommon in individuals with stroke to present with concomitant underlying respiratory conditions, monitoring of oxygen saturation may provide valuable clinical information regarding the patient's ability to tolerate the respiratory work of ingestion. Desaturation may not imply aspiration, but it may suggest that the apnea associated with swallowing is taxing to the underlying respiratory system. More research is required to determine additional information in which pulse oximetry can provide to the CSE.

CERVICAL AUSCULTATION

Executing Cervical Auscultation

Cervical auscultation to amplify either swallowing sounds or airway sounds during direct oral intake may be employed by clinicians. Generally, a simple stethoscope is used, but a microphone (Cichero & Murdoch, 2002) or accelerometer (Takahashi, Groher, & Michi, 1994) may be added for improved fidelity and signal recording. Various stethoscope placements have been proposed. One suggested placement is the lateral border of the trachea just inferior to the cricoid cartilage (Takahashi et al., 1994), whereas the lateral portion of the thyroid cartilage with the larynx at rest is suggested by others (Hamlet, Nelson, & Patterson, 1990). To amplify breath sounds, the stethoscope is placed on the lateral side of the neck around the laryngeal area (Zenner, Losinski, & Mills, 1995).

Interpreting Cervical Auscultation

When measuring swallowing sounds with auscultation, the clinician is listening for a "double click," which is associated with pressure changes involved in upper esophageal sphincter opening and closing (Hamlet et al., 1990). Although it is suggested that patients with dysphagia will not produce this sound, no data are available to support this. Cervical breath sounds are hollow or "tubular" (Zenner et al., 1995). Normal swallowing has a brief apneic period followed by exhalation after the swallow with clear breath sounds. If deviant from this, impairment in the pharyngeal phase of swallowing is suspected. Aspiration is suspected when a "flushing sound of material" is evident prior to initiation of the swallow or when breath sounds are changed, for example, wet, after the swallow.

Two studies recently evaluated the reliability of cervical auscultation for detecting aspiration in stroke patients (Borr, Hielscher-Fastabend,

& Lucking, 2007; Leslie, Drinnan, Finn, Ford, & Wilson, 2004). Participants underwent cervical auscultation and a videofluoroscopic swallowing evaluation in both studies. Results suggest reduced reliability among raters, which in turn yielded reduced ability to distinguish between stroke patients with and without aspiration. Until inter-rater reliability is established, cervical auscultation cannot be assumed to provide additional value to the CSE.

COUGH REFLEX TESTING[1]

Researchers and clinicians in respiratory medicine have utilized inhalation cough challenge testing for well over 50 years in the assessment of patients with underlying respiratory disease. First introduced in the 1950s (Bickerman & Barach, 1954; Bickerman, Cohen, & German, 1956), the cough challenge involves the delivery of tussive or chemoreactive agents into the upper airways with a recording of behavioral response, most readily observed as a cough reflex. The importance of a cough response to airway protection and consequently pulmonary integrity has long been acknowledged, particularly in the neurogenic population. Patients with weak cough have an increased risk of developing aspiration pneumonia (Smith Hammond et al., 2001). Absence or delayed recovery of a cough reflex after stroke has been postulated to increase morbidity and mortality (Addington, Stephens, & Gilliland, 1999). Laryngeal cough reflex has been identified in the stroke population to be impaired for up to one month or longer with permanent impairment in some patients (Kobayashi, Hoshino, Okayama, Sekizawa, & Sasaki, 1994). Despite this, the explicit testing of cough in the dysphagia diagnostic armamentarium has only recently emerged.

---

[1]The authors acknowledge the effort of LiPyn Leow for her contributions to this section.

The first reported clinical use of inhalation cough challenge in the neurogenic population with dysphagia was published by Addington, Stephen, and Gilliland (1999). A prospective study of 400 patients in the acute poststroke population was conducted to identify those patients at risk for developing aspiration pneumonia. Participants were administered a single dose of tartaric acid with subsequent cough response scored as normal, weak or absent. Recommendations for oral feeding were based heavily on outcome of cough challenge testing with those presenting a normal cough response fed orally, and those with absent or weak scores fed either nonorally or on a restricted diet. Incidence of pneumonia was compared to a sister hospital which did not employ cough challenge testing in determining management. Results demonstrated that 5 of 400 patients who received cough challenge ultimately developed pneumonia, whereas in the stroke population of the sister hospital without cough testing, 27 of 204 developed pneumonia ($p < .001$). In a subsequent study of 818 consecutive stroke patients, 35 (4.3%) developed pneumonia. Of the 736 (90%) patients who had a normal cough response, 26 (3.5%) developed pneumonia, and of the 82 (10%) patients with an abnormal cough response, 9 (11%) developed pneumonia despite preventive interventions ($p < .005$).

The preceding work lends support to the inclusion of inhalation cough testing as a valuable adjunct to the clinical assessment. To date, similar research has not been conducted to evaluate the influence of this test on outcomes when it is included as a component of more traditional clinical and diagnostic assessments, rather than used as a sole determinant of oral intake. One might speculate that outcomes would be substantially improved. Swallowing diagnosis is based largely on subjective interpretation of both behavioral presentation and instrumental visualization; there are very few quantitative clinical measures of swallowing associated behaviors. When a quantitative measure is available and preliminary data support that it is effective for identifying patients at risk, it would be wise to integrate it into clinical protocol.

Executing the Cough Reflex Test

A variety of stimuli have been utilized for cough reflex testing including citric acid (Kastelik et al., 2002), capsaicin (Midgren, Hansson, Karlsson, Simonsson, & Persson, 1992), and tartaric acid (Addington, Stephens, & Goulding, 1999). In a comparison of agents, Morice, Kastelik, and Thompson (2001) documented that only capsaicin and citric acid can be considered reproducible across time and thus are considered reliable for clinical use. Additionally, a number of protocols have been described including that by Addington, Stephens, and Gilliland (1999). However, given the wide variety of tussigenic agents, concentrations and delivery methods, universal standards for cough challenge testing are unavailable. The following suggested protocol is adapted from research by Morice and colleagues (2001). Citric acid is diluted in 0.9% sodium chloride to prepare samples of stimuli at 1.4 M and 2 M concentrations. These concentrations represent levels at which healthy elders produce a natural cough and suppressed cough. The clinician may wish to consult professionals in the pharmacology department of their facilities for assistance in preparing the stimuli. Delivery of citric acid is presented via nebulized air utilizing a full exhalation-full inhalation method (Pounsford & Saunders, 1985). With a nose clip in place, participants are instructed to place the mouthpiece of the nebulizer kit into their mouths to form a good seal. When the nebulizer is turned on, they should fully exhale to functional residual capacity then fully inhale to vital lung capacity. For the lower concentration, participants are instructed to cough "when you feel the need to cough." Once this is completed, the higher concentration is presented with the instruction to "try to suppress the cough, and cough only when you have to." By using both methods, the clinician is assessing not only the natural cough but also suppressed cough.

The method used by Addington, Stephens, and Gilliland (1999) prescribes a 20% solution of l-tartaric acid dissolved in 2 ml of sterile normal saline. With a nose clip in place, the single concentration of nebulized stimulus is delivered for a maximum of three trials. The test is terminated when a cough response is elicited or no response is generated after all three trials.

Interpreting the Cough Reflex Testing

For the protocol based on the work by Morice et al. (2001), cough within the first 10 seconds of inhalation is documented. The test is repeated four times and positive cough response is documented when the participant coughs at least twice on 50% of presentations. For the protocol suggested by Addington, Stephens, and Gilliland (1999), the test is terminated when a cough response is elicited or no response is generated after all three trials.

Identification of cough sensitivity may help expand on the diagnostic picture. Addington, Stephens, and Gilliland (1999) advocate a somewhat binary approach, with those passing the test able to assume oral intake and those failing the test being restricted or non-orally fed. However, integration of these data into the overall clinical picture may help identify patients that are appropriate for subsequent diagnostic clarification of swallowing physiology and may then augment clinical decision making.

Unfortunately, normative data are unavailable for either tussive agent described above. The concentrations of citric acid presented are based on as-yet unpublished data for threshold levels in elderly adults.[2] No justification is provided for the selection of stimuli concentrations advocated by Addington, Stephens, and Gilliland (1999). Past research has documented gender differences in cough response, with women having greater sensitivity, hence lower cough thresholds, compared to men (Dicpinigaitis & Rauf, 1998; Kastelik et al., 2002). Children are documented to respond at lower thresholds

---

[2]From the dissertation of L. Leow, The University of Canterbury (2007), data collected from a small sample of 16 elder adults.

than adults (Chang, Phelan, Roberts, & Robertson, 1996). Additionally, asthma (Chang, Phelan, & Robertson, 1997) and gastroesophageal reflux disease (Ferrari et al., 1995) lead to increased sensitivity of cough receptor sensitivity whereas smoking (Dicpinigaitis, 2003) diminishes airway sensitivity.

Thus, considerable research is required before inhalation cough challenge can be fully integrated into the clinical assessment. The absence of normative data is a major limitation to incorporating this as a clinical adjunct. However, given the ramifications of an absent cough response on airway protection and the high incidence of "silent" aspiration that hinders accurate clinical assessment, emergence of this modality in the diagnostic armamentarium is well overdue.

10 The Instrumental Examination

The Videofluoroscopic Swallow Study

THE NEED FOR DIAGNOSTIC SPECIFICITY

Once the clinical swallowing examination (CSE) has been completed and the need for an instrumental examination is determined, the clinician must decide which procedure will provide the greatest information for a particular patient. In acute stroke, it is believed that the videofluoroscopic swallow study (VFSS) provides the most comprehensive information as it provides the clearest view of the integration of the different phases of swallowing. Findings from the VFSS will detail bolus flow and biomechanics. However, the VFSS may not provide all of the diagnostic information needed to fully understand the nature of swallowing physiology. This is of significant consequence. By not understanding the specific nature of the swallowing disorder, management of the dysphagia can, in fact, exacerbate the disorder rather than facilitate recovery.

It is increasingly clear that diagnostic precision is a mandate of rehabilitative effectiveness. As an example, early research into the technique of thermal tactile stimulation is not compelling to support its efficacy (Rosenbek, Robbins, Fishback, & Levine, 1991). However, a careful examination of much of that literature reveals that inclusion criteria for those studies were based on symptoms of preswallow pharyngeal pooling. We now understand that this symptom can be due primarily to either a motor or sensory based disorder. It would not be surprising that outcome data for this technique are unconvincing if a proportion of participants possessed primarily a motor deficit and thus would not demonstrate response to a sensory treatment. Basing practices on symptoms is shortsighted; careful definition of pathophysiology is required.

The complexities of swallowing cannot be understood based solely on clinical examination and frequently can defy understanding based on a single diagnostic tool. We want to emphasize the need for multimodality assessment when appropriate and highlight the unique contribution of emerging techniques. Frequently the information obtained from a single examination will provide general information on biomechanics, but a subsequent assessment may be needed to identify the underlying specifics of pathophysiology. Indeed, new information about both compensatory and rehabilitative techniques suggests substantial potential for harm with misidentification of physiology.

Although there are additional tools available, such as pharyngeal manometry, to facilitate identification of pathophysiology, further development in diagnostic procedures will facilitate greater understanding and more precise diagnosis. Our understanding of swallowing and the underlying nature of dysfunction is dynamic. What is known has changed considerably over the last 30 years since health professionals have addressed dysphagia as a diagnostic entity. The process will continue to evolve, and in another 30 years the current diagnostic and management approaches likely will appear inadequate.

The instrumental examination has many purposes in the diagnosis of dysphagia in stroke:

- Evaluate biomechanical and physiologic function and dysfunction
- Determine swallowing safety
- Identify effects of compensatory management
- Determine appropriate diet.

Three types of instrumental evaluations are discussed: videofluoroscopic swallowing study, videoendoscopy, and manometry. The advantages and disadvantages of each evaluation method are presented in Table 10–1.

Table 10–1. Advantages and Disadvantages of Each Instrumental Examination Method

Instrumentation	Strengths	Weaknesses	When to Use
Videofluoroscopic Swallowing Study	Direct assessment of oral, pharyngeal, and esophageal stages. Evaluate bolus flow, temporal and spatial structural measurements. Determine the effects of compensatory strategies.	Radiation exposure that limits the length of the examination. Difficulty with patient positioning, especially patients with hemiplegia. Non-natural environment—may exacerbate cognitive problems. Use of barium as opposed to real food.	Preferred evaluation for stroke patients, especially the initial assessment.
Videoendoscopic Evaluation of Swallowing	Completed at bedside. Use of real food. No time constraints. No radiation exposure. Direct visualization of the larynx.	No visualization of the oral stage. No visualization of the actual swallow due to "whiteout", thus details of oral and pharyngeal motility must be inferred. No ability to assess esophageal functioning. Limited to no ability to evaluate bolus flow, and analyze structural movement.	Physical or cognitive limitations would significantly restrict videofluoroscopic findings. Patient is ventilator dependent or in the intensive care unit. Follow-up assessments to restrict radiation exposure.
Manometry	Quantification of observed pharyngeal biomechanics. No time constraints. No radiation exposure. Not subjective.	Does not visualize anatomic structure or biomechanical movement. Scope of evaluation limited to pharyngeal pressure	For differential diagnosis of pharyngeal motility disorders when primary diagnostic tests have already been completed.

THE VIDEOFLUOROSCOPIC SWALLOWING STUDY

Executing the Videofluoroscopic Swallowing Study

VFSS Setup

The ideal setup for obtaining VFSS is to record the study for later viewing. Swallowing is a rapid event with many features occurring simultaneously or within milliseconds of each other; thus, it is ideal to review the study, preferably with the opportunity to view in slow motion or frame-by-frame. Additional options that are strongly recommended for recording the VFSS are a microphone and a counter timer. By having audio input, the clinician may verbally identify the volumes and consistency provided to the patient and the compensatory strategy employed. As stroke patients may have cognitive and/or attentional impairments, the microphone will capture the amount of verbal cuing provided to the patient and any extraneous verbalization by the patient. The counter timer encodes digital time in hundredths of a second on each video frame. This, in turn, allows the clinician to make objective and precise temporal measurements.

Patient Positioning

Obtaining adequate patient positioning for the VFSS can be challenging in stroke patients due, in part, to hemiplegia and cognitive deficits. The advent of specially designed VFSS chairs that can be positioned from stretcher to chair have facilitated patient transfer and positioning. The VFSS is initiated with the patient in the lateral position. This view allows a clear view of the upper aerodigestive tract. Ideally, the clinician should be able to view the oral cavity, larynx, pharynx, and cervical esophagus. This allows for documentation of bolus flow and structural movement through the oropharyngeal swallowing system. The clinician may find, however, that the stroke patient does not maintain optimal positioning and moves out of the fluoroscopic view or cannot be positioned properly due to hemiplegia. In these cases, findings from the CSE are extremely important in identifying the possible area of focus for the VFSS. Moreover, the stroke patient may shift positions throughout the evaluation. As such, it is important that radiology personnel be prepared to move the fluoroscopic tube as the patient moves in order to capture the swallow. Having the patient hold the bolus in the oral cavity until verbally cued to swallow may assist in obtaining a higher quality view of the swallowing. Verbal cue, however, does impact swallowing in healthy adults (see Table 3–1); the effect on swallowing in stroke patients is currently unknown.

Obtaining an anterior-posterior (A-P) view is optional in the evaluation of swallowing in stroke patients and dependent on findings obtained from the lateral view. Fortunately, specially designed VFSS chairs allow for easy rotation of patients into the A-P position. Generally, this view is obtained if the clinician identifies postswallow residual in the piriform sinuses. After identifying postswallow residual in the lateral plane, the patient is turned to the A-P position. The patient's chin is slightly lifted to clearly view the hypopharynx thereby allowing for identification of postswallow residual location. By obtaining an A-P view, the clinician can determine if the residue is unilateral or bilateral. Unilateral pharyngeal hemiparesis frequently results in residue in the contralesional piriform sinus and often is evident in stroke patients. It is important to distinguish between unilateral or bilateral residual as specific management strategies are designed for each. The A-P view also helps identify unilateral vocal fold paresis, which is not uncommon in lateral medullary stroke. In the A-P view, the patient phonates "ah" and movement of the true vocal folds can be seen. If unilateral vocal fold paresis is identified, a referral to otolaryngology should be made.

Nasogastric Feeding Tubes

Many stroke patients, particularly those patients evaluated acutely, may have a nasogastric feeding tube (NGT) present for the VFSS. Changes in bolus flow with a NGT present have been identified in healthy adults and stroke patients. In healthy young adults, large-bore NGTs significantly affected durational measures such as stage transit duration (STD) and upper esophageal sphincter (UES) opening with similar trends evident with small-bore NGTs (Huggins, Tuomi, & Young, 1999). Although most durational measures were increased with the NGT present, STD was decreased. The authors suggest that earlier evocation of the pharyngeal swallow with the NGT in place may be a result of: (1) anticipatory behavior to avoid pharyngeal discomfort, (2) compensatory behavior yielding earlier hyolaryngeal elevation, or (3) pharyngeal wall stimulation. The presence of a large-bore NGT also has been shown to increase bolus flow timing measures in stroke patients, although findings were not statistically significant (Wang, Wu, Chang, Hsiao, & Lien, 2006). Moreover, the presence of a manometric catheter in the pharynx was associated with increased airway invasion in healthy older adults (Robbins et al., 1992). If an NGT is present during the VFSS, the clinician must determine if the feeding tube is contributing to the dysphagia. In facilities where it is the purview of the clinician to do so, obtaining physician orders for removal of the NGT during the VFSS will allow the clinician the opportunity to remove the feeding tube if it is determined that the NGT is causing or exaggerating any swallowing problem.

Bolus Presentation Guidelines

There is no set protocol for liquid and food administration for the VFSS. The VFSS may be defined as protocol-driven or patient-driven

(Campion, Haynos, & Palmer, 2007). In the protocol-driven assessment, the clinician administers the same volumes and consistency without considering a patient's needs. In the patient-driven assessment, the VFSS is tailored to a patient's specific needs. For stroke patients a combination of the two approaches is recommended. Like the CSE, it is ideal to start with small volumes of thin liquid, particularly in the initial evaluation. This limits the amount of aspiration should it occur and any postswallow residual, which is less with thin liquids, thereby reducing the effects on subsequent swallows. Self-administration with a cup or straw is preferred to mimic real-life eating situations. The influence of ingestion of liquids via cup versus straw on bolus flow has not been studied empirically in healthy adults or stroke patients; thus, it is unclear if there are positive or negative aspects of using either a cup or straw in which to ingest liquid. The use of a cup or straw in which to administer the liquid should be determined from the CSE. If the patient has difficulty with oral containment and anterior bolus loss is identified, use of a straw may be preferred.

In addition to considering the effect of liquid ingestion via cup or straw, the clinician must also consider the impact of verbal cue on swallowing. Frequently, verbal cue to swallow arbitrarily is applied in the VFSS, yet recent research indicates that verbal cue affects swallowing in healthy adults (Daniels et al., 2007) (see Chapter 3, Table 3–1). Currently, it is unknown if cue to swallow has a facilitory or deleterious effect on swallowing in stroke patients. Anecdotal evidence suggests that cue to swallow may contribute to "apraxia of swallowing" in patients with left hemisphere damage (Logemann, 1998; Robbins & Levine, 1988; Robbins et al., 1993); however, this has not been empirically confirmed. Conversely, cue to swallow may increase volition in the act of swallowing by allowing the patient an opportunity to organize and execute bolus transfer thus facilitating swallowing. By using a cue to swallow, the clinician must consider the potential for positive and negative effects.

Calibrated volumes may be used for the VFSS, or as with the CSE, a structured but still carefully regulated examination may be undertaken. By using calibrated volumes, the clinician can identify the precise volume in which swallowing difficulty begins. This may prove beneficial when recommending oral intake. For example, if a patient demonstrates a functional swallow with a 5-ml volume but significant dysfunction with a 10 ml volume, 5-ml liquid volumes for pleasure or during treatment may be recommended. Furthermore, subsequent re-evaluations can begin at the volume of difficulty. By using specific volumes, at least initially, the clinician can compare patients and results thereby creating a database in which to report possible clinical research findings. Generally, a clinician may initiate the study with a thin liquid volume (3 or 5 ml) and progress to a larger volume up to 20 ml, which is the normal single-bolus volume in healthy adults (Adnerhill, Ekberg, & Groher, 1989). Two to three trials of each volume or consistency are recommended to reliably judge swallowing function (Lazarus et al., 1993). If dysphagia is identified with resulting aspiration, the examination is not necessarily terminated, but rather, appropriate compensatory techniques are initiated to facilitate swallowing. If aspiration is evident on the first swallow, the clinician may want to repeat the swallow using the same volume and consistency. It may be that the patient required a "warm-up" period and swallowing improves after the first or second swallow.

If dysphagia and aspiration persist with liquids, compensatory techniques should be employed. Determining the appropriate compensatory technique is determined by the specific swallowing problem. (Compensatory management is discussed in detail in Chapter 17.) Generally, it is ideal to begin with posture compensation and if a specific posture does not facilitate swallowing, altering the consistency should then be attempted. The patient's comprehension and memory function may dictate the type of compensatory strategy employed. For example, in a patient with a right hemispheric stroke and poor attention, the clinician may have the patient attempt a chin tuck posture for a delayed pharyngeal swallow to determine benefit of this posture. The clinician can determine the extent of cuing necessary for the patient to implement and maintain the posture. Even if improvement is seen, the clinician also should determine the impact of consistency manipulation, for example, thickened liquid. If successful, thickened liquid may be the compensatory strategy recommended for this patient due to the extent of cognitive deficits. However, if chin tuck was also successful, in addition to addressing rehabilitative techniques to facilitate elicitation of the pharyngeal swallow, the clinician also can train in maintaining the chin tuck posture. Thickened liquids, however, are not part of the routine VFSS and are administered as indicated as a compensatory strategy.

If liquid aspiration cannot be prevented by employing the appropriate compensatory strategy, administration of liquids should be discontinued; however, evaluation of semisolid and solid swallowing should be considered if postswallow residual is not significant. To evaluate ingestion of semisolids, the barium paste may be administered alone or mixed with semisolid food such as pudding or mashed potatoes. It is optimum to have the patient self-feed; however, for some stroke patients, particularly those patients evaluated in the acute phase, the clinician may need to administer the semisolid. To evaluate mastication and swallowing of a solid bolus, a solid such as part of a cookie, is coated with barium paste. If the stroke patient has reported difficulty with a particular food-type, it is ideal to mix the barium with that type of food.

All food types cannot and should not be assessed during the instrumental examination due to time constraints secondary to radiation exposure and attentional limitations of the stroke patient. In addition, the clinician must allow enough time in the VFSS to pursue management strategies. Thus, it is imperative that astute clinicians infer swallowing function across food types from a limited number of consistencies administered during the VFSS.

If large single volumes of liquid can be safely swallowed by the patient, sequential swallowing should be evaluated as this is a more typical pattern of swallowing compared to single, discrete swallows. For sequential swallowing, the patient is provided with a large volume, for example, 100 ml, and instructed to continually swallow. The patient self-regulates the volume and pace of ingestion. The use of straw or cup delivery is dependent on results of the earlier single swallows.

If significant aspiration is not observed, esophageal motility should be screened. Research documenting esophageal motility following stroke is limited with results indicating that propagation of distal esophageal peristalsis, percent of completed peristaltic events (Aithal, Nylander, Dwarakanath, & Tanner, 1999), and resting pressures of upper and lower esophageal sphincters (Lucas, Yu, Vlahos, & Ledgerwood, 1999) are reduced following stroke. To screen for esophageal motility, a liquid bolus and a semisolid bolus should be followed as each progresses through the esophagus to the stomach. It is important for the clinician to have a cursory understanding of esophageal motility as esophageal dysfunction may contribute to pharyngeal dysfunction (Martin-Harris & Easterling, 2006). Consultation with a radiologist concerning results of the esophageal screening can facilitate identification of dysmotility and determine the need for further radiographic evaluation and/or gastroenterology consultation.

Interpreting the Videofluoroscopic Swallowing Study

The clinician must integrate numerous components of the VFSS in order to obtain a complete and accurate determination of swallowing function and safety. The components of the VFSS include:

■ Anatomic abnormalities

- Bolus flow
- Temporal coordination of structural movement relative to bolus flow
- Extent of structural movement
- Response to compensatory strategies and determining treatment plan.

Although the VFSS may be interpreted on-line during the assessment, it is best to record and review the study after the examination is completed. In this fashion, swallowing motility can be viewed in various speeds to facilitate identification of dysfunction. A narrative may be written directly following viewing of the VFSS or an evaluation sheet may be used to document dysfunction with the narrative taken from the score sheet. Table 10–2 provides an example of a detailed score sheet. As with the CSE, it is strongly recommended that clinicians working together at various sites, such as hospitals, or nursing homes, determine specific parameters to define dysphagia and work together as a team to establish inter- and intrarater reliability on these variables within their respective institutions. Until this is completed, diagnosing dysfunction on VFSS will not be consistent across or within individual clinicians (Kuhlemeier, Yates, & Palmer, 1998; McCullough et al., 2001; Scott, Perry, & Bench, 1998; Stoeckli, Huisman, Seifert, & Martin-Harris, 2003; Wilcox, Liss, & Siegel, 1996).

Anatomic Abnormalities

Judgment of the integrity of anatomic structures should be completed with all patients. Although anatomic abnormalities such as cervical osteophytes are unrelated to stroke, their incidence, like stroke, may increase with aging. The identification of any anatomic abnormality should be noted as well as its effect on swallowing. Deviation in anatomy may exaggerate the swallowing problem that occurs following stroke.

Table 10–2. An Example of a Videofluoroscopic Swallowing Study Score Sheet

VIDEOFLUOROSCOPIC SWALLOWING STUDY

Name: _____   ID#: _____

STUDY CONDITIONS:

View: _____ Lateral _____ A-P   **Presentations:** _____ Cup _____ Straw _____ Syringe

Code: L1 = liquid trial 1; L2 = liquid trial 2; P1 = pudding trial 1; P2 = pudding trial 2; S1 = solid trial 1; cont = continuous drinking 100 ml

Circle appropriate consistency/sequence	3 ml	5 ml	10 ml	20 ml	pudding	solid	cont
	Normal						

ORAL STAGE:

	3 ml	5 ml	10 ml	20 ml	pudding	solid	cont
A. Anterior loss	L1 L2	L1 L2	L1 L2	L1 L2	P1 P2	S1	L1
B. Premature spillage	L1 L2	L1 L2	L1 L2	L1 L2	P1 P2	S1	L1
Spillage to: valleculae	L1 L2	L1 L2	L1 L2	L1 L2	P1 P2	S1	L1
pyriform sinus	L1 L2	L1 L2	L1 L2	L1 L2	P1 P2	S1	L1
C. Delayed initiation	L1 L2	L1 L2	L1 L2	L1 L2	P1 P2	S1	L1
D. Uncoordinated initiation	L1 L2	L1 L2	L1 L2	L1 L2	P1 P2	S1	L1
E. Multiple lingual gestures	L1 L2	L1 L2	L1 L2	L1 L2	P1 P2	S1	L1
F. Piecemeal deglutition	L1 L2	L1 L2	L1 L2	L1 L2	P1 P2	S1	L1
G. Residue	L1 L2	L1 L2	L1 L2	L1 L2	P1 P2	S1	L1

PHARYNGEAL STAGE:

	Normal						
A. Delayed swallow	L1 L2	L1 L2	L1 L2	L1 L2	P1 P2	S1	L1
Pooling: valleculae	L1 L2	L1 L2	L1 L2	L1 L2	P1 P2	S1	L1
piriform sinus	L1 L2	L1 L2	L1 L2	L1 L2	P1 P2	S1	L1
B. ↓ velopharyngeal closure	L1 L2	L1 L2	L1 L2	L1 L2	P1 P2	S1	L1
C. ↓ tongue base retraction	L1 L2	L1 L2	L1 L2	L1 L2	P1 P2	S1	L1
D. ↓ vocal fold closure	L1 L2	L1 L2	L1 L2	L1 L2	P1 P2	S1	L1
E. ↓ laryngeal movement	L1 L2	L1 L2	L1 L2	L1 L2	P1 P2	S1	L1
F. ↓ epiglottic inversion	L1 L2	L1 L2	L1 L2	L1 L2	P1 P2	S1	L1
G. ↓ supraglottic closure	L1 L2	L1 L2	L1 L2	L1 L2	P1 P2	S1	L1
H. Mistimed laryngeal closure	L1 L2	L1 L2	L1 L2	L1 L2	P1 P2	S1	L1
I. ↓ pharyngeal contraction	L1 L2	L1 L2	L1 L2	L1 L2	P1 P2	S1	L1
J. ↓ UES opening	L1 L2	L1 L2	L1 L2	L1 L2	P1 P2	S1	L1
K. Penetration (P-A 2–5)*	L1 L2	L1 L2	L1 L2	L1 L2	P1 P2	S1	L1
L. Aspiration (P-A 6–8)*	L1 L2	L1 L2	L1 L2	L1 L2	P1 P2	S1	L1
M. Residue: valleculae**	L1 L2	L1 L2	L1 L2	L1 L2	P1 P2	S1	L1
piriform sinus**	L1 L2	L1 L2	L1 L2	L1 L2	P1 P2	S1	L1
aryepiglottic folds	L1 L2	L1 L2	L1 L2	L1 L2	P1 P2	S1	L1
pharyngeal wall	L1 L2	L1 L2	L1 L2	L1 L2	P1 P2	S1	L1

*Penetration-Aspiration Scale

**Rate severity   1—Mild (coating)   2—Moderate (1/2 filling)   3—Severe (>1/2 filling)

Cognitive status during testing (circle all that apply): Alert   Cooperative   Drowsy   Inattentive   Neglect   Agitated
Confused   Anosognosia

Comments/Recommendations: _____

continues

131

Table 10–2. *continued*

THERAPEUTIC TECHNIQUES (page 2)

_____ Chin Tuck   _____ Head turn (Right/Left)   _____ Cyclic ingestion

_____ Thick liquids (nectar/honey)   _____ Effortful swallow   _____ Breath hold

_____ Mendelsohn maneuver   _____ Combination (list)

STUDY CONDITIONS:

View: _____ Lateral _____ A-P   **Presentations:** _____ Cup _____ Straw _____ Syringe

Circle appropriate consistency/sequence   3 ml   5 ml   10 ml   20 ml   pudding   solid   cont

ORAL STAGE:

	Normal						
A. Anterior loss	L1 L2	L1 L2	L1 L2	L1 L2	L1 L2	P1 P2	S1 L1
B. Premature spillage	L1 L2	L1 L2	L1 L2	L1 L2	L1 L2	P1 P2	S1 L1
Spillage to: valleculae	L1 L2	L1 L2	L1 L2	L1 L2	L1 L2	P1 P2	S1 L1
piriform sinus	L1 L2	L1 L2	L1 L2	L1 L2	L1 L2	P1 P2	S1 L1
C. Delayed initiation	L1 L2	L1 L2	L1 L2	L1 L2	L1 L2	P1 P2	S1 L1
D. Uncoordinated initiation	L1 L2	L1 L2	L1 L2	L1 L2	L1 L2	P1 P2	S1 L1
E. Multiple lingual gestures	L1 L2	L1 L2	L1 L2	L1 L2	L1 L2	P1 P2	S1 L1
F. Piecemeal deglutition	L1 L2	L1 L2	L1 L2	L1 L2	L1 L2	P1 P2	S1 L1
G. Residue	L1 L2	L1 L2	L1 L2	L1 L2	L1 L2	P1 P2	S1 L1

PHARYNGEAL STAGE:

	Normal						
A. Delayed swallow	L1 L2	L1 L2	L1 L2	L1 L2	P1 P2	S1	L1
Pooling: valleculae	L1 L2	L1 L2	L1 L2	L1 L2	P1 P2	S1	L1
piriform sinus	L1 L2	L1 L2	L1 L2	L1 L2	P1 P2	S1	L1
B. ↓ velopharyngeal closure	L1 L2	L1 L2	L1 L2	L1 L2	P1 P2	S1	L1
C. ↓ tongue base retraction	L1 L2	L1 L2	L1 L2	L1 L2	P1 P2	S1	L1
D. ↓ vocal fold closure	L1 L2	L1 L2	L1 L2	L1 L2	P1 P2	S1	L1
E. ↓ laryngeal movement	L1 L2	L1 L2	L1 L2	L1 L2	P1 P2	S1	L1
F. ↓ epiglottic inversion	L1 L2	L1 L2	L1 L2	L1 L2	P1 P2	S1	L1
G. ↓ supraglottic closure	L1 L2	L1 L2	L1 L2	L1 L2	P1 P2	S1	L1
H. Mistimed laryngeal closure	L1 L2	L1 L2	L1 L2	L1 L2	P1 P2	S1	L1
I. ↓ pharyngeal contraction	L1 L2	L1 L2	L1 L2	L1 L2	P1 P2	S1	L1
J. ↓ UES opening	L1 L2	L1 L2	L1 L2	L1 L2	P1 P2	S1	L1
K. Penetration (P-A 2–5)*	L1 L2	L1 L2	L1 L2	L1 L2	P1 P2	S1	L1
L. Aspiration (P-A 6–8)*	L1 L2	L1 L2	L1 L2	L1 L2	P1 P2	S1	L1
M. Residue: valleculae**	L1 L2	L1 L2	L1 L2	L1 L2	P1 P2	S1	L1
piriform sinus**	L1 L2	L1 L2	L1 L2	L1 L2	P1 P2	S1	L1
aryepiglottic folds	L1 L2	L1 L2	L1 L2	L1 L2	P1 P2	S1	L1
pharyngeal wall	L1 L2	L1 L2	L1 L2	L1 L2	P1 P2	S1	L1

*Penetration-Aspiration Scale

**Rate severity   1—Mild (coating)   2—Moderate (1/2 filling)   3—Severe (>1/2 filling)

Bolus Flow

Bolus flow generally is evaluated in terms of timing, direction, and clearance. Timing is discussed in terms of transit times, for example, oral transit time, stage transit duration (STD), and so forth. Timing may be characterized in general terms such as slow or delayed or it can be objectively quantified. Using the various playback speeds of the recording the clinician can make subjective judgments of oral and pharyngeal transit times and time to onset of the pharyngeal swallow. Additionally, with a time code generator, the clinician can capture onset and offset points for each timing measure of interest to obtain objective measures of bolus timing (Table 10-3).

Table 10-3. Calculation of Durations for Bolus Timing Measures		
Bolus Timing	*Onset*	*Offset*
Oral Transit Time	Beginning of anterior or posterior movement of the bolus head or tail	Leading edge of the bolus at the posterior angle of the ramus of the mandible
Stage Transit Duration	Leading edge of the bolus at the posterior angle of the ramus of the mandible	Initiation of maximum superior movement of the hyoid
Pharyngeal Transit Time	Leading edge of the bolus at the posterior angle of the ramus of the mandible	Bolus tail passed through the upper esophageal sphincter
Pharyngeal Response Time	Initiation of maximum superior movement of the hyoid	Bolus tail passed through the upper esophageal sphincter
Total Swallowing Duration	Beginning of anterior or posterior movement of the bolus head or tail	Bolus tail passed through the upper esophageal sphincter

When determining onset of evocation of the pharyngeal swallow, or as it is measured in research studies, STD, it is important that the clinician distinguish between onset of *maximum* hyolaryngeal complex (HLC) elevation and movement of the tongue and HLC in an attempt to initiate the swallow. Onset of maximum HLC elevation is characterized by smooth, continual superior and anterior movement of the HLC. Whereas, when the pharyngeal swallow is notably delayed or absent, repetitive oral and base of tongue movement is evident yielding HLC movement; however, this movement does not progress toward maximum, and the subsequent pharyngeal events in swallowing do not occur.

Bolus direction is described in terms of laryngeal penetration or aspiration. Direction of bolus flow can be determined using either a global notation of laryngeal penetration and aspiration or the more detailed Penetration-Aspiration (P-A) Scale (Rosenbek, Robbins, Roecker, Coyle, & Wood, 1996). The P-A Scale is a validated ordinal scale to measure bolus direction by focusing on depth of airway invasion, clearance, and the patient's response (e.g., cough) to airway invasion (Table 10–4). A score of 1 indicates no airway invasion (i.e., no laryngeal penetration or aspiration). Scores 2 to 5 indicate laryngeal penetration using depth and clearance to determine the specific score. Scores 6 to 8 indicate aspiration using response and clearance to determine the specific score. As the P-A Scale was developed to capture airway invasion during all points of time during the swallow, VFSS is the instrumentation of choice in which to use the P-A Scale.

Timing of airway invasion is classified as either preswallow, during the swallow, or postswallow. Preswallow airway invasion is identified by entry of material into the larynx prior to onset of maximum hyolaryngeal excursion. Airway invasion during the swallow is determined by entry of material into the larynx during the course of the pharyngeal swallow. Airway invasion during the swallow can be visualized only with VFSS. Postswallow airway invasion is determined

Table 10–4. The Penetration-Aspiration Scale

Airway Invasion	Score	Description
	1	Material does not enter the airway
Laryngeal Penetration	2	Material enters the airway, remains above the vocal folds, and is ejected from the airway
	3	Material enters the airway, remains above the vocal folds, and is not ejected from the airway
	4	Material enters the airway, contacts the vocal folds, and is ejected from the airway
	5	Material enters the airway, contacts the vocal folds, and is not ejected from the airway
Aspiration	6	Material enters the airway, passes below the vocal folds, and is ejected into the larynx or out of the airway
	7	Material enters the airway, passes below the vocal folds, and is not ejected from the trachea despite effort
	8	Material enters the airway, passes below the vocal folds, and no effort is made to eject

From "The Penetration-Aspiration Scale," by J. C. Rosenbek, J. Robbin, E. B. Roecker, J. L. Coyle, and J. L. Wood, 1996, *Dysphagia, 11*, p. 94. Copyright © by Springer-Verlag. Adapted with permission.

by entry of material into the larynx following return of the structures to rest.

Bolus clearance is judged by postswallow residual in the oral cavity, valleculae, piriform sinuses, as well as along the base of tongue and aryepiglottic folds. The clinician should note changes in residue over multiple swallows or with increased bolus consistency. The amount of residue cannot be objectively determined during any instrumental swallowing examination used for clinical purposes. Clinicians, however, can subjectively judge the amount of residue by using a

Likert scale with 1 indicating none to minimum bolus retention, 2 indicating moderate retention with residue encompassing up to half of the pharyngeal recess, and 3 indicating severe bolus retention with residue encompassing over half of the pharyngeal recess. Spontaneous response to postswallow residual such as repeated swallows should be identified before the patient is instructed to dry swallow.

Temporal Coordination and Extent of Structural Movement

Timing and distance of structural movement can be obtained with VFSS. As with bolus timing, temporal and spatial structural measures can be made subjectively and are traditionally used in the clinical setting as more objective measures are labor intensive. Objective measurement of timing of structural movement in relation to bolus flow may be calculated when employing the onset and offset of movement of specific structures such as the UES opening duration. Spatial measurement of structural movement can be determined only by employing special software to determine exact distances, such as extent of hyolaryngeal elevation. Regardless of whether the clinician is employing subjective or objective measures, one should note velar elevation, base of tongue retraction, superior and anterior hyolaryngeal movement, closure of the laryngeal vestibule, and UES opening in terms of coordination of movement relative to bolus flow and extent of structural movement.

Response to Compensatory Strategies and Determining the Treatment Plan

By the end of a thorough VFSS, the clinician should have objective confirmation of the effects of specific compensatory swallowing strategies that were evaluated and should be able to make recommendations concerning dysphagia management as well as diet recommendations. As discussed earlier, the recommendation for a particular compensatory strategy, as well the types of rehabilitative techniques, will depend on the patient's cognitive status.

Assignment of Severity

With few exceptions, most of our diagnostic tests for swallowing impairment rely on subjective interpretation of objective information. The VFSS provides a clear representation of swallowing events, but its value in the diagnostic process is dependent on the skill and experience of the clinician. Interpretation of dynamic radiographic data is not simple. Thus, clinicians have sought to develop methods for structuring interpretation of this information.

There is an inherent tradeoff in these methods between specificity and utility. Many scales provide some organization and definition of various parameters of swallowing. The sample VFSS score sheet provided in Table 10-2 is an excellent example. This type of scale covers a lot of ground quickly and can be very helpful to classify and diagnosis. However, scales of this type typically are based on binary assessment (presence or absence) of a pathophysiologic feature and, therefore, do not offer a mechanism for quantifying severity. Thus, they are unable to measure anything but very large increments of change in post-treatment repeated studies. In response, assignment of severity may be included (as in item M in Table 10-2). However these are problematic due to lack of objectivity. What is mild to an experienced clinician may be perceived as quite severe to a less experienced clinician.

When specific and unambiguous definitions are provided, the scales tend to address only a limited number of swallowing features, such as the P-A Scale (see Table 10-4) or a scale developed by Murray, Langmore, Ginsberg, and Dostie (1996) for documenting pharyngeal secretions observed with videoendoscopy. Tools such as these are very valuable in clinical quantification of the feature under observation and in standardizing the language that clinicians use to communicate regarding swallowing impairment. However, they do not help to define other complex features of impaired swallowing that may not present with aspiration as a symptom.

However, increasing the complexity of this type of scale may render it cumbersome to all but the most seasoned clinician. An example of this type of scale is the New Zealand Index for the Multidisciplinary Evaluation of Swallowing (NZIMES) (Appendix). This Index was developed in an attempt to provide the level of detail in severity assignment used in the P-A Scale across many measures of swallowing. In doing so, clinicians would be availed of a tool that allows the sensitive measures of smaller increments of change as a function of rehabilitation. The NZIMES Subscale One is a clinical evaluation tool that categorizes swallowing parameters into five broad phases (Oral Parameters, Oral Pharyngeal Transit, Pharyngeal Parameters, Cricoesophageal Parameters, and Laryngeal Parameters). For each parameter grouping, there are 5 graded severity level categories, ranging from 0 (no significant impairment) to 4 (profound impairment). To guide assignment of an aggregated severity score for each phase of swallowing, the NZIMES Subscale 1 provides between 2 and 5 specific physiologic characteristics that define each parameter grouping. Each physiologic characteristic is further defined by a detailed description of swallowing physiology at various degrees of impairment. For example, the phase grouping of Pharyngeal Parameters is further described by three primary physiologic features that contribute to pharyngeal swallowing: velopharyngeal closure, pharyngeal contraction/bolus propulsion, and laryngeal excursion. Each of these physiologic features subsequently is characterized by detailed severity descriptors at each level of severity. Midpoint intervals can be selected to extend the 5-level scale (no impairment, mild, moderate, severe, profound) to 9 levels (including slight, mild to moderate, moderate to severe, severe to profound). Determination of the categorical phase rating would represent an estimated, clinical "average" of the severity scores ascribed to each subcategory within that phase. The NZIMES includes a separate subscale that address the multidisciplinary evaluation of clinical features associated with swallowing. NZIMES Subscale 2 addresses nursing status, nutritional status, cognitive status, and self-feeding ability and was designed for completion by members of an interdisciplinary swallowing team during clinical assessment or screening. Ratings from both subscales can then be recorded on a Dysphagia Profile Summary Sheet. Several inter- and intrarater reliability studies have been completed using a large sample of clinicians and a large number of VFSS, but these have yet to be submitted for publication. Thus, as with the VFSS score sheet in Table 10–2, this tool can, at this point, only be considered a nonvalidated guide for clinical assignment of severity levels.

11 The Instrumental Swallowing Examination

Evaluation of Swallowing Respiratory Coordination—An Auxiliary to the Videofluoroscopic Swallow Study

As discussed in Chapter 3, the pharynx serves a dual role as a conduit for both ingested food and ventilatory air; therefore, several functional adaptations of the aerodigestive tract have developed to protect the airway during swallowing (Preiksaitis & Mills, 1996). The epiglottis directs an oncoming bolus to the lateral channels away from the airway and into the esophagus. Adduction of the true vocal folds and the ventricular folds shields the airway from pulmonary invasion (Hadjikoutis, Pickersgill, Dawson, & Wiles, 2000). This represents one of the earliest airway protection mechanisms, and has been reported to precede the onset of hyoid movement associated with onset of the pharyngeal swallow (Martin-Harris et al., 2005; Shaker et al., 1990). The momentary cessation in respiration during deglutition is termed swallowing apnea (SA) and is considered a key feature of airway protection (Palmer & Hiiemae, 2003).

Although SA appears as a biomechanical component of the pharyngeal swallow, there is evidence that a distinct swallowing apneic reflex exists that is centrally integrated (Broussard & Altschuler, 2000; Miller, 1999; Widdicombe, 1986). Evidence for this central integration is provided through studies of laryngectomized (Hiss, Strauss, Treole, Stuart, & Boutilier, 2003) and intubated patients (Nishino & Hiraga, 1991) where biomechanical apnea is prevented.

Regardless, these patients continue to demonstrate measurable SA in the absence of glottic closure, thus suggesting that this apnea is not driven by the biomechanical interruption of respiration but is centrally initiated. This central control mechanism is confounded by biomechanical factors, and thus potentially places the patient with neurologic impairment at significant risk.

As such, recent research has focused on the importance of swallowing respiratory coordination in airway protection. Although more frequently engaged as a research tool, the development of preliminary normative databases and the substantial implications for swallowing safety in stroke suggest that this evaluation may emerge as a standard adjunct to the instrumental assessment.

Acquisition of instrumental techniques in isolation, as described above, allows us to clinically investigate, and sometimes carefully quantify, features of the deglutitive process. However, these techniques in isolation may bias our view of the complex relationships involved in the deglutitive process. A multimodality assessment may be required to fully grasp the intricacy of relationships between oral, pharyngeal, laryngeal, esophageal, and respiratory structures and functions. This is particularly true for the assessment of swallowing respiratory coordination.

Executing the Evaluation of Swallowing Respiratory Coordination

Measurement of swallowing respiratory coordination requires instrumentation for monitoring of the respiratory waveform, as well as some measure of swallowing onset or execution. Respiration can be monitored using a nasal thermister, which measures temperature at the entrance to the nares, or a respiratrace, which monitors expansion and contraction of the thoracic dimension (Selley, Flack, Ellis, & Brooks, 1989a). Although these techniques provide the information required, they are fairly specialized pieces of equipment and thus not readily available in clinical settings. More often reported in the literature is a system of evaluating nasal airflow using standard nasal prongs, as used to deliver oxygen in health care settings. This plastic tubing is simply placed at the entry to the nares and secured over the ears. The patient must be instructed to breathe through the nose. Those with habitual mouth breathing may require an alternative measure of respiration.

Respiratory tracings can be acquired synchronously with several other types of instrumental techniques. Onset of swallowing can be easily documented with the use of surface electromyography of the floor of mouth muscles. These muscles are chosen as they provide a proxy measure of onset and peak hyolaryngeal excursion, which is considered the leading complex of the pharyngeal swallow. After the skin surface is cleaned to remove any excess oil, makeup, or loose epithelial tissue, standard surface electrodes are placed longitudinally over this muscle group. Outputs from these sensors are fed into any digital recording system that will display ongoing waveform data.

For more detailed information regarding coordination of respiration with specific biomechanical features of airway protection and pharyngeal motility, the clinician may wish to couple the respiratory tracing with either radiographic or endoscopic evaluation of swallowing. To accomplish these integrated evaluations, respiratory recordings are required during the completion of diagnostic protocols described in prior sections of this chapter. Figure 11–1 represents a combined assessment of respiration and swallowing biomechanics using videofluoroscopy.

Once the instrumentation is in place, regardless of the nature of the paired assessment, swallowing respiratory coordination can be monitored during naïve swallows of secretions or during bolus swallows of increasing size and consistency as are acquired during other assessment protocols. In order to ensure temporal specificity, an integrated hardware software system that allows for synchronized acquisition from multiple digital data sources is required. This type

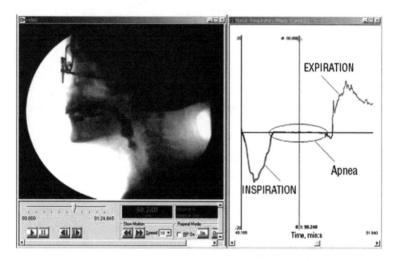

Figure 11–1. Simultaneous diagnostics incorporating VFSS (*on the left*) and swallowing respiratory coordination (*on the right*). VFSS = videofluoroscopic swallow study.

of system can be custom designed by professionals in biomedical engineering or can be purchased as packaged systems by manufacturers of medical devices.

Interpreting the Evaluation of Swallowing Respiratory Coordination

Interpretation of data from the evaluation of swallowing respiration coordination focuses on the temporal relationships between apnea and other biomechanical features of swallowing and the duration of swallowing apnea. Phase relationships generally are coded using the classification provided in Figure 11–2. In these figures, the downward moving component of the tracing negative to the abscissa represents inspiration, the upward moving component positive to the

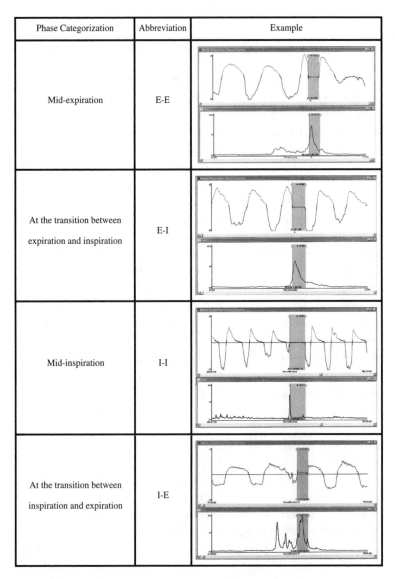

Phase Categorization	Abbreviation	Example
Mid-expiration	E-E	
At the transition between expiration and inspiration	E-I	
Mid-inspiration	I-I	
At the transition between inspiration and expiration	I-E	

Figure 11–2. Phase categorization descriptions for classifying swallowing respiratory coordination. E-E = expiration-expiration, E-I = expiration-inspiration, I-I = inspiration-inspiration, I-E = inspiration-expiration.

abscissa represents expiration, and the flat line of the waveform represents SA.

The surface electromyography tracing (in the lower windows of Figure 11–2) is a proxy for anterior hyoid movement and assists in identifying a swallowing event. Swallowing apnea duration (SAD) is represented by the gray shaded area; most commercially available data acquisition systems would offer a similar utility for waveform measurement. Martin-Harris et al. (2005) operationally define SAD as a "plateau in respiratory tracing along the abscissa" for the onset and "departure from plateau in respiratory tracing along abscissa in positive or negative direction" for offset.

Data are emerging that will aid the clinician in determining pathophysiology based on these measurements by first documenting variance in these swallowing respiratory measures in healthy adults and elders, and then in patients with neurologic disorders, including stroke. It is clear that SA occurs most frequently in the mid-expiratory phase of respiration in healthy adults (Klahn & Perlman, 1999; Preiksaitis & Mills, 1996). This is considered to be the most effective phase relationship for clearing postswallow residual in supraglottic airways and thus inhibiting postswallow aspiration (Hadjikoutis et al., 2000). However, reported frequencies vary. For example, Hiss, Treole, and Stuart (2001) reported greater than 62% of apneic periods during mid-expiration, whereas Martin, Logemann, Shaker, and Dodds (1994) reported between 94 to 100% of mid-expiratory swallows. Methodological differences such as size of bolus and method of bolus delivery may account for these differences. Considerable research has investigated the variance in measures of swallowing respiratory coordination. Hiss and colleagues (2001) evaluated the effects of age, gender, bolus volume, and trial on SAD and swallowing respiratory phase relationships in 60 healthy adults. The pattern of mid-expiratory swallowing apnea was demonstrated in 62% of participants' swallows. However, age, gender, or bolus volume did not predict the pattern of exhale-swallow-exhale. Significant main effects of age, gender, and bolus volume were identified with elders demonstrating prolonged SAD as compared to young and middle-aged adults. Women had longer SAD than men, and SAD increased as bolus volume increased. Preikasaitis and Mills (1996) found that the inspiration following swallowing was documented at 5% for single bolus swallows, but this phase pattern increased for ingestion of 200 ml of fluid to 23% when taken by cup and 27% by straw. Postswallow inspiration increased to 16% when eating solid textures. Thus, the clinician will need to take these factors into account when interpreting clinical data.

More recently, data have emerged that document changes in swallowing respiratory coordination as a function of age. Martin-Harris et al. (2005) evaluated swallowing respiratory coordination across the life span using simultaneous videofluoroscopy and nasal respiratory airflow. As with prior research, the most common respiratory phase category was expiration-expiration (E-E) (75%); this was followed by inspiration-expiration (I-E) (18%), expiration-inspiration (E-I) (4%), and inspiration-inspiration (I-I) (3%). When comparing collapsed postapnea expiratory patterns (E-E, I-E) to postapnea inspiratory patterns (E-I, I-I), a significant age effect was also seen, with post-deglutitive inspiration seen more frequently in elder participants. SAD was also influenced by age. SAD increased from 0.6 seconds to 1 second, respectively, when comparing younger to elder adults in a study by Selley, Flack, Ellis, and Brooks (1989a). Hiss et al. (2001) likewise reported that the overall duration of SA in elderly adults (>60) was significantly longer than young and middle age adults (<60). In the Martin-Harris et al. (2005) study, SAD during ingestion of 5-ml water bolus ranged from 0.5 to 10.02 seconds with a median duration of 1.0 seconds. Outliers all were from the oldest participants. As many individuals who are evaluated for swallowing impairment poststroke are in this age group, recognition that age influences swallowing respiratory coordination is critical.

Aberrant patterns of swallowing respiratory coordination have been reported in patients with neurologic disorders (Selley, Flack, Ellis, & Brooks, 1989b). These authors reported that 43% of a population of patients with mixed neurologic disorders demonstrated postswallow inspiration, whereas Hadjikoutis et al. (2000) reported this finding in up to 91% of his population studied. Specific to stroke, Leslie, Drinnan, Ford, and Wilson (2002) studied a relatively small sample of 18 stroke patients with mixed site of lesion and stroke severity and 50 healthy controls. Individuals with dysphagia subsequent to stroke were found to present fewer instances of postswallow expiration than those in the control group. SAD was not significantly different in patients with and without stroke; although in both groups, SAD increased with advancing age. Disparate findings for SAD were identified in a recent study by Butler, Stuart, Pressman, Poage, and Roche (2007) who described swallowing respiratory relationships in patients with dysphagia subsequent to stroke who aspirate and those who do not aspirate, and compared these data to healthy elders. Those patients with documented aspiration demonstrated significantly longer SAD than those without aspiration. Additionally, they demonstrated SAD that was twice as long as that in healthy elder adults. In reference to patterns of swallowing respiratory coordination, stroke patients with documented aspiration demonstrated a greater percentage of swallows within mid-inspiration (9%) with increasing percentage of this pattern with increased dysphagia severity. Nonaspirating patients with swallowing impairment presented this pattern on 3% of swallows with healthy elders documented at only 0.1%.

As with many of our emerging diagnostic tools, the evaluation of swallowing respiration coordination is hindered by incomplete and/or conflicting normative data. As research in this area continues, clinicians will be in a better position to assign diagnostic criteria to the data gleaned from this assessment. Until that time, the assessment of swallowing respiratory coordination can be cautiously compared to existing data and used as a supportive measure of diagnosing swallowing impairment and aspiration risk.

12 The Instrumental Swallowing Examination

Videoendoscopic Evaluation of Swallowing

Although the videofluoroscopic swallow study (VFSS) is generally the evaluation of choice for stroke patients, the videoendoscopic evaluation of swallowing does have particular strengths (see Table 10–1) that make it well-suited for certain stroke patients. Due to its portability, videoendoscopy may be advantageous for critically ill stroke patients, that is, patients in the intensive care unit or those who are ventilator dependent. For those patients with significant cognitive impairment and for whom the radiology environment may decrease cooperation and performance, videoendoscopy may be a good alternative to VFSS. In addition, videoendoscopy is ideal for directly evaluating airway protection.

EXECUTING THE VIDEOENDOSCOPIC EVALUATION OF SWALLOWING

Videoendoscopic Setup

When using videoendoscopy to evaluate swallowing, a flexible laryngoscope and light source are required. As with the VFSS, it is ideal to have the evaluation recorded, to have a microphone to capture audio, and to use a counter timer to record time. A clinician may piece together a videoendoscopic setup or choose predesigned models.

Patient and Videoendoscope Positioning

Patients may be evaluated while sitting in bed or when seated in a chair or wheelchair. Unlike VFSS, patient positioning is not an issue and little time and effort are required to achieve optimal viewing of pharyngeal and laryngeal structures. The scope, however, will constantly need to be repositioned as the velum elevates and lowers during speech and swallowing and the pharynx changes dimensions during the swallow. The clinician also should be prepared to reposition the scope as stroke patients may move thereby disrupting optimal scope positioning.

The use of topical anesthesia is not imperative for videoendoscopy. No difference in patient comfort has been identified with or without the use of a topical anesthetic (Leder, Ross, Briskin, & Sasaki, 1997), although stroke patients were not the particular focus of the study. The need for anesthesia depends on the patient and the experience of the clinician in handling the endoscope. If desired, topical anesthesia, such as 2% viscous lidocaine may be used to anesthetize the nares. Aerosol anesthetic should be avoided due to the potential for affecting pharyngeal sensation.

The endoscope is placed transnasally generally alongside or under the inferior turbinate. If a small-bore nasogastric feeding tube (NGT) is in place, the scope can usually be passed on the same side following the same route. If a large-bore NGT is present, the scope may need to be passed through the other nares. The scope is inserted continuously until the nasopharynx is visualized. If velopharyngeal closure incompetence is suspected and the stroke patient can produce volitional speech, evaluation of palatal functioning should be completed at this point. Velopharyngeal functioning is determined by having the patient repeatedly contrast oral plosives and nasal resonance sounds, that is., "duh-nuh." Following evaluation of velopharyngeal competence, the scope is inserted further until the distal end is placed above the uvula (Figure 12–1). This position should be maintained prior to each swallow as it allows a view of the epiglottis,

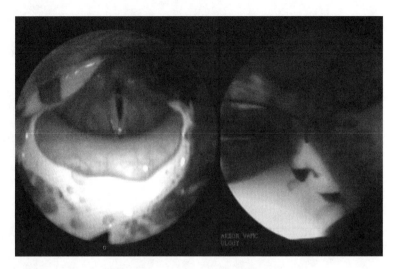

Figure 12–1. Correct placement of the endoscope to view the pharynx and larynx for swallowing. (Figure courtesy of Dr. Joseph Murray.)

base of tongue, hypopharynx, and larynx. After each swallow, the clinician should quickly advance the scope further to determine if residual material is in the larynx or the trachea. The scope then is retracted to the more superior position before the next swallow.

Preswallow Observations

Numerous observations in addition to the evaluation of velopharyngeal competence should be completed prior to administration of food and liquid (Table 12–1). The appearance and symmetry of structures and recesses (valleculae, piriform sinuses) should be observed with any deviations noted. Integrity of true vocal fold (TVF) functioning is completed by having the patient phonate /ee/. The clinician should note the magnitude and symmetry of TVF movement and closure as well as vocal quality. As with velopharyngeal incompetence,

Table 12–1. Features to Assess with Videoendoscopy Prior to the Administration of Food or Liquid

- Velopharyngeal competence
- Appearance and symmetry of structures
- True vocal fold adduction
- Breath holding
- Cough
- Secretions
- Sensation

unilateral vocal fold paresis frequently may be seen in patients with a lateral medullary stroke.

Breath holding is assessed by having the patient hold his or her breath with notation of: (1) ability to achieve breath holding, (2) the duration of breath holding, and (3) the adduction of true and ventricular vocal fold closure. Cough is evaluated by volitional production. Components of the volitional cough include: inspiration (glottic abduction), supraglottic closure with increased tracheal pressure, and glottic abduction with release of pressure (Murray, 1999). Although volitional cough may not relate to the effectiveness of a spontaneous cough, it will provide information on the ability to use volitional cough as part of therapeutic intervention and is a good indicator for poor performance when it is weakly produced.

Evaluation of secretion management is completed by documenting the collection of secretions in the pharyngeal recesses and in the laryngeal vestibule. The amount and location of secretions should be noted as well as any response from the patient in an attempt to clear the material. Does the patient spontaneously swallow, throat clear, or cough in attempt to clear, or is there no response to the accumulation of secretions? Is the patient successful in attempts to clear secretions? Pooling of secretions in the laryngeal vestibule is associated with wet vocal quality and may be evident following stroke. Pooling of secretions in the laryngeal vestibule is strongly associated with aspiration of food and liquid (Murray et al., 1996).

Sensation initially may be evaluated by noting the patient's response to pooled secretions, postswallow residual, and aspiration. That is, does the patient repeatedly swallow or cough to clear secretions or residue; does the patient cough in response to aspiration? Although not a quantitative measure, the patient's response to material in the larynx and pharynx is the most clinically relevant measure of laryngopharyngeal sensation in the context of ingestion.

Fiberoptic endoscopic evaluation of swallowing with sensory testing (FEESST) may be used to quantitatively evaluate laryngopharyngeal sensation. FEESST is completed by using a specially designed endoscope with an attached port to allow delivery of air-puff stimulation to the medial surface of the pyriform sinuses and the aryepiglottic folds in order to evoke a laryngeal adductor reflex (LAR) (Aviv et al., 1999). LAR results in brief adduction of the TVF. The tip of the scope is placed 2 mm from the target site and air pulses are delivered in durations of 50 msec with the intensity varying from 1 to 10 mm Hg. Three blocks of ascending stimulus presentation (beginning at a minimal intensity level with 1 mm Hg increases until LAR is evoked) and three blocks of descending stimulus presentation (beginning at a high intensity level and decreasing by 1 mm Hg until no LAR is evoked) are presented in random order (Langmore & Aviv, 2001). The patient's sensory threshold is defined as the mean of the lowest detected pressures following completion of the six blocks of stimulus presentation. Both the right and left sides of the laryngopharynx should be tested in a patient. Sensory thresholds may be classified as normal (<4.0 mm Hg), moderately impaired (4.0–6.0 mm Hg), or severely impaired (>6.0 mm Hg) (Aviv et al., 1996).

Although increased thresholds have been associated with pooled secretions, laryngeal elevation, and aspiration (Aviv, 1997;

Link, Willging, Miller, Cotton, & Rudolph, 2000), the association of the LAR and *response* to airway invasion during swallowing (e.g., repeated swallows, cough), however, has not been empirically determined. Studies have shown that supraglottic penetration can occur in healthy young and older adults without elicitation of a response (Daniels et al., 2004; Robbins et al., 1999). The clinician should note that FEESST data are based on the use of a specialized endoscope with air delivery through an indwelling port as described earlier. These data may not translate to newer systems that rely on air delivery through a sleeve on a standard endoscope.

Bolus Presentation Guidelines

The same guidelines suggested with the clinical swallowing examination or VFSS should be followed for videoendoscopic evaluation of swallowing. As with these other evaluations, initiating the videoendoscopic evaluation with small liquid volumes is strongly encouraged with stroke patients to reduce the amount of aspiration and to prevent contamination of subsequent swallows with significant postswallow residual. Murray (1999) recommends beginning the examination with ice chips for those patients who demonstrate accumulation of secretions in the laryngeal vestibule or who have been without oral feedings for an extended period. This will prevent a large amount of aspiration in those patients who are at high risk of aspiration and may help "alert" the swallowing system in those patients who have been without oral intake for a period of time.

As the videoendoscopic evaluation of swallowing does not involve ingestion of barium, the clinician is free to use any food or liquid. At a minimum, the clinician should consider assessing swallowing of liquids, semisolids, and solids, but as with the other evaluation methods, progression to larger volumes and thicker consistencies depends on the patient's response to small liquid volumes. Early in the use of videoendoscopy to evaluate swallowing, food coloring was added to material ingested to facilitate visualization of the bolus. Recent research, however, suggests that nondyed food (milk, pudding) is as reliable as dyed material for completing critical swallowing measures (Leder, Acton, Lisitano, & Murray, 2005). The authors suggest that the ability of a bolus to reflect light is the critical feature for determining the visibility of a bolus in laryngopharyngeal region. Thus, milk-based products, particularly liquids, are frequently suggested in the videoendoscopic evaluation of swallowing.

By having no time constraints on the length of the videoendoscopic evaluation of swallowing, the clinician can extend the assessment to evaluate the effects of fatigue or swallowing behavior over time. The repeated use of a compensatory strategy can be evaluated; this is important for the stroke patient in whom the clinician has concern for continuous employment of a posture without clinician cue. Videoendoscopy also may be used to provide visual feedback during the initial assessment or in treatment to instruct the patient on the implementation of such compensatory strategies such as the supersupraglottic swallow.

INTERPRETATING THE VIDEOENDOSCOPIC EVALUATION OF SWALLOWING

Interpreting the videoendoscopic evaluation can be challenging as the oral cavity is not viewed and the view is obscured during velar elevation or when the base of tongue contacts the posterior pharyngeal wall, both of which will trap the lens with light from the endoscope reflecting back into the lens. The obscuring of the view is frequently termed "whiteout" and results in loss of view of critical portions of the swallowing event. Thus, judgments of oral and pharyngeal motility must be inferred by viewing observable bolus flow patterns such as preswallow pharyngeal pooling and postswallow residual patterns.

Anatomic Abnormalities

Detailed information concerning pharyngeal and laryngeal anatomy can be obtained with videoendoscopy. The superior view of mucosa covering the structures obtained with videoendoscopy may provide more detail about anatomic deviations, particularly evidence of a mass, in the pharynx and larynx as compared to the lateral view with VFSS. Abnormality in appearance and symmetry should be reported as well as the effects on swallowing. The preswallow observations on secretions, breath holding, and so forth, will provide the clinician with information on glottic function and sensation, which are important for swallowing and can assist in forming an impression as to how well the patient may perform during subsequent presentations of food and liquid.

Bolus Flow

Information on bolus timing through the oral cavity and pharynx cannot be obtained with videoendoscopy as the oral cavity is not visualized and whiteout obscures the actual swallow. Although different from VFSS, information concerning stage transit duration can be determined by observing the entry of the bolus into the pharynx (onset) through the point of whiteout (offset). In this fashion, delay in evocation of the pharyngeal swallow can be determined.

Timing of airway invasion can only be measured if it occurs preswallow or postswallow. Determining intraswallow aspiration is determined if material is visualized in the airway after the period of whiteout is over. Unlike VFSS, the clinician will not be able to view intraswallow airway invasion as it happens. Distinguishing between preswallow laryngeal penetration and aspiration may be difficult at times if whiteout occurs before visualization of entry of material into the trachea. Only by inspecting the trachea for residual material once the swallow is completed can intraswallow aspiration be identified. The Penetration-Aspiration (P-A) Scale, as reviewed in the VFSS section, was designed for use during VFSS (Rosenbek et al., 1996); however, reliability in scoring has been demonstrated with videoendoscopy (Colodny, 2002). Again, the clinician is cautioned that depth of airway invasion in the larynx, one of the measures of the P-A Scale, may be difficult to determine using videoendoscopy. Furthermore and not surprisingly, assignment of higher P-A scores using endoscopy as compared to videofluoroscopy has been identified (Kelly, Drinnan, & Leslie, 2007).

Postswallow residue can be viewed in the pharynx using videoendoscopy. Unlike VFSS, which provides a lateral or A-P view of the depth of residual, the clinician must identify residual material and subjectively determine amount from a superior view. The piriform sinuses and valleculae are easily viewed with videoendoscopy. As with VFSS, it is ideal for clinicians to have a working knowledge of what is normal residue for various consistencies before judging abnormal clearance. Recent research has suggested that pharyngeal residue is judged to be greater in a videoendoscopic examination as compared to VFSS (Kelly, Leslie, Beale, Payten, & Drinnan, 2006). Thus, it is critical that clinicians new to the use of videoendoscopy in the evaluation of swallowing internally calibrate their judgment of postswallow residual with experienced endoscopists and against VFSS findings.

Temporal Coordination and Extent of Structural Movement

Aside from airway protection, any dysfunction in swallowing biomechanics must be inferred using videoendoscopy. That is, the clinician must use information gleaned from swallowing function prior to the onset of whiteout as well as information obtained after the swallow, for example, postswallow residual, to determine the area of dysfunction. For example, entry of material into the pharynx before onset of whiteout may be due to premature spillage or to delayed elicitation of the pharyngeal swallow. Without viewing the oral cavity, this may be very difficult to distinguish. Oral dysmotility or delayed initiation of oral transfer also may be inferred by delayed appearance of the bolus in the pharynx or delayed whiteout. The presence and location of postswallow residual must be used to judge pharyngeal motility. Vallecular residue may indicate decreased base of tongue retraction and/or reduced epiglottic inversion. Piriform sinus residue may indicate reduced anterior hyolaryngeal movement and/or decreased upper esophageal sphincter opening.

Response to Compensatory Strategies and Determining the Treatment Plan

The implementation and use of specific management techniques is the same with videoendoscopy as it is with VFSS. As time is not an issue with videoendoscopy, the clinician may spend more time instructing and having the patient practice various compensatory techniques. Although persistence or resolution of the signs of dysphagia, that is, postswallow residual or aspiration, is viewed with videoendoscopy, the effect on the swallowing biomechanics is not observed. For example, the Mendelsohn maneuver is implemented in a patient with reduced hyolaryngeal movement and postswallow piriform sinus residual. The clinician would see reduced residual using videoendoscopy, whereas with VFSS, the clinician could observe improved hyolaryngeal excursion as well as reduced postswallow residual.

13 The Instrumental Swallowing Examination

Manometric Evaluation of Swallowing

As discussed in previous chapters, the videofluoroscopic swallow study (VFSS) provides critical information about swallowing biomechanics through observations of structural and mucosal movement and bolus flow. The endoscopic evaluation of swallowing nicely augments this information by providing optimal visualization of airway closure mechanisms. These are undoubtedly very valuable and irreplaceable tools, but can be limited by the subjective nature of interpretation of some aspects of swallowing biomechanics, resulting in compromised reliability and thus questionable validity (Kuhlemeier et al., 1998; McCullough et al., 2001; Scott et al., 1998; Stoeckli et al., 2003; Wilcox et al., 1996).

Esophageal manometry is well established in the diagnostic armamentarium of gastroenterologic medicine for the evaluation of esophageal pressure systems. Pharyngeal manometry as a means to assess pressure systems underlying pharyngeal motility is slowly transitioning from the research laboratory into clinical application. Manometry provides a measure of pressure and in so doing will offer to the diagnostic dysphagia evaluation information about the amplitude and timing of pressure events within the pharyngeal cavity and cricopharyngeal sphincter. Although this technique provides no direct visualization of swallowing events, the issue of subjectivity and subsequent reliability is minimized through the provision of quantitative measures of swallowing biomechanics. Pharyngeal manometry should be considered not a primary evaluation tool, rather an augmentation of the comprehensive diagnostic workup. The technique can provide clarification and quantification of diagnostic features identified through other techniques. Pharyngeal manometry has limitations that have hindered its widespread acceptance. Manometric catheters are not standardly manufactured. As a result, a broad range of custom-made catheters have been designed for use in research to answer specific questions. The result is that currently there are no large sample normative values on which to base diagnostic interpretation of the objective output of amplitude and sequencing of pharyngeal events.

The more traditional method for esophageal manometry using a hydraulic system of perfused water-filled catheters largely has been replaced for pharyngeal manometry by solid-state recordings. Using this method, the manometry catheter, which is inserted through the oral cavity or nare, houses multiple transducer elements. The information received by these transducers is amplified and displayed generally through computerized recording systems. Salassa, DeVault, and McConnel (1998) present a valuable review of manometric methods and should be requisite reading for any clinician who wishes to include manometry in their diagnostic workup. They propose optimal "standard" catheter design for pharyngeal manometry, or manofluorography. The ideal standard pharyngeal manometry catheter is recommended to:

- be 2 × 4 mm (or smaller) in diameter, ovoid in shape, and 100 cm long.
- be marked in cm with anterior to posterior orientation.
- have a slightly malleable, 3- to 4-cm length of catheter without sensors beyond the most distal sensor.
- use solid-state transducers with one sensor each in three or four locations:
  - cricopharyngeus
  - hypopharynx

- tongue base
- with esophagus as optional 4th sensor
- sensor spacing should be 3 cm between cricopharyngeus and hypopharynx and 2 cm between hypopharynx and tongue base.

Pharyngeal manometry is best completed in conjunction with other diagnostic assessments. Perhaps the best option is joint manometry with videofluoroscopy, termed in the literature "manofluorography." With visualization of bolus flow time-locked to pressure recordings, the clinician is able to gain greater insights into the relationships between pressure and pharyngeal biomechanics. The clinician thus is able to quantify the observed pharyngeal events with an objective measure. This provides great advantages over videofluoroscopy in isolation. Manofluorography is the only method that allows for measurement of intrabolus pressure, or the amount of pressure exerted on the bolus as it is transported through the pharynx, as interpretation of this measurement requires visualization of bolus flow. This technique also allows for confirmation of sensor placement through observation. To complete this examination the manometric catheter must be placed prior to or during the study (radiographically guided) and the recording equipment for both techniques integrated into a single acquisition system. As such, this type of recording can be cumbersome, requires considerable staffing and expertise, and is not readily available.

Another option for completing manometry is to pair this technique with endoscopy, termed manovideoendoscopy by Butler (2006). This option has benefits in flexibility and portability and allows the clinician to visually confirm placement of pharyngeal sensors. Execution of the pharyngeal swallow produces a "whiteout" on endoscopy; thus, the period of bolus flow over the manometric sensors is not visualized using this technique. Intrabolus pressure can only be inferred and loses the precision gained from manofluorography. Regardless, in patients who are unable to transfer to the videofluoroscopy suite and require examinations performed at bedside, the manovideoendoscopic study will provide valuable information.

Finally, the "bare-bones" approach to manometry consists of pharyngeal manometry completed in isolation. This type of assessment would only be appropriate when prior diagnostic studies have been completed and there is a specific differential diagnosis required. Placement of the catheter must be inferred by waveform interpretation and requires the clinician to be meticulous in monitoring placement throughout the study. Intrabolus pressure cannot be measured, but only weakly inferred. Thus, the examination relies on investigation of pharyngeal contact pressure, or the approximation of pharyngeal structures behind the bolus that constitute clearing pressure.

EXECUTING THE MANOMETRIC EVALUATION

The American Speech-Language-Hearing Association has included pharyngeal manometry, in conjunction with videofluoroscopy, in the document on Instrumental Diagnostic Procedures for Swallowing (American Speech-Language-Hearing Association, 1992). The manometric evaluation in clinical settings is completed jointly by the gastroenterologist and the swallowing clinician. Although manofluorography and/or manoendoscopy are recommended, instructions are provided below for "blind" manometry, or manometry completed in isolation as described in prior research (Gumbley, Huckabee, Doeltgen, Witte, & Moran, in press; Hiss & Huckabee, 2005; Huckabee, Butler, Barclay, & Jit, 2005; Huckabee & Steele, 2006; Steele & Huckabee, 2007; Witte, Huckabee, Doeltgen, Gumbley, & Robb, in press). Certainly with the augmentation of the procedure using other techniques, the protocol below will require adaptation.

As the procedure requires contact with potentially infectious bodily fluids via intraoral or intranarial catheter placement, facility approved infection control procedures should be adhered to. After calibrating the catheter to the manufacturers' specifications, the clinician should prepare the catheter by rinsing with warm water and coating the distal end with a water-based lubricant to facilitate ease of transfer through the nasal cavity. As with all diagnostic procedures, clear instructions should be given to the patient prior to initiation of the examination. With the sensors facing the ceiling, the catheter is passed into and through the nasal cavity, taking care to maintain position below the inferior turbinate. Anesthetic typically is not required. The clinician will feel slight resistance as the catheter abuts the posterior pharyngeal wall. If the catheter does not easily pass from the horizontally oriented nasal cavity into the more vertically oriented pharyngeal cavity, asking the patient to look up to the ceiling will reduce the angle at the nasopharyngeal junction and allow transfer. As the catheter enters the pharynx, the sensors will now be oriented toward the posterior pharyngeal wall. During blind placement, care must be taken to avoid laryngeal irritation or invasion with the tip of the catheter. To accomplish this it is best to let the patient control placement by executing either dry, or if tolerated, water swallows. In this case, the patient "swallows" the catheter into the esophagus, thus protecting the airway as the tip of the catheter moves through the hypopharynx. If resistance is encountered in passing the catheter through the upper esophageal sphincter (UES), a slight quarter-turn rotation of the catheter may facilitate guidance through the lateral channels and esophageal entry.

After the catheter enters the esophagus and the uppermost sensor is placed within the esophagus (up to 40 cm from the tip of the nose), the clinician must correctly position the catheter. This is accomplished using a "pull through" technique. With the waveform display running, the catheter is slowly withdrawn. As the uppermost sensor passes through the high-pressure zone of the UES, pressure recordings in this channel will increase and then subsequently decrease as the sensor exits into the hypopharyx. Similarly, the mid-pharyngeal sensor will produce a waxing and waning amplitude as it passes through the cricopharyngeus and into the pharynx. As the lowermost sensor passes through the UES, the clinician will pull through the pressure zone and then push the catheter very slightly back into the zone of high pressure, approximately 1 cm in after peak pressure is achieved. In so doing, the lowermost sensor is resting near the top of the cricopharyngeus muscle. During swallowing, if the catheter is appropriately positioned, the clinician will observe a typical "M" wave (Castell, Dalton, & Castell, 1990; Richter & Castell, 1989) as displayed in Figure 13–1. Baseline pressure, although not maximal resting pressure, is evident at rest. As hyolaryngeal excursion is initiated, the cricopharyngeus muscle is pulled fully over the lowermost sensor, resulting in peak amplitude, or the first peak in the "M." Cricopharyngeal relaxation then produces a substantive drop in pressure as the UES is maximally opened; this pro-

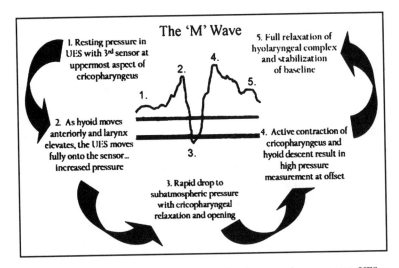

Figure 13–1. The characteristic M wave in pharyngeal manometry. UES = upper esophageal sphincter.

duces the middle drop in the "M" wave. The cricopharyngeus then contracts after bolus transfer with again a maximal rise in pressure then subsequently returns to a lower resting average as passive return of hyolaryngeal excursion drops the cricopharyngeus back to the inferior aspect of the lowermost sensor.

When the catheter is appropriately positioned, the clinician should ensure that the guide numbers on the catheter are facing up at the nose, indicating that the sensors within the pharynx are posteriorly oriented. The catheter then should be secured to the nose with standard medical tape, and the patient is allowed time to adjust to the catheter *in* vivo. Figure 13–2A displays a catheter in vivo at rest; Figure 13–2B displays a manometry catheter in vivo during pharyngeal swallowing with the pharynx fully closed around the catheter.

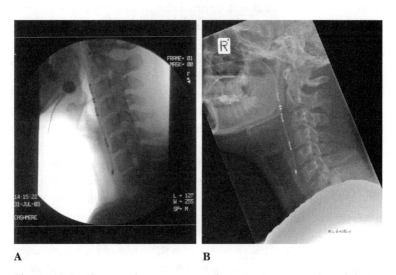

A   **B**

Figure 13–2. Pharyngeal manometric catheter in vivo at rest (**A**) and during swallowing (**B**).

INTERPRETING THE MANOMETRIC EVALUATION

As a measurement of pressure, pharyngeal manometry provides quantitative information about the amplitude and duration of pressure events within the pharyngeal cavity and cricopharyngeal sphincter. Typically, pressures are measured in the oropharynx, hypopharynx, and within the cricopharyngeal sphincter. Perhaps more importantly, valuable information can be gained about the sequencing of pharyngeal events. Figure 13–3 represents three manometry waveforms acquired with a 2.1-mm diameter round catheter with posteriorly facing sensors. The waveforms were acquired during secretion swallows in a healthy individual.

The uppermost waveform represents pressure generation in the proximal pharynx, at approximately the level of base of tongue to posterior pharyngeal wall approximation. The middle waveform represents pressure generation in the mid-pharynx, at approximately the level of the laryngeal additus. For both waveforms, at rest there is a flat baseline at approximately atmospheric pressure. During swallowing, a short peak is visualized. The point of a sharp increase in pressure is subtracted from the return to baseline postswallow for calculation of duration of pharyngeal pressure. Peak pressure is identified as the nadir amplitude during swallowing. The lowermost sensor rests at the upper margin of the cricopharyngeus muscle. At rest the baseline is measured with positive pressure. As the hyoid elevates and pulls the cricopharyngeus over the sensor, there is a peak in amplitude that represents peak pressure within the cricopharyngeus before relaxation. The waveform then drops dramatically to atmospheric or subatmospheric pressure levels as the UES is pulled open. Peak negative pressure is the nadir of pressure during this drop. As the cricopharyngeus contracts at conclusion of swallowing, there is again a sharp rise in pressure that represents peak offset. Subtracting onset time from offset time derives duration of

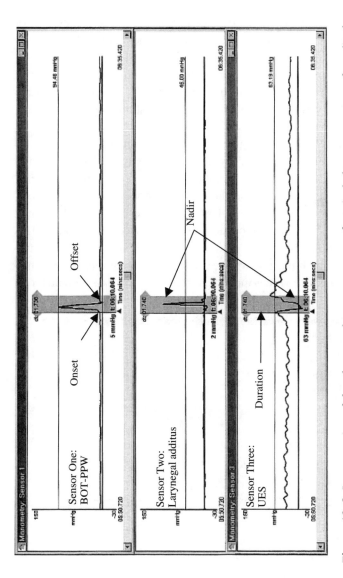

Figure 13–3. Interpretation of the pharyngeal manometry waveform includes measurement of amplitude at nadir, as well as time of onset and offset which allows calculation of duration. BOT = base of tongue; PPW = posterior pharyngeal wall; UES = upper esophageal sphincter.

UES opening. In addition to peak and durational measures, it is of interest to evaluate sequencing of pressure generation. This is easily visualized by using overlapping waveforms as shown in Figure 13–4. Onset of pressure in the upper pharynx should precede onset of pressure in the lower pharynx. The onset of UES opening appears somewhat variable. Offset of UES opening should occur after peak pressure in the mid-pharynx.

The waveform in Figure 13–4 is an example of contact pressure. It is important that the clinician differentiate contact pressure from intrabolus pressure. Intrabolus pressure is defined as brief, moderate pressure increase elicited by the bolus passing the pharyngeal sensors (Cerenko et al., 1989; Kahrilas et al., 1992; McConnel, 1988). This is a measure of the pressure exerted *on* the bolus. This measure is reliably identified only with manofluorography, as visualization of the bolus relative to sensors is a prerequisite to determining whether pressure is indeed exerted from the passing bolus. This

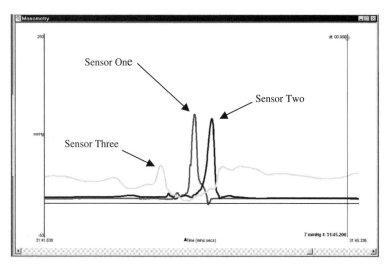

Figure 13–4. Overlapping waveforms acquired through pharyngeal manometric evaluation allow for clear visualization of sequencing of pharyngeal pressure generation.

is contrasted with pharyngeal contact pressure, which is the pressure exerted by approximation of pharyngeal structures after the bolus passes. This constitutes clearing pressure to strip the bolus from the pharyngeal cavity. Ingestion of a bolus swallow will allow the clinician to visualize not only intrabolus pressure but also contact pressure. On swallowing, there is a brief, moderate pressure increase at the pharyngeal sensors, prior to the pronounced and fast pressure rise. The pronounced and fast pressure rise reflects pharyngeal wall contact, whereas the preceding pressure increase is elicited by the bolus passing the pharyngeal sensors, thus measuring intrabolus pressure (Cerenko et al., 1989; Kahrilas et al., 1992; McConnel, 1988). This also can be observed on some secretion swallows, although intrabolus pressure is very subtle. The distinction between intrabolus and contact pressure is an important one as contact pressure is considerably higher than intrabolus pressure in unimpaired swallowing. Research by Olsson, Nilsson, and Ekberg (1995) has documented a mean intrabolus pressure of 33.2 mm Hg at the inferior pharyngeal constrictor; whereas contact pressure generates a mean of 137.1 mm Hg at the same location.

VARIABLES INFLUENCING PHARYNGEAL PRESSURE MEASUREMENT

Swallowing biomechanics, and thus the measured pharyngeal pressures supporting those biomechanics, can be influenced by several variables in the nonimpaired population, and thus quite likely in the patient with stroke. Data are beginning to emerge that document measurement characteristics and variances in manometric recordings. These studies often differ in focus, design, methods, and catheter type and are based on relatively small numbers of subjects. As such, there is still considerable uncertainty in the literature.

Several researchers have documented differences in pharyngeal pressure generation based on gender. Perlman, Schultz, and VanDaele (1993) identified that pressure duration was longer in men than women in the hypopharynx; although amplitude was invariant. When evaluating the UES rather than hypopharynx, van Herwaarden et al. (2003) found conflicting results with shorter duration of UES relaxation in men than women and lower UES resting pressure. Findings of both studies were confirmed by Robbins and colleagues (1992) who identified longer UES relaxation duration in women and no gender differences for pharyngeal pressure generation.

Recent data by Witte and colleagues (in press) evaluated the influence of bolus on contact pressure in the pharynx and UES in nonimpaired research participants, aged 20 to 40 years. Amplitude of pharyngeal pressure was greater for saliva swallows than 10 ml water swallows in the upper pharynx only, suggesting that greater lingual contribution in the dry swallow condition contributed to pharyngeal pressure generation. Duration of pressure was longer in both pharyngeal sensors for saliva swallows. Thus, those performing clinical manometry should be cognizant of the bolus as an influencing variable for both pressure and duration. Pressure within the UES did not vary as a function of bolus.

Bolus size has also been the subject of research in interpretation of manometric findings. Within the hypopharynx, Shaker et al. (1993) evaluated both intrabolus and pharyngeal contact pressure from a small subject group. Results demonstrated that bolus volume had no significant effect on the amplitude or duration of pharyngeal contact pressure in both young and elderly age groups. These results were confirmed in a larger study by Gumbley et al. (in press), which identified no hypopharyngeal differences in contact pressure between boli of 5, 10, and 20 ml. Kahrilas et al. (1992) studied contact pressure in the hypopharynx and identified that the only effect between 5 and 10-ml water boluses was sequentially later pharyngeal pressure with larger bolus size. Castell and colleagues (1990) evaluated temporal sequencing of contact pressure within the pharynx and UES during 5, 10, and 20-ml water swallows. Increases in the duration of pharyngeal contraction were evident as bolus size increased from 5 to 20 ml.

Bolus volume affects not only the extent of UES opening, but also duration (Castell et al., 1990; Jacob et al., 1989; Kahrilas, Dodds, Dent, Logemann, & Shaker, 1988; Kahrilas, Lin, Chen, & Logemann, 1996). Gumbley et al. (in press) have identified that negative pressure in the UES is inversely proportionate to bolus volume; however, in contrast to previous work, durational measures of UES relaxation were not significantly different.

WHAT CAN MANOMETRY OFFER TO CLINICAL PRACTICE? CASE EXAMPLES

Pharyngeal manometry offers quantification of observed biomechanics that have been documented from other diagnostic tests. This will aid the clinician in differential diagnosis of pharyngeal motility disorders by providing objective measures of pharyngeal events. Unfortunately, data have not yet emerged that quantify pharyngeal motility disorders in stroke. Several clinical cases are presented below that highlight the clinical utility of this technique; however, until a thorough normative data set is established, application in clinical practice will be limited. Mr. N is a 72-year-old male admitted to the acute hospital with a pontine stroke. He was evaluated clinically for dysphagia secondary to intermittent coughing during meals during his brief 4-day hospitalization. VFSS revealed significant postswallow pharyngeal residual with intermittent aspiration that was cleared with a reflexive cough. The treating clinician was unsure from the examination if the residual was secondary to overall poor pharyngeal motility, or specific impairment of bolus transport through the UES. The patient was being considered by the head and neck surgery service for a cricopharyngeal myotomy. A manovideoendoscopy study was completed with three primary findings (Figure 13–5). First, although resting pressure in the cricopharyngeus was variable, impaired opening of the UES was ruled out. The lowermost cricopharyngeal

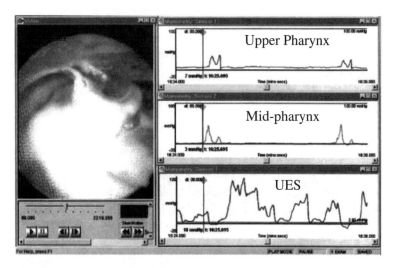

Figure 13–5. Patient example Mr. N. Results of manovideoendoscopic evaluation reveal very low pressure generation, paired with mis-sequencing of pharyngeal pressure within the pharynx.

sensor documented appropriate relaxation to negative pressure during swallowing. Second, the uppermost and middle pharyngeal sensors documented overall reduced pharyngeal contact pressure generation during swallowing. Average pressure of 17.2 mm Hg (standard deviation = 8.1) in the upper pharynx and 32.3 mm Hg (standard deviation = 21) in the lower pharynx was compared to local normative values taken from 40 healthy individuals of 99.44 mm Hg (standard deviation = 41.0) at the upper pharyngeal sensor and 116.32 mm Hg (standard deviation = 48.06) at the lower sensor using the same methods and catheter. Finally, and perhaps most interestingly, the patient presented an inconsistent mis-sequencing of pharyngeal events. On 67% of swallows pressure generation was initiated in the lower pharynx an average of 123 msec *before* pressure in the upper pharynx. Based on local normative values, unimpaired individuals will consistently generate pressure in the upper pharynx on average 201 msec before pressure in the lower pharynx. Given this pattern of pharyngeal pressure generation, cricopharyngeal myotomy was determined not to be the appropriate treatment course. Fortunately for this patient, the dysphagic presentation resolved within 2 weeks and he returned to a normal diet.

This patient can be contrasted to Ms. N who is a 40-year-old female referred for swallowing rehabilitation with a 4-year history of chronic pharyngeal phase dysphagia subsequent to brainstem stroke. Shortly postonset, she underwent surgical true vocal fold medialization secondary to asymmetry in vocal fold closure. She was initially fed via gastrostomy tube but this was discontinued at approximately 3 years postonset. At the time of referral, the patient was ambulatory and independent with significant left-sided weakness and gait disturbance. She was consuming a soft, moist, or minced diet with thin liquids. A VFSS completed at the time of referral revealed presumed overall reduced pharyngeal motility with postswallow residual, particularly for heavier textures, paired with nasal redirection of liquids in the presence of adequate velopharyngeal closure. As a young woman with an active social life, the patient expressed a treatment goal of reducing nasal redirection, as this impacted her socially.

Manometric evaluation on this patient revealed a consistent pattern of pharyngeal motility as shown in Figure 13–6. Although amplitude was mildly reduced (again compared to limited normative data collected using the same catheter and method), this patient generated pressure simultaneously in the upper and lower pharynx. Thus, instead of a smooth superior to inferior propulsion of the bolus, pharyngeal motility was characterized by "slapping" the bolus at mid-pharynx, thus presumably directing some of the bolus inferiorly and some superiorly into the nasal cavity. This finding explains her radiographic presentation of pharyngeal residual and nasal redirection. Unfortunately for this patient, rehabilitation efforts were only partly effective. She was able to increase diet level tolerance, but did not positively effect nasal redirection. At this time, no rehabilitation techniques have been developed to address the phenomenon

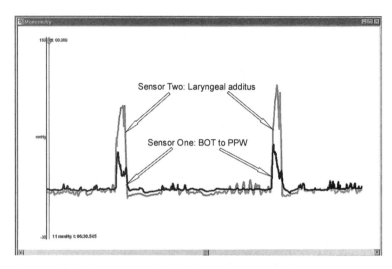

Figure 13–6. Patient example Ms. N reveals an atypical pattern characterized by the absence of superior to inferior pressure distribution. Clinically, this correlated with nasal redirection and postswallow residual.

of "pharyngeal mis-sequencing," perhaps in large part because our diagnostic tools have not allowed for identification of this pathophysiologic feature.

Considerable work remains before pharyngeal manometry can emerge as a standard diagnostic tool. More specific and objective measurement of pharyngeal biomechanics will help us identify pathophysiologic features of swallowing that are poorly defined based on existing diagnostic techniques. Identification of these features consequently will increase the demand for availability and incorporation of these techniques into standard clinical practice.

14 Professional Responsibilities

Dysphagia Diagnosis in Stroke

A medical diagnosis, although hypothesized through careful history, observation, and noninstrumental assessment by a health care provider, requires instrumental or laboratory assessment for confirmation. Dysphagia is a medical diagnosis and, as such, instrumental assessment is presumed to follow a clinical swallowing examination (CSE) in patients with suspected dysphagia following stroke. Indeed, more than one assessment may be required to explicitly define the nature of pathophysiology and develop efficacious and cost-efficient treatment. Failure to do so carries serious consequences for patient outcomes and consequent professional integrity. However, this standard of practice does not always appear to be accepted or acted on in many clinical settings. So what impedes best practice? Based on our earlier model, rather than accepting this symptom of clinical impairment, an exploration of the underlying etiology is appropriate. In this medical arena of clinical practice, we appear to be plagued by either underconfidence or overconfidence, both of which are complicated by resource issues and both of which can hinder our work.

For the speech pathologist comfortable and confident in the health care arena, the medical model of diagnosis and the implications of this are apparent. However, as a profession, our uneasiness in this setting sometimes becomes noticeable when approaching diagnosis of swallowing impairment. Speech-language pathology is a profession that historically has provided diagnoses based on a careful history, astute observation, and critical listening. Additionally, early

175

on, speech pathologists were lacking appropriate instrumental techniques and a detailed recognition of the complexities of swallowing pathophysiology. Times have changed and clinical practice must change with it. Instrumentation for swallowing is an accepted and necessary component of practice (American Speech-Language-Hearing Association, 1992). However, it appears that as a profession, speech pathologists have been accustomed to practicing with limited resources without insisting on what is required for optimal patient management. Timidity in requiring orders for instrumental assessment does not benefit anyone. It fails the patient through inadequate diagnosis. It fails the profession by perpetuating the myth that clinicians can gather the necessary information through observation. The provision of optimal assessment and care of the dysphagic patient is the responsibility of the clinician. All clinicians will require confidence in their professional problem-solving and negotiation skills to ensure this responsibility is met. Anything less is unacceptable and unethical. Speech pathologists have earned a place in the health care system and should maintain that place as a confident and contributing member of the health care team.

Equally hindering the management of the dysphagic patient is overconfidence in our clinical skills and techniques. Many of the wisest clinicians have learned the hard way that overestimation of our clinical abilities or overconfidence in clinical assessment procedures can have adverse effects. Our data and clinical evidence support this. Certainly every single referral cannot have an instrumental assessment. There will be some who are culled for very justifiable reasons; they may not be appropriate for oral intake regardless of what the instrumental assessment reveals. But caution should be exercised in exaggerating clinical accuracy under the guise of "judicious use of clinical resources," particularly in patients with stroke who, because of potential sensory deficit and cognitive impairment, cannot assist with detection of dysphagia. Sparing resources by deferring diagnostic examination may ultimately cost the health care system more in the long term. As above, if the clinician proposes that they can infer a diagnosis for one stroke patient without instrumental assessment, then they weaken the argument for instrumental assessment in the next. The bottom line is one cannot see what cannot be seen. This does not reflect on the clinician, rather it reflects on the nature of the disorder and limitations of observational assessment.

Although this text presents a "hard line" on the use of instrumentation, it is acknowledged that resourcing issues are ever present in health care settings. The current reality is that the videofluoroscopic swallow study (VFSS) or other diagnostic techniques may not be currently and readily available in some rural regions. In this case, the following are recommended:

1. In the short term:
   a. Maximize the accuracy of the clinical assessment through a thorough investigation, rather than a cursory observation of oral intake. Pay close attention to history and cranial nerve findings in the stroke population to provide guidance of the underlying pathophysiology. Use less invasive and less expensive instrumental adjuncts to the clinical assessment such as pulse oximetry and auscultation.
   b. Document the need for diagnostic assessment and the limitations of clinical assessment.
   c. Make it clear in notes to the health care team and to the patient, that clinical impressions are not diagnostic in nature but are speculations based on observable behavior.
   d. Make it clear in notes to the health care team and to the patient, that any recommended management approach has the potential for a positive effect, a neutral effect, or even an adverse effect without the benefit of diagnostic examination for clarity.
2. In the long term:
   a. Advocate for patients. No one will provide resources if clinicians do not argue strongly for their necessity. Prepare

proposals for resources that are strongly substantiated by the literature.

b. Once again, the clinician must document. In order to effect a change in practice, it may be necessary to perpetually document what is needed to do the job well. Accepting less will not change practice, attitudes, or resources.

c. Investigate all diagnostic options. If VFSS is clearly not available, then look into alternatives such as the emerging mobile VFSS. Budgeting for this service may not be prohibitive for your system.

d. As well, if VFSS is not available, enhance collaborations with colleagues in gastroenterology and otolaryngology. Pooled financial and skill resources may facilitate the establishment of pharyngeal manometry or endoscopy clinics. Although in the stroke population, these may be considered adjunctive instrumental examinations, something is better than nothing to support the clinical examination.

CASE EXAMPLE

MF, a 76-year-old female, was admitted from her internist's office to the hospital with a right parietal stroke. Neurologic impairments documented in her admission notes included mild left-sided weakness, decreased left sensation, left visual and sensory neglect, impaired balance, mild oropharyngeal dysphagia, and mild dysarthria. Her past medical history was significant for mitral valve repair, type II noninsulin-dependent diabetes, afibrillation, and osteoporosis. Although the patient reported to the health care team an acute onset of dysphagia for solids, no formal clinical or diagnostic swallowing evaluation was initiated. She completed her acute hospitalization with no indication of nutritional or pulmonary compromise.

Not long after admission, the patient was transferred to an acute inpatient rehabilitation setting. Again, no swallowing evaluation was included as part of her admission workup. Some time following rehab admission, the speech pathologist was consulted to evaluate the patient for dysphagia. After clinical assessment and observation of a meal, the clinician concluded "MF finished her meal without difficulties. No oral or pharyngeal phase swallowing problems were apparent. The patient is apprehensive about eating solids. Recommend: soft diet, thin liquids." Ten days later, nursing notes included the following comment: "the patient is apprehensive about eating lunch, yet appeared to manage a soft diet." Two weeks later: "the patient choked on solids at lunch; plan to supervise meals." At this point her albumin levels suggested potential undernutrition. However, speech pathology was not reconsulted for a follow-up evaluation. She demonstrated no evidence of pulmonary compromise.

Approximately 2 months poststroke, the patient was transferred to a nursing home. One month later, she was visited by a dietician through a home health care agency who documented "the patient prefers minced, pureed food. She has self-selected a pureed diet due to difficulty swallowing solids." Again, no further evaluation was recommended.

A referral for outpatient swallowing evaluation was sought by the patient's family one year later due to increasing dysphagic symptoms. On evaluation, she continued to complain of increasing dysphagia for solids with more recent difficulty managing liquids. Rigorous coughing during meals was frequent and discomforting. She experienced a substantial weight loss since her onset admission. No strongly lateralizing cranial nerve findings were present. However, vocal quality was weak and wet. Speech was mildly dysarthric of the flaccid type. VFSS revealed a moderate pharyngeal phase dysphagia with overall poor pharyngeal motility and diffuse residual. Of note was the presence of a pronounced filling Zenker's diverticulum with backflow of contents into the pharynx on completion of the swallow and postswallow aspiration.

The patient was referred for surgical evaluation of diverticulum excision but was deemed an unsuitable candidate due to complicating cardiac factors. Rehabilitation of dysphagia at this point was unlikely to be effective due to the size of the pouch; thus, conservative compensatory management was implemented to decrease risks. Despite this, the patient developed pulmonary infection and expired within 8 months.

There are several possibilities with this patient. It is possible that she had a long-standing dysphagia that was not recognized until the onset of her stroke, although the patient reported acute onset. It is possible that the diverticulum would have developed regardless of her stroke; that is, it represented a coincidental occurrence. From her history however, the most likely scenario is that her neurologic impairment led to specific dysfunction of the cricopharyngeus with an acute-onset dysphagia for solids secondary to impaired upper esophageal sphincter opening. This was not diagnosed acutely or subacutely and within the ensuing year resulted in the development of the pouch. Unfortunately for this patient, there are many options for rehabilitation of cricopharyngeal abnormalities that were not made available to her because of a failure to diagnose. Whether the responsibility for this failure is on the shoulders of the clinician, the physician, or the health care system is irrelevant to the patient and her family. By treating without optimal information, the clinician may undermine not only the outcomes possible for the patient but also the advancement of clinical practice. It is acknowledged that sometime restraints of resources and support may inhibit optimal practice. However, if the clinician proceeds down this route, the potential consequences must be recognized.

15 Diagnosis of Dysphagia in Stroke

Establishing an accurate dysphagia diagnosis is a process of problem-solving through what is inferred from the clinical assessment and what is visualized on the instrumental evaluation. This information is then compared with normative data and the limited etiology-specific data available. The diagnosis of dysphagia frequently is initiated from a consideration of the symptoms presented, for example, postswallow residue. However, the thorough examination is incomplete if the clinician fails to identify the underlying physiologic basis of the dysfunction. Both components are of substantial importance. Symptoms of dysphagia more often are addressed through compensatory management, whereas the physiologic abnormality is targeted by direct rehabilitative exercise. Elucidation of one without the other leaves the dysphagic patient with an incomplete treatment plan and reduced potential for positive outcome. Table 15–1 describes dysphagic symptoms and their physiologic etiologies.

In this chapter, we present a format for diagnosis of oropharyngeal dysphagia by identifying symptoms and then determining the underlying basis of each symptom through an understanding of physiology. This methodical approach suits the nature of data available from many of our instrumental examinations. The signs or symptoms of dysphagia (e.g., preswallow pooling, postswallow residual) are more often static and thus, frequently easier to visualize. The clinician can observe these features over a longer period of time. In comparison, underlying physiologic abnormalities (e.g., hyoid movement, epiglottic deflection) are frequently dynamic and require a 'quick eye' to visualize. Thus, direct observation can be

Table 15–1. Differentiation Between Symptoms and Physiologic Abnormalities Underlying Dysphagia

Symptoms	*Physiologic Abnormalities*
• Inadequate bolus preparation	• Oral motor impairment
• Anterior leakage	• Delayed pharyngeal swallow
• Postswallow oral residual	• Inadequate BOT to PPW approximation
• Premature spillage	
• Preswallow pharyngeal pooling to the level of the _____	• Weakened pharyngeal contraction/poor stripping
• Inadequate epiglottic deflection*	• Inadequate epiglottic to arytenoid deflection*
• Inadequate opening of the UES*	
• Postswallow vallecular residual	• Inadequate hyolaryngeal excursion
• Postswallow piriform sinus residual	• Incomplete velopharyngeal closure
• Aspiration	• Impaired opening of the UES
• Penetration	

*May be both symptom and physiologic abnormality; UES = upper esophageal sphincter; BOT = base of tongue; PPW = posterior pharyngeal wall.

more challenging. A structured approach to problem-solving will focus the clinician toward an accurate diagnosis without distraction from the dynamic array of diagnostic data. At the conclusion of the examination and based on the identified sign or symptom, the clinician should be able to present a diagnostic summary that reflects the sequence of problem-solving in the following format:

"The patient presents *[which phase]* dysphagia characterized by *[symptoms]* secondary to *[physiologic abnormality]*."

Frequently a single physiologic abnormality can result in a number of observed signs and symptoms. Thus, written presentation of written data may be facilitated by structuring the diagnostic summary with the physiologic abnormality first.

"The patient presents *[which phase]* dysphagia characterized by *[physiologic abnormality]*, resulting in *[symptoms]*."

To facilitate understanding and clinical carryover, two table formats are presented. The first, Table 15–2 supports the approach that clinical problem-solving starts at the symptoms and works its way into the physiologic abnormality. The second, Table 15–3, may aid the clinician in clear documentation by presenting physiologic abnormalities followed by their consequent symptoms.

ORAL PHASE

Within the oral phase of swallowing, an array of symptoms can be visualized on both clinical and diagnostic examination. These are summarized in Table 15–3, and all are a consequence of the primary physiologic abnormality of **poor orolingual control**. Unfortunately, a more specific and objective definition of this physiologic abnormality is difficult with our current instrumentation and, thus, requires more subjective speculation. Poor orolingual control may feasibly be secondary to bilateral or hemiweakness, spasticity, or a discoordinated quality characteristic of apraxia. The term "apraxia of swallowing" has been applied to patients with "the inability to organize the front-to-back lingual and bolus movement normally characteristic of a swallow or . . . simply holding the bolus without initiating any oral activity" (Logemann, 1998, p. 83). Describing this disorder as "apraxia," however, implicates specific principles in the act of swallowing. It suggests that swallowing is learned, skilled movement and that the abnormal movement pattern observed is not attributable to sensory or elemental motor deficits. The similarities and differences of apraxia of swallowing with more traditional disturbances of the praxis system (limb apraxia, buccofacial apraxia, apraxia of speech) have previously been reviewed (Daniels, 2000).

Table 15–2. Swallowing Symptoms Associated with Specific Physiologic Abnormalities

The Symptoms of	Occurring	Can be Secondary to	In Which Phase
Anterior leakage	Preswallow	Poor orolingual control	Oral
Inadequate bolus preparation	Preswallow		
Inadequate bolus formation			
Oral residual	Postswallow		
Pharyngeal pooling to the level of ___	Preswallow	Delayed pharyngeal swallow	Pharyngeal
Nasal regurgitation	During the swallow	Poor pharyngeal motility	
		Decreased anterior hyoid movement	
Inadequate epiglottic deflection	During the swallow	Intrinsic structural changes in supportive tissue	
Vallecular residual	Postswallow	Decreased base of tongue to posterior pharyngeal wall approximation	
		Inadequate epiglottic deflection*	
Inadequate opening of the UES*	During the swallow	Decreased anterior hyoid movement*	
		Intrinsic structural functional changes in cricopharyngeus	

Symptom	Timing	Physiologic abnormality	
Piriform sinus residual	Postswallow	Inadequate opening of the UES*	Pharyngeal
	Preswallow	Pharyngeal pooling*	Oral
			Pharyngeal
			Oral
Penetration	During the swallow	Inadequate epiglottic deflection*	Pharyngeal
		Inadequate supraglottic shortening/laryngeal elevation*	
	Postswallow	Oral residual*	Oral
		Pharyngeal residual*	Pharyngeal
Aspiration	Preswallow	Pharyngeal pooling*	Oral
	During the swallow	Inadequate true vocal fold closure	Pharyngeal
	Postswallow	Oral residual*	Oral
		Pharyngeal residual*	Pharyngeal

*Occasionally a symptom will be caused by another symptom, which requires the clinician to problem-solve through to the initial presenting physiologic abnormality.

UES = upper esophageal sphincter.

Table 15–3. Physiologic Abnormalities with Their Consequent Symptoms

The patient presents oral phase dysphagia characterized by poor oral lingual control resulting in:

Preswallow	• Anterior leakage • Inadequate bolus preparation • Premature spillage with pharyngeal pooling to the level of _____ • Inadequate mastication • Supraglottic penetration of preswallow pooling • Aspiration of preswallow pooling
During the swallow	• Supraglottic penetration of pooled material • Aspiration of pooled material
Postswallow	• Anterior leakage of postswallow oral residual • Postswallow oral residual • Postswallow pharyngeal pooling of oral residuals to the level of _____ • Supraglottic penetration of postswallow oral residual that pools into pharynx • Aspiration of postswallow oral residual that pools into pharynx

The patient presents pharyngeal dysphagia characterized by delayed pharyngeal swallow resulting in:

Preswallow	• Pharyngeal pooling to the level of _____ • Supraglottic penetration of preswallow pooling • Aspiration of preswallow pooling
During the swallow	• Supraglottic penetration of pooled material • Aspiration of pooled material
Postswallow	• None

The patient presents pharyngeal dysphagia characterized by inadequate anterior hyoid movement resulting in:

Preswallow	• None
During the swallow	• Decreased epiglottic deflection[1] • Decreased traction force for UES opening[2] • Supraglottic penetration
Postswallow	• Vallecular residual >piriform sinus as a secondary effect[1] • Piriform sinus residual >vallecular as a secondary effect[2]

Table 15–3. *continued*

Postswallow *continued*	• Supraglottic residual
	• Aspiration of supraglottic or pharyngeal residual

The patient presents pharyngeal dysphagia characterized by inadequate base of tongue to posterior pharyngeal wall resulting in:

Preswallow	• None
During the swallow	• Impaired bolus transport through proximal pharynx
Postswallow	• Postswallow vallecular residual (>piriform sinus residual)
	• Supraglottic penetration of residual
	• Aspiration of supraglottic or pharyngeal residual

The patient presents pharyngeal dysphagia characterized by impaired UES opening in the presence of substantial anterior hyoid movement resulting in (implies intrinsic cricopharyngeus abnormality or timing issue):

Preswallow	• None
During the swallow	• Impaired bolus transport through cricopharyngeus
Postswallow	• Postswallow piriform sinus residual (>vallecular residual)
	• Supraglottic penetration of residual
	• Aspiration of supraglottic or pharyngeal residual

The patient presents pharyngeal dysphagia characterized by poor pharyngeal motility resulting in:

Preswallow	• None
During the swallow	• Impaired bolus transport throughout the pharynx
	• Nasal redirection
	• Supraglottic penetration
Postswallow	• Diffuse (nonspecific) pharyngeal residual
	• Nasal residual
	• Supraglottic penetration of residual
	• Aspiration of supraglottic or pharyngeal residual

[1,2]The physiologic abnormality results in a symptom during the swallow that consequently results in another symptom postswallow.

UES = upper esophageal sphincter.

Regardless of the semantic or theoretical issues, however, there *is* an oral dysmotility disturbance that is characterized by repetitive, disorganized anterior-posterior bolus movement in the oral cavity, which prolongs oral transfer and is evident in stroke patients (Daniels et al., 1999; Robbins & Levine, 1988; Robbins et al., 1993).

Oral physiologic abnormality may also be disguised as, or exacerbated by, decreased attention. In these cases, the prolonged and inefficient oral phase of swallowing is not solely physiologically based but is complicated by cognitive factors. Augmentative instrumental assessments, such as oral manometry (e.g., Iowa Oral Pressure Instrument), or the more invasive intramuscular electromyography (EMG) may provide valuable information; however, these techniques are rarely incorporated into clinical practice. Normative data using these measures are not available, the availability is limited, and specific expertise may be required (in the case of intramuscular EMG), thus discouraging clinical application. Integration of cranial nerve findings will assist in differential diagnosis of oral inefficiency. A patient with no evidence of hypoglossal nerve damage on assessment but who demonstrates oral inefficiency during ingestion more likely may present with cognitive inattention as the primary etiology.

PHARYNGEAL PHASE

Preswallow Pooling

A common symptom of dysphagia in stroke is the presentation of **preswallow pooling** in the pharynx. Table 15–3 presents this symptom, as well as aspiration and penetration, which are produced by the sensory deficit of **delayed pharyngeal swallow**. At first glance, this appears rather straightforward; however, working from the symptoms of preswallow pooling to delayed pharyngeal swallow, in practice, is quite complicated.

The conclusion of oral parameters of swallowing is marked by volitional transfer of the prepared bolus into the oropharynx and, thereby, outside the reach of voluntary control. The transition between oral and pharyngeal components of the swallowing process is heavily influenced by the integrity of neurosensory response systems and subsequent timing of onset of the pharyngeal swallow in relation to voluntary transfer. The videofluoroscopic swallow study (VFSS) can provide an image of bolus transfer and swallowing onset marked by hyoid movement. However, VFSS cannot provide specific measures of sensory thresholds; for diagnosis of pharyngeal onset disorders, the clinician must infer sensory deficit based on biomechanical data. This is a difficult and perhaps imprecise task. Augmentative instrumental assessments are emerging for evaluation of sensory systems. Fiberoptic endoscopic evaluation of swallowing with sensory testing and cough reflex testing are two of these (see Chapters 9 and 12 for review). However, these procedures are more heavily focused on laryngeal, rather than pharyngeal, sensitivity. The clinical technique of assessing gag reflex is considered to be a direct evaluation of glossopharyngeal sensory integrity; however, as previously discussed, it lacks diagnostic sensitivity.

One complication in diagnosing delayed pharyngeal swallow arises from the fact that the primary symptom of this disorder, that of preswallow pharyngeal pooling, is shared by the physiologic abnormality of poor orolingual control. Differential diagnosis of these two disorders is difficult based on VFSS and has substantive clinical consequences. A misdiagnosis may result in the clinician providing a sensory-based treatment for a motor-based disorder, or vice versa, with consequent treatment failure. This represents a waste of health care resources, and frustration for both patient and clinician. Several observations, summarized in Table 15–4, may guide the clinician toward a physiologic diagnosis based on the symptom of preswallow pooling; however, none of these in isolation can be considered an undisputed feature of either diagnosis. There exists no peer-reviewed research to document the sensitivity and specificity

Table 15–4. Differential Diagnosis of the Etiology of Preswallow Pooling: Delayed Pharyngeal Swallow Versus Premature Spillage Due to Poor Orolingual Control

Clinical Question	Poor Orolingual Bolus Control	Delayed Pharyngeal Swallow
As the bolus approaches the oral cavity (preoral), what does the base of tongue do?	Does not approximate soft palate for protective glossopalatal seal	Arches to approximate soft palate for protective glossopalatal seal
How does the bolus enter the pharynx?	In noncohesive, unformed bits as it falls off of base of tongue during bolus preparation	As a cohesive, single bolus unless the patient volitionally segments the transfer
Is there a pronounced drop of the base and push of the blade of the tongue to transfer the bolus?	No	Yes, although there will be a significant temporal delay between this movement and onset of pharyngeal swallow
On which consistency is the pooling most pronounced?	Heavier consistencies, solids	Liquids

of these radiographic features, in part, because we lack reliable sensory data on which to validate the observations.

The second major complication inhibiting accurate assignment of a diagnosis of delayed pharyngeal swallow is the innate variability in temporal relationships in nonimpaired individuals and the associated flexibility provoked by consistency adaptation. Specific measures of swallowing onset include the temporal measures of stage transit duration (STD), which is measured from the point where the bolus head reaches the ramus of the mandible to the onset of maximum hyolaryngeal elevation. Strict interpretation of STD is discouraged as this may lead to overdiagnosis. As discussed in Chapter 3, recent research has indicated that the bolus may be inferior to the ramus of the mandible at onset of maximum hyolaryngeal elevation during sequential swallowing and single swallows in healthy adults (Chi-Fishman & Sonies, 2000; Daniels et al., 2004; Daniels & Foundas, 2001; Martin-Harris et al., 2007; Stephen et al., 2005). This indicates that hypopharyngeal bolus location at onset of the pharyngeal swallow cannot be interpreted as abnormal if all other physiologic components of swallowing are intact. That is, clinicians must understand that although onset of the pharyngeal swallow may occur deep in the pharynx, for this to be classified as "normal" swallowing, airway protection must be maintained and risk of pulmonary invasion must be consistently low.

Postswallow Residual

The pharyngeal swallow is signaled by the onset of hyolaryngeal excursion, particularly anterior movement of the hyoid, which plays an important role in pharyngeal dynamics as discussed in Chapter 3. As such, **inadequate anterior hyoid movement** is a common symptom of dysphagia in stroke and can lead to a cascade of pharyngeal events and symptoms, as outlined in Table 15-3. Of note is that the impaired anterior hyoid movement is the etiology of other impaired biomechanical events, which subsequently cause other observable symptoms. Working backward from the symptoms (see Table 15-2), the presentation of postswallow **vallecular residual** is a consequence of (1) **decreased epiglottic deflection**, thus "trapping" the bolus in the superior pharynx, or (2) **decreased base of tongue to posterior pharyngeal wall approximation** with resulting inadequate positive pressure to drive the bolus into the hypopharynx. VFSS is not the appropriate instrument to comment directly and objectively on base of tongue to posterior pharyngeal wall pressure generation; pharyngeal manometry would be the technique of choice. Thus, observation of epiglottic deflection and a diagnosis by exclusion is the more usual course of clinical problem-solving for determining the source of vallecular residual. If epiglottic deflection has failed, then the etiology of this biomechanical movement must consequently be questioned. Failure to deflect the epiglottis may be a consequence of either (1) intrinsic **tissue changes** in the cartilaginous tissue of the epiglottis as in irradiated patients or those with connective tissue disease, or (2) inadequate anterior hyoid movement, which fails to pull the base of the epiglottis anteriorly and shift the apex over the airway. Tissue characteristics cannot be directly evaluated with our clinical tools and in uncomplicated stroke are unlikely. Therefore, observation of hyoid movement is imperative for understanding the underlying basis of epiglottic deflection.

Decreased anterior hyoid movement also contributes indirectly to the symptom of postswallow **piriform sinus residual**. Again working backward from the symptom, if a patient presents with pyriform sinus residual greater than vallecular residual, this would typically signal an isolated impairment of upper esophageal sphincter (UES) opening. **Impaired UES opening** can logically be a consequence of (1) decreased anterior hyoid movement, (2) intrinsic **structural functional changes of cricopharyngeus muscle**, or (3) a **mistiming of biomechanical events** with neurophysiologic relaxation of the muscle. Of these three potential etiologies, VFSS is the technique of choice to visualize hyoid movement. Pharyngeal manometry with or without intramuscular EMG may be required to optimally evaluate the other two possible sources of piriform sinus residual. Manometry will aid in documentation of the relationships between pressure in the pharynx and cricopharyngeus and the amplitude of pressure drop in the cricopharyngeus. EMG will provide specific objective information about cricopharyngeal activation and deactivation.

Nasal Redirection

The presenting symptom of **nasal redirection** of the bolus is one of controversy as we lack substantive data to guide our practice. Invasion of the bolus into the nasal cavity is not simply an issue of impairment of velopharyngeal closure, but this symptom, more importantly, requires impairment of pressure systems that provide the driving force behind the bolus. Therefore, this is likely to be presented in cases of pharyngeal dysmotility, where pressure systems are disrupted or mistimed. Although VFSS reveals bolus flow patterns, more specific information about pharyngeal pressure systems would best be obtained through pharyngeal manometry. Using this instrumentation, the clinician may obtain objective measures of dysmotility patterns that underlie the symptom of nasal redirection.

Reduced Pharyngeal Motility

In the prior section, specific biomechanical characteristics that are subject to impairment in stroke and a method for problem-solving from symptom to specific physiologic etiology were discussed. In many individuals with stroke, the dysphagic presentation is much more extensive with multiple components of impairment with diffuse postswallow residual. The categorical term of **poor pharyngeal motility** may be applied when either all components of the process are collectively impaired or a specific etiology is not able to be identified. Poor motility may be a result of any number of neuromuscular or temporal deficits, characterized with terms such as weakness, spasticity, slowness, reduced pharyngeal shortening, or discoordination. Again, VFSS reveals bolus flow patterns and allows for assessment of timing measures; pharyngeal manometry would be required to provide specific objective measures of pressure systems or very detailed pressure sequences. Neuromuscular substrates such as weakness and spasticity are only presumed in our current practice due to inadequately developed clinical instrumentation.

Airway Invasion

Supraglottic penetration can be a symptom of any number of physiologic abnormalities and can occur preswallow from pooled material, postswallow from oral or pharyngeal residual, or during the swallow secondary to either impaired epiglottic deflection and pharyngeal/supraglottic shortening or overflow of pooled material that enters the airway as the larynx elevates. Aspiration, as well, can occur before or after the pharyngeal swallow, but only occurs during the swallow in the case of specific impairment of either the degree or timing of vocal fold closure. It is not an uncommon finding for stroke patients to present with supraglottic penetration during pharyngeal swallowing and then proceed to aspirate on postprandial glottic opening. VFSS and videoendoscopy will allow for detection of supraglottic penetration and aspiration. Videoendoscopy may more optimally visualize vocal fold closure and identify impairments of adduction. Multimodality assessment using more standard techniques paired with respiratory airflow will be required to evaluate swallowing respiratory coordination.

ORAL AND PHARYNGEAL DYSMOTILITY IN STROKE

Given this overview of diagnosing dysphagia, what can research and clinical observation teach us about swallowing following stroke? Any clinician who has worked with stroke patients knows there is no "prototypical" swallowing pattern in this population, aside perhaps from patients with lateral medullary syndrome (LMS). Research findings (Table 15-5) when integrated with clinical observations can, however, help focus clinicians on particular patterns of pathophysiology that may be evident following stroke.

To facilitate discussion, stroke is discussed in terms of supratentorial (cortical, subcortical) and brainstem lesions. Research has suggested that dysphagia following stroke primarily is secondary to large cortical lesions, for example, middle cerebral artery territory infarcts (Alberts et al., 1992; Robbins et al., 1993). Other studies, however, have demonstrated that changes in swallowing can occur with small subcortical lesions (Daniels & Foundas, 1999; Logemann et al., 1993) with some proposing that swallowing generally is functional with small subcortical lesions, albeit different from age-matched controls (Logemann et al., 1993). As no study has identified specific dysmotility patterns distinguishing swallowing between cortical and subcortical lesions, cortical and subcortical lesions are discussed under the umbrella term, supratentorial.

Dysphagia in Supratentorial Stroke

Oral dysmotility is a common problem following supratentorial stroke characterized by longer transfer and possibly discoordination in oral transfer. Stroke research has focused on defining oral stage impairment primarily by measuring oral transit time (OTT). This is defined as the time from onset of bolus movement to the point where the bolus head reaches the ramus of the mandible. OTT is increased for stroke patients as compared to healthy controls (Robbins & Levine, 1988; Robbins et al., 1993). "Apraxia of swallowing" also has been described in a subset of patients with left hemisphere damage (LHD) and has been characterized by a "lack of labial, lingual, and mandibular coordination" with OTT of over 10 seconds (Robbins et al., 1993, p. 1298).

Table 15–5. Research Detailing Dysphagia in Stroke Patients

Authors	Subjects	Time Post-Onset	Trials/Stimuli
Butler et al. (2007)	26 stroke with dysphagia (11 aspirators, 15 nonaspirators) 20 healthy adults	N/A	Two trials: 5, 10 15, 20 ml thin and thick liquid
Chen, Ott, Peele, & Gelfand (1990)	46 stroke	1 month	3 and 5 ml thin and thick liquid; 3 ml paste; ¼ cookie
Daniels et al. (1999)	59 stroke	5 days	Two trials: 3, 5, 10, 20 ml; 1 tsp paste; ½ cookie
Daniels & Foundas (1999)	54 stroke	5 days	Two trials: 3, 5, 10, 20 ml; 1 tsp paste; ½ cookie
Daniels et al. (2006)	13 healthy adults 9 stroke	2 days 33 days	Two trials: 5 ml liquid

Techniques	Measures	Results
Simultaneous VFSS and respiratory measure	Objective	– ↑ SAD and variability of duration in stroke patients as compared to controls – ↑ SAD in aspirators as compared to non-aspirators – ↑ in I-I respiratory pattern in aspirators and greater dysphagia severity
VFSS	Subjective	– 39 oral and pharyngeal dysmotility – 5 isolated pharyngeal dysmotility – 2 isolated oral dysmotility – 18 mild dysphagia – 23 moderate dysphagia – 5 severe dysphagia – Dysmotility pattern not associated with hemisphere
VFSS	Subjective and Objective	– Equal incidence of lingual discoordination in RHD and LHD
	Subjective and Objective	– Equal incidence of dysmotility patterns (subjectively measured) and aspiration between in LHD and RHD – 19 oral and pharyngeal dysmotility – 20 isolated pharyngeal dysmotility – 3 isolated oral dysmotility
VFSS	Objective	– Dysphagia defined as dysfunction on 2 of 6 swallowing measures: OTT, STD, PTT, P-A Scale, vallecular residual, piriform sinus residual – 2 SD above normal means to determine dysfunction – 5 stroke patients presented with dysphagia acutely – 2 presented with continued dysphagia at 1 month.

continues

Table 15–5. *continued*

Authors	Subjects	Time Post-Onset	Trials/Stimuli
Irie & Lu (1995)	74 stroke	2 to 59 days	3 ml liquid and paste; mouthful liquid
Leslie et al. (2002)	18 stroke patients with clinically determined dysphagia 50 healthy adults	4 to 28 days	5, 20 ml liquid; 5 ml pudding
Logemann et al. (1993)	8 LHD (basal ganglia/internal capsule) 8 healthy adults	21 to 28 days	Two trials; 1, 3, 5, 10 ml liquid; 1 ml paste; ½ cookie
Mann et al. (2000)	128 stroke	10 days	5, 10 ml thin liquid, thick liquid, paste; 20 ml thin liquid
Nilsson, Ekberg, Bulow, & Hindfelt (1997)	33 neurologically impaired (including stroke) patients with clinically determined dysphagia	N/A	Mouthful thick liquid barium

Techniques	Measures	Results
VFSS	Objective	– 33 oral and pharyngeal dysmotility – 8 isolated pharyngeal dysmotility – 24 isolated oral dysmotility – stroke isolated oral dysmotility in LHD – ↑ in both oral and pharyngeal dysfunction in RHD
Simultaneous VFSS and respiratory measure	Objective	– ↑ inspiration after swallow in stroke group
VFSS	Subjective and Objective	– ↑ OTT – ↓ OPSE* – ↓ PRT
VFSS	Subjective and Objective, ordinal scale for severity; weighted median score determined dysphagia and severity	– 36 oral and pharyngeal dysmotility – 22 isolated pharyngeal dysmotility – 3 isolated oral dysmotility – 37 mild dysphagia – 39 moderate dysphagia – 6 severe dysphagia
Simultaneous VFSS and respiratory measure	Objective	– Airway invasion associated with lower SSI** – Postswallow respiratory phase not associated with airway invasion

continues

Table 15–5. *continued*

Authors	Subjects	Time Post-Onset	Trials/Stimuli
Perlman et al. (1994)	330 (101 stroke)	N/A	N/A
Robbins & Levine (1988)	8 LHD 8 RHD 8 healthy adults	3 wks	Two trials: 2 ml liquid and paste
Robbins et al. (1993)	20 LHD 20 RHD 20 healthy adults	3 wks	Two trials: 2 ml liquid and paste
Robbins et al. (1999)	15 multi-infarct 98 healthy adults	mean—146 days	Two trials: 3 ml liquid
Selley et al. (1989b)	21 neurologically impaired patients with complaints of dysphagia (11 stroke)	N/A	5 ml liquid
Smithard et al. (1997)	121 stroke (only 95 had VFSS)	3 days 29 days	Thin and thick liquid
Teasell et al. (2002)	20 medullary stroke (only 9 had VFSS) 8 healthy adults	4 to 77 days	Thin and thick liquid, pudding, solids
Veis & Logemann (1985)	38	<1–4 months	Two trials: 1/3 tsp liquid and paste

$\uparrow$ = increase; $\downarrow$ = decrease; I-I = inspiration-inspiration, LHD = left hemisphere damage, N/A = not available, OPSE = oropharyngeal swallowing efficiency, OTT = oral transit time, P-A = penetration-aspiration, PRT = pharyngeal response time, PTT = pharyngeal transit time, RHD = right hemisphere damage, SAD = swallowing apnea duration, SSI = swallowing severity index, STD = stage transit duration, VFSS = videofluoroscopic swallow study.

Techniques	Measures	Results
VFSS	Subjective and Objective	– Deviant epiglottic inversion, delayed pharyngeal swallow, vallecular residue, hypopharyngeal residue, decreased hyoid elevation; Linear trend between incidence of aspiration and severity of postswallow residual and delayed pharyngeal swallow
VFSS	Objective	– ↑ OTT and "apraxia of swallowing" in LHD – ↑ PTT and aspiration in RHD
VFSS	Objective	– ↑ OTT and "apraxia of swallowing" in LHD – ↑ STD, PTT and aspiration in RHD
VFSS	Objective	– ↑ in P-A scale scores – ↑ silent aspiration – ↑ within subject variability
Nasal airflow	Subjective and Objective	– ↑ inspiration after swallow
VFSS	Objective	– ↑ aspiration acute LHD/RHD – ↑ aspiration RHD at 1 month
VFSS	Subjective and Objective	– Postswallow residual – Delayed pharyngeal swallow – Aspiration – Reduced epiglottic deflection – Reduced hyoid movement
VFSS	Subjective and Objective	– Delayed onset of the pharyngeal swallow – Reduced pharyngeal peristalsis – Reduced lingual control

*OPSE—calculated by dividing the percentage of the bolus swallowed (minus percentage of oral residue, pharyngeal residue, and aspiration) by oral plus pharyngeal transit times.

**SSI—calculated by dividing SAD by PTT.

Daniels and colleagues (1999) describe lingual discoordination in patients with LHD as well as right hemisphere damage (RHD) ranging from durations of 1 to 3 seconds (mild), 4 to 10 seconds (moderate), or greater than 10 seconds (severe). Verbal cue to swallow has been reported to exacerbate this oral dysmotility pattern (Logemann, 1998; Robbins & Levine, 1988; Robbins et al., 1993) with resolution of oral dysfunction during the normal mealtime environment. Conversely, others note persistent oral dysmotility in the natural environment in patients with LHD as well as RHD (Daniels et al., 1999).

Although preswallow pooling is common following supratentorial stroke, research has not attempted to identify if the etiology of the pooling is more related to oral dysmotility or delayed evocation of the pharyngeal swallow. As noted previously, oral dysmotility yielding preswallow pooling is prominent following stroke. Stroke patients, however, frequently demonstrate increased STD (Daniels et al., 1996; Robbins & Levine, 1988; Robbins et al., 1993), which yields pharyngeal pooling. Increased STD has been identified as an independent predictor of aspiration, with increased delay associated with an increasing likelihood of aspiration (Perlman, Booth, & Grayhack, 1994). In this study, STD was rated on a Likert scale from 1 (STD between 1 and 2 seconds) to 3 (STD >5 seconds). Although this study consisted of a heterogeneous population, one-third of the patients had a stroke etiology.

The study of bolus flow has been the primary focus in stroke research; however, pharyngeal biomechanics can be impaired. No study has compared objective temporal and spatial structural measures in patients with supratentorial strokes and age-matched healthy participants. Only one study has detailed pharyngeal biomechanical events in a homogeneous cohort which included stroke patients (Perlman et al., 1994); however, the measure of these events was qualitative more than quantitative. This study, however, focused on the relationship between swallowing biomechanics and aspiration.

Dichotomous yes/no scores were used to define abnormal structural movement, whereas depth of postswallow residual was measured on a scale of 1 (mild) to 3 (severe). Abnormal epiglottic inversion and reduced hyoid elevation as well as bolus flow measures of vallecular residual and diffuse hypopharyngeal residual were strongly related to aspiration. As with STD, as severity of the residue increased, the number of patients who aspirated increased. As discussed earlier, reduced extent of structural movement can lead to postswallow residual. Patients with supratentorial stroke may present with unilateral pharyngeal hemiparesis, which yields postswallow residual on the contralesional side of the pharynx.

Increased airway invasion (laryngeal penetration and aspiration) has been documented in patients with supratentorial stroke (Alberts et al., 1992; Mann et al., 2000; Robbins et al., 1993). When using the Penetration-Aspiration Scale to rate airway invasion, stroke patients generally have higher scores as compared to healthy controls (Robbins et al., 1999). Aspiration in stroke patients, particularly those with supratentorial stroke, may not be hallmarked by a cough or voice change and is frequently termed as "silent." In a study of consecutive acute stroke patients, aspiration was identified in 38% of the patients, with 33% of these patients aspirating overtly, that is, coughing, and 67% aspirating silently (Daniels et al., 1998). Although lesion location (supratentorial or brainstem) was not specified, the increased incidence of inspiration after swallowing in stroke patients (Leslie et al., 2002; Selley et al., 1989b) has been shown to be associated with increased aspiration in this population (Butler et al., 2007).

Although stroke can impact all phases of swallowing, the clinician must also consider the impact of reduced cognition on swallowing. Cognitive deficits, particularly neglect, have been correlated with dysphagia. Hemispatial inattention has been associated with increased nonoral intake in acute stroke patients (Schroeder et al., 2006). Reduced awareness of dysphagia results in lack of self-modification of swallowing behavior and increased medical complications as compared to patients who are aware of dysphagia symptoms (Parker et al., 2004). Moreover, rehabilitation of swallowing is longer in stroke patients with neglect (Neumann, 1993).

Although hemispatial inattention and other cognitive disorders are not totally lateralized, they generally occur more frequently in patients with RHD as compared to patients with LHD (Heilman et al., 2003). These cognitive deficits may yield greater functional impairment in patients with RHD even though swallowing pathophysiology may be similar in patients with RHD and LHD. Greater functional impairment may lead the clinician to impose greater restrictions on oral intake for patients with RHD. Thus, in addition to rehabilitating swallowing, it is critical that clinicians also address cognitive deficits in treatment.

Dysphagia in Brainstem Stroke

Research is limited concerning swallowing in brainstem stroke. Studies are generally limited to single case reports that have outlined the progression of swallowing recovery in patients with brainstem stroke (Logemann & Kahrilas, 1990; Martino, Terrault, Ezerzer, Mikulis, & Diamant, 2001; Robbins & Levine, 1993) or focused on aspiration in case series (Kim, Chung, Lee, & Robbins, 2000; Teasell et al., 2002). Clinicians, however, are probably aware of the patients with LMS presenting with classic features. These are the patients who in the acute stage are expectorating saliva into a container due to inability to swallow. The clinical swallowing examination generally is characteristic of intact cognition and language and the presence of dysphonia and dysarthria. Unilateral true vocal fold paresis is not uncommon in patients with LMS. Patients are fully aware of swallowing deficits with intact sensation and immediate coughing with attempts to swallow the smallest of volume.

The preoral and oral stages of swallowing generally are intact. Although attempts at evocation of the pharyngeal swallow are present (on the clinical swallowing evaluation, the clinician may palpate multiple lingual hyolaryngeal gestures), the pharyngeal swallow is frequently never evoked or, if evoked, it is significantly delayed with limited extent of superior and anterior hyolaryngeal movement and UES opening (Logemann, Kahrilas, Kobara, & Vakil, 1989; Martino et al., 2001; Teasell et al., 2002). Unilateral pharyngeal hemiparesis is not uncommon in patients with LMS and is characterized by post-swallow residual on one side of the pharynx (Logemann & Kahrilas, 1990; Logemann et al., 1989). Airway invasion may be evident before, during, or after the pharyngeal swallow. Although swallowing is severely impaired in patients with LMS and recovery frequently is slow, they make the ideal client for swallowing rehabilitation due to intact sensation, cognition, and motivation.

Patients with brainstem stroke not involving the lateral medulla or with pontine stroke also may present with dysphagia, but characteristics are not as circumscribed as those with LMS. Given the close proximity to the medullary swallowing center and the multiple neural networks involved with swallowing, these patients warrant swallowing evaluation.

SUMMARY

The analysis of swallowing biomechanics and physiology is a complex process of integrating what is known of normal swallowing processes, paired with amalgamation of both subjective and objective evaluation of instrumental and clinical data. Given the complexity of this task and the substantive consequences of inaccurate or incomplete diagnosis, the astute clinician will develop a methodical approach for problem-solving relying on the easily observable symptoms to lead to the physiologic source of the impairment.

16 Diet Considerations

To Feed or Not to Feed

AN OVERVIEW OF OPTIONS FOR FEEDING THE DYSPHAGIC PATIENT

Management of the stroke patient with dysphagia should reflect on several primary goals: to ensure pulmonary safety, to promote nutritional integrity, to normalize swallowing physiology, and to maximize patient quality of life. Certainly, one would hope in the best circumstance for a resolution of the dysphagic symptoms and a return to a full, satisfying oral diet that realizes these goals. However, in the short term, and unfortunately for some in the long term, alternative routes of nutritional intake are required to address the goals of management.

Wise decisions regarding the route of nutritional intake are multifaceted, complex, and demand an interdisciplinary approach. Although the speech pathologist may be in the best position to understand risks of aspiration and oropharyngeal ingestion better than many others on the team, the complexities of pulmonary clearance and resilience to infection as well as the intricacies of nutritional digestion, absorption, and assimilation generally are well beyond standard clinical training. Historically in dysphagia management, our strong focus has been on prevention of aspiration, almost to the neglect of all else. Fortunately for our patients, we are learning that inhibition of aspiration may not be the key in the effective management of the dysphagic patient. Langmore and colleagues (1998) published a landmark study that has served our clinical thinking well. In an effort to identify true risk factors for development of aspiration pneumonia, this research group followed 189 elderly patients for 4 years to monitor for the outcome of aspiration pneumonia as it relates to a variety of risk factors. The best predictors of pneumonia were dependence for feeding, dependence for oral care, number of decayed teeth, tube feeding, more than one medical diagnosis, number of medications, and current smoking. Dysphagia, although identified as posing some risk, was not sufficient to cause pneumonia unless other risk factors were present as well.

Using this information, clinicians may now develop a more intelligent approach that weighs the hazards of aspiration more realistically against other consequences of diet manipulation. A thoughtful balance of risks to the pulmonary system, the nutritional system, and the sociocultural systems that underlie oral intake may not always have pulmonary safety as the priority. With increased attention to patient rights and quality of life, this may be particularly true in the elderly patient with substantial disability.

Thus, decisions regarding route of oral intake should be make through collaborative discussion between the patient, family, and a variety of other skilled health care professionals. In most clinical settings, this is the standard of practice but, unfortunately, this is not the case in all. Relative to percutaneous endoscopic gastrostomy (PEG) insertion, Sinha, James, and Hasan (2001) documented that 87% of physicians they surveyed always involved speech pathology input. However, Hasan, Meara, Bhowmick, and Woodhouse (1995) documented that the decision to use PEG feedings was reached through a multidisciplinary team approach for only 64% of their survey respondents.

There are data that suggest that these decisions should be made sooner rather than later. An interesting study by Davalos and colleagues (1996) sought to determine the prevalence of malnutrition after 1 week of hospitalization for acute stroke. Of significant concern was the finding that malnutrition increased progressively during hospitalization with malnutrition evident in 16.3% at admission, 26.4% after 1 week, and 35% after 2 weeks. Certainly many factors would be predicted to contribute to this trend, but it is suggested that nutrition, in whatever form, should be addressed promptly after admission. This finding was confirmed in a study of 62 stroke patients, most of whom demonstrated marked and significant deterioration in nutritional status within 4 weeks of hospitalization (Gariballa, Parker, Taub, & Castleden, 1998). After adjusting for an array of logical covariates, low serum albumin (a measure of protein) was a strong and independent predictor of death following acute stroke. Others have provided data that support the role of nutrition in positive patient outcomes. Finestone, Greene-Finestone, Wilson, and Teasell (1996) evaluated 49 consecutive patients admitted to an inpatient rehabilitation unit. Their data suggest that when adjusted for stroke severity, overall nutrition was an independent predictor of length of stay and therefore functional improvement rate. They conclude by commenting that nutrition is "likely the most potentially modifiable variable relating to length of stay and functional outcome" (p. 340).

NONORAL, ENTERAL FEEDING OPTIONS

Adaptation of diet consistency for both food and liquid is a common approach in dysphagia management and is discussed at length in Chapter 17. The decision to withhold oral feeding leaves the patient and medical team with several options. Presuming that nutrition can be taken enterally (i.e., utilizing the gastrointestinal system), the primary decision most often is a selection between nasogastric tube (NGT) feedings and PEG feeding.

Nasogastric Tube (NGT)

An NGT ensures the provision of enteral nutrition and hydration via a flexible tube which enters through the nasal cavity (or oral cavity in the case of an orogastric tube), passes through the pharynx and UES, and enters the stomach. NGT generally is considered to be a short-term option for nonoral enteral feeding. The effect of an NGT in situ has been studied by two research groups. Huggins and colleagues (1999) presented the first study, which compared the conditions of no NGT, a fine-bore NGT, and wide-bore NGT on swallowing function in young healthy participants. The wide-bore NGT was found to significantly alter several temporal features of swallowing, including stage transition, pharyngeal response, and UES opening. Similar, although nonsignificant, trends were seen for the fine-bore tube. This study presents an important question: Are we creating an iatrogenic dysphagia through our management approaches?

This study was followed by videofluoroscopic swallow study (VFSS) evaluation of 22 stroke patients by Wang et al. (2006). These researchers report that transit times were reduced from 0.2 to 0.6 sec after removing the tube. However, in contrast to the Huggins et al. study, this finding was not significant and, indeed, no other temporal or spatial measures were found to be significantly impacted by the presence of the tube. Clinicians can take some comfort in this finding; however, despite these findings, there may be some isolated patients in which the NGT indeed obstructs bolus flow and evaluation would be best using the tube-in and tube-out conditions.

Other complications of NGT feeding were reported by Mullan, Roubenoff, and Roubenoff (1992) through an evaluation of 276 tube fed patients over a 6-month period. Twelve aspiration events were documented (prevalence 4.4%, incidence 2.4 per 1,000 tube feeding days); however, no increase in mortality was associated with aspiration. The major risk factors for aspiration were patient age and hospital location with more frequent development on the wards rather than in the intensive care unite. A broader range of complications were reported by Ciocon, Silverstone, Graver, and Foley (1988). Seventy tube fed patients were followed across 11 months. Early complications of NGT included agitation and self-extubation in 67% and a notable 43% with aspiration pneumonia. Late complications were the same, but with aspiration pneumonia at 44% and agitation seen in 39%.

Percutaneous Endoscopic Gastrostomy (PEG)

Gastrostomy tube feeding consists of enteral nutrition and hydration via surgically placed tubing through the abdominal wall and directly into the stomach. The surgical gastrostomy has largely been replaced, except when contraindicated, by the PEG in which the tube is placed through the abdominal wall using endoscopic guidance. Sinha and colleagues (2001) sought to investigate practice patterns surrounding PEG insertion using a questionnaire completed by 88 physicians. NGT was reported typically to precede PEG placement in 76% of respondents with 45% waiting more than 2 weeks before PEG insertion. The use of PEG was strongly preferred by the surveyed physicians with only 7% preferring long-term NGT feeding to PEG.

PEG historically has been considered the procedure of choice when the nonoral status of the patient is considered to be longer term or permanent. However, it should be clear from the following studies that placement of a PEG does not implicate permanence. James, Kapur, and Hawthorne (1998) completed a retrospective review of 126 patients fed via PEG for dysphagia secondary to stroke. Median duration of PEG across all participants was 127 days; however, for patients with PEG inserted within 2 weeks of onset, the average duration of placement was 52 days. At long-term follow-up, 29% of patients had the PEG removed, 57% had died, and only 12% continued with PEG feedings. Aspiration pneumonia was found to be the most common complication in patients fed via PEG.

A later study by Yim, Kaushik, Lau, and Tan (2000) consisted of a clinical audit of 50 PEG placements to evaluate practice patterns.

Stroke was the etiology for placement in 80% of the population. PEG was placed within the first month in 46% of the population, within 1 to 2 months in another 16%, with the final 38% receiving their tube greater than 2 months postonset. Post-PEG infection was documented in 14% of patients receiving routine antibiotics and in 39% not provided antibiotics. Infection was also found to be an earlier complication is a study by Anis and colleagues (2006); however, this was only reported in 3% of 191 patients. Late complications of PEG were infection at the tube site in 15% and dislodgement or blocking of the tube in 13.6%. Ciocon et al. (1988) also reported on complications with placement of PEG. Early complications included 56% of patients developing aspiration pneumonia, 50% with tube dysfunction, and 44% with agitation and self-extubation.

DECISION-MAKING FOR NONORAL NUTRITION

Oral Versus Nonoral Intake

Several studies have sought to identify characteristics of patients requiring nonoral feeding. Wojner and Alexandrov (2000) evaluated clinical differences in age, stroke severity scores, length of stay, and cost per case between the tube feeding and control group patients. Seven dependent risk factors were identified; four were found to be independent risk factors. These included wet voice after swallowing water, hypoglossal nerve dysfunction, National Institutes of Health Stroke Scale score, and incomplete oral labial closure. A subsequent study by Lin et al. (2005) identified biomechanical features of swallowing on VFSS that were associated with feeding dependency at discharge in 189 patients with dysphagia subsequent to stroke. In the final logistic regression analysis model, advanced age, recurrent stroke, confinement to a wheelchair at discharge, long duration from stroke onset to VFSS, and stasis in valleculae or piriform sinuses and aspiration on VFSS were independently associated with tube feeding dependency at discharge.

The assumption that feeding tube placement attenuates the risk of aspiration and subsequent pneumonia has been evaluated by several research groups. As referenced earlier in this section, seminal work by Langmore and colleagues (1998) identified that tube feeding in nonoral patients was one of the highest predictors of aspiration pneumonia in a group of 189 elderly patients of mixed etiology followed for 4 years. This assumption was also questioned in the individuals with stroke by Nakajoh et al. (2000). They studied three groups of poststroke patients: those who were oral feeding without dysphagia ($n = 43$), those on oral feeding with dysphagia ($n = 48$); and NGT feeding with dysphagia ($n = 52$), using cough reflex testing and swallowing physiology on initial evaluation and by documenting pneumonia development within the first year postonset. Results of this study support that nonoral feeding may reduce pulmonary complications. The incidence of pneumonia was found to be related to suppressed cough and was higher in patients with oral feeding than those with tube feeding. Dziewas and colleagues (2004) also sought to address this question, but with conflicting results. They evaluated 100 patients with acute stroke fed via NGT secondary to dysphagia. Logistic regression was used to identify variables significantly associated with the occurrence of pneumonia and those related to a poor outcome at 3 months. Pneumonia was diagnosed in 44% of the tube fed patients with most acquiring pneumonia within 3 days of onset. Independent redictors for the occurrence of pneumonia were a decreased level of consciousness and severe facial palsy. The authors concluded that NGTs offer only limited protection against aspiration pneumonia in patients with dysphagia from acute stroke; however, this study did not offer a comparison group to those with NGT. Mamun and Lim (2005) supported these data with a comparative study of 122 patients in two groups: those on NGT feedings and those orally fed. The rate of aspiration pneumonia and death were greater in patients fed via NGT than those who were orally fed. However, the authors concede that patients requiring NGT were more cognitively and functionally impaired than those on an oral diet; indeed, when they compared those on NGT to those who were recommended for NGT but refused, no statistically significantly differences were identified.

This limitation was addressed in a project in which morbidity, mortality, and functional recovery of patients admitted to rehabilitation with PEG in situ were studied using a retrospective case-matched study (Iizuka & Reding, 2005). Patients with a PEG admitted for stroke rehabilitation ($n = 193$) were matched with case controls without PEG ($n = 193$). Participants were within 90 days of stroke onset, and were matched for age, sex, type of stroke, functional independence measure (FIM) score, duration from onset to stroke unit admission, and year of admission. Patients with PEG more often required transfer back to acute hospital and had a poorer survival status. However, those patients with PEG that survived were no different relative to length of rehabilitation admission, improvement in total FIM score from admission to discharge, and final discharge destination (home versus institution), compared to those with poor survival.

Perhaps the most comprehensive approach to addressing decision making relative to provision of nutrition was completed by researchers in the United Kingdom. The FOOD trial (Dennis, Lewis, Cranswick, & Forbes, 2006) consisted of three randomized controlled trials which recruited over 5000 patients from 131 hospitals. The first study evaluated the benefits of nutritional supplements when added to a normal hospital diet and identified a reduction in risk of death of 0.7% as well as an increase in the risk for death or negative outcome of 0.7%; thus, the recommendation for oral supplements is ambiguous. The second study investigated whether early tube feeding within the first week of admission compared to holding tube feeding for 1 week improves outcomes in dysphagic stroke patients. Early tube feeding was associated with a reduction in risk of death of 5.8%. This provides clear evidence in a large population of patients that early tube feeding may substantially decrease mortality and supports the early quoted study by Garaballa and colleagues (1998). The third investigation compared the method of NGT to PEG placed during the first 30 days on patient outcomes. PEG was associated with an increase in absolute risk of death of 1.0% and an increased risk of death or poor outcome of 7.8%. This finding is contrary to other studies comparing PEG to NGT as outlined below.

NGT Versus PEG

Park and colleagues (1992) evaluated 40 patients with dysphagia of at least 4 weeks duration who were randomized to receive either NGT or PEG. No complications occurred in the NGT group but three (16%) of the PEG group developed what the authors considered to be minor problems, aspiration pneumonia (two patients) wound infection (one). However, the patients with PEG received a significantly greater proportion of their prescribed nutritional intake (93%) compared with those receiving NGT (55%) and consequently gained significantly more weight after 7 days of feeding. The average duration of NGT feeding was quite brief (5.2 days); thus, longer term comparisons were not possible.

Norton, Homer-Ward, Donnelly, Long, and Holmes (1996) evaluated 30 acute stroke patients who were randomized to receiving gastrostomy or NGT feedings at 14 days postonset. Contrary to the FOOD trial results, mortality at 6 weeks was significantly lower in the gastrostomy group with two deaths (12%) compared with eight deaths (57%) in the NGT group. Patients on NGT received a significantly smaller proportion of their prescribed nutrition (78%) compared with the gastrostomy group (100%). In the gastrostomy group, the mean albumin concentration increased; whereas there was a reduction of albumin in patients fed via NGT. Six patients from the gastrostomy group were discharged from hospital within 6 weeks of the procedure compared with none from the NGT group.

Bath, Bath, and Smithard (2000) completed a review of the literature to assess the effect of different management strategies for dysphagic stroke patients, in particular, how and when to feed, whether to supplement nutritional intake, and how and whether to treat dysphagia. Based on their review through March 1999, it was concluded that PEG reduces end-of-trial case fatality and treatment failures, and improves nutritional status, including weight, mid-arm circumference, and serum albumin as compared with NGT feeding. This overall conclusion is supported by more recent work by Hamidon and colleagues (2006) who published a small randomized study of 22 patients which compared NGT and PEG for nutritional outcomes. PEG tube feeding was found to be more effective than NG tube feeding in improving the nutritional status (in terms of the serum albumin level) of patients with dysphagic stroke. As with the study by Norton et al. (1996) NGT feeding resulted in decreased serum albumin level within 4 weeks of initiation of tube feedings.

Clearly further research is required to fully evaluate relative risks and benefits of oral versus nonoral and NGT versus PEG feedings. The smaller randomized studies tend to support PEG feedings over NGT. However, this is in stark contrast to the very large FOOD trial (Dennis et al., 2006).

Ethical Considerations

Much of the research relative to risks and benefits of nonoral feeding in patients with stroke has addressed nutritional and pulmonary safety. Much less has been written regarding the ethical and quality of life dilemmas that emerge when approaching decisions regarding nonoral feeding in the dysphagic stroke patient. Two studies have been identified that sought to evaluate the perception of patients and caregivers in regards to PEG placement. Callahan, Haag,

Buchanan, and Nisi (1999) gathered information from patients or surrogate decision makers through face to face interview; in addition, 82 primary care physicians completed a written questionnaire. Although not limited to stroke, the most common etiology necessitating the need for PEG was stroke. Several adverse factors were reported by patient or their surrogates, including the confusion of having multiple discussants, incomplete information, and considerable distress in arriving at the decision to proceed with artificial feeding. According to these consumers, the decision for gastrostomy often appeared to be a "nondecision" in the sense that decision-makers perceived few alternatives. Physicians also reported considerable distress in providing recommendations for PEG, including perceived pressures from families or other health care professionals. Although most health care workers reported having a clear method for selecting patients appropriate for PEG placement, the assumptions underlying clinical practice were not well supported by the medical literature.

Anis and colleagues (2006) studied a mixed population of patients who had undergone PEG. Using a questionnaire to address psychological, social, and physical performance status, of the health related quality of life issues, they interviewed 126 patients/caretakers. Sixty percent of those surveyed would agree to have the PEG tube again if required; 83% felt ease in feeding, and 60% felt that the PEG tube helped in prolonging their survival. Regarding negative opinions, 39% felt that the feeding was too frequent, 36% felt apprehensive about dependency for feeding, and 49% were concerned about the cost of care.

FREE WATER

The use of free water has been recommended for patients with liquid aspiration who are either on tube feeding or receiving thickened liquids, and was initially put forth by the Frazier Rehabilitation Institute in Louisville, Kentucky (for review, Panther, 2005). The premise behind the free water protocol is that water has a neutral pH, which is innocuous to the lungs if aspirated in small amounts. The free water protocol is suggested to promote compliance, improve hydration, and increase quality of life.

The guidelines for the Frazier free water protocol include:

- Unrestricted water access for patients on oral diets—water pitchers are in the room (successful compensatory strategies are encouraged during ingestion of water)
  - Patients with cognitive deficits such as impulsiveness or excess coughing during water ingestion are provided water under supervision
  - Patients with significant choking during water ingestion are not eligible to receive water
- Water intake is discontinued for 30 minutes after a meal to allow clearing of postswallow residual
- Aggressive oral care is undertaken
- Medications are not provided with water.

It is noted that use of a water protocol should be tailored for individuals in acute care settings as the original protocol is designed for patients in a rehabilitation unit (Panther, 2005).

Only one study has been completed to evaluate a free water protocol (Garon, Engle, & Ormiston, 1997). In this study, 20 patients in a stroke rehabilitation unit who had documented aspiration of thin liquids were randomized to one of two groups: (1) thickened liquids only, or (2) thickened liquids with free access to water. Patients were within 3 weeks of stroke and were followed until resolution of thin liquid aspiration. Slightly different than the Frazier protocol, participants completed a prerinse prior to water ingestion and the patient had to request water; it was not available for uncontrolled access. Results revealed that no patient in either group developed dehydration or pneumonia. Patients with thickened liquids only averaged approximately 1 week longer to resolution of thin liquid aspiration as compared to the patients receiving free water. In addition, patients in the thickened liquid group averaged slightly less fluid intake (1210 ml) per day as compared to the thickened liquid plus free water group (1318 ml). As expected, patient satisfaction was higher in those receiving free water compared to those who only received thickened liquids.

Although results of this study are positive, the reader must look closely at the study methods to fully interpret results, particularly in regard to stroke patients.

- Exclusion criteria included:
  - poor cognition
  - severe coughing with aspiration
  - aspiration of thickened liquids or food
  - inability to rinse and expectorate
  - inability to hold a cup or self-feed
  - impulsive behavior
- 94 patients did not meet criteria
- 5 patients assigned to the thickened liquids only group demonstrated aspiration on >50% of swallows evaluated as compared to only 1 patient assigned to the free water group
- 3 patients assigned to the thickened liquids only group demonstrated aspiration on <10% of swallows evaluated as compared to 6 patients assigned to the free water group
- Patients had to request water.

Results may be related to participant selection. Longer recovery for those patients receiving only thickened liquids may be related to more significant dysphagia as demonstrated by >50% aspiration. Moreover, the vast majority of patients admitted to the rehabilitation facility were excluded, yet these are frequently the stroke patients who present with dysphagia. Until large randomized controlled studies are completed incorporating all stroke patients with thin liquid aspiration, an individualized approach must be undertaken in recommending free water to stroke patients with dysphagia and aspiration.

SUMMARY

Our approaches to diet manipulation in patients with swallowing impairment are maturing. Clinicians are now in a better position to more intelligently judge the real risks of developing pneumonia and therefore can more judiciously balance the needs of pulmonary safety, nutrition, and patient quality of life. Certainly, there will be times when complete nonoral nutrition is the only wise option either in the short term until rehabilitative potential is reached or in the long term for patients with poorer prognosis.

17 Compensatory Management

Compensatory management does not change the physiology of the swallow; rather, bolus flow is altered. Compensatory strategies provide immediate benefit by eliminating the patient's symptoms, for example, aspiration, postswallow residual. Benefits are seen immediately but are not permanent. That is, when the compensatory strategy is removed, the previously noted swallowing dysfunction prevails. These strategies are frequently manipulated by the clinician and many require only limited cognitive ability. Compensatory strategies should be thought of as short term to maintain oral intake with long-term management focusing on rehabilitative intervention, which changes swallowing physiology. Only in those patients with significant cognitive deficits should management stop with compensatory strategies.

Before implementing compensatory strategies, most should be proven effective during the instrumental examination (e.g., during the videofluoroscopic swallow study [VFSS], aspiration is eliminated with a chin tuck posture). When attempted during the clinical swallow examination (CSE), the clinician cannot be certain that the compensatory strategy accomplished its goal. That is, a patient may no longer cough when thickened liquid is employed, but the clinician does not know if aspiration ceased or it is no longer overt. Although not addressing thickened liquids as a compensatory technique, Daniels et al. (1998) noted increased silent aspiration with barium during VFSS as opposed to overt aspiration with water in these same patients during the CSE. This may suggest that lack of cough cannot be equated with resolution of aspiration. Other types of compensatory strategies, such as airway management, may require additional training outside the instrumental evaluation with subsequent re-evaluation to determine effectiveness.

It is not the role of the clinician to instruct implementation of the compensatory strategy at every meal. Rather, the clinician should apply the best compensatory strategy based on the patient's swallowing pathophysiology and cognitive ability, instruct and document competency in implementation by either the patient or caregiver, and reassess as indicated. Once the compensatory strategy is effectively employed, the clinician should devote management to rehabilitative techniques. Compensatory strategies and the physiologic abnormalities and resulting symptoms for which they are indicated are listed in Table 17–1. The reader will find this a more basic table in which to understand the variety of disorders for which compensatory techniques are applied. Table 17–2 takes a symptom-based approach and lists the multiple compensations that can be applied to a single presenting symptom. This is the approach that most clinicians would use based on the results on the instrumental examination.

Table 17–1. Compensatory Strategy Approach to Management

Compensation	*Physiologic Abnormality*	*Symptom*
Thickened liquid	Reduced oral control yielding premature spillage Delayed pharyngeal swallow	Pharyngeal pooling
Chopped or puree diet	Poor mastication	Ingestion of large, unmasticated food particles
Cyclic ingestion	Reduced lingual or buccal strength Reduced BOT retraction Reduced HLC elevation yielding reduced UES opening Reduced pharyngeal contraction	Postswallow residual

Table 17–1. *continued*

Compensation	Physiologic Abnormality	Symptom
Volume regulation	Primarily: Reduced oral control yielding premature spillage Delayed pharyngeal swallow	Aspiration with large liquid volumes
3-second prep	Discoordinated oral transfer	Repetitive A-P or random movement of the bolus in the oral cavity
	Delayed pharyngeal swallow	Pharyngeal pooling
Chin tuck	Reduced oral control yielding premature spillage Delayed pharyngeal swallow	Pharyngeal pooling
	Reduced BOT retraction	Vallecular residue
	Reduced airway closure	Aspiration during the swallow
Head turn to the weaker side	Pharyngeal hemiparesis	Unilateral piriform sinus residue
Carbonation	Not specified	Postswallow residual Aspiration
Increased taste—sour bolus	Delayed onset of oral transfer	No movement or delayed movement of the bolus in the oral cavity
	Delayed pharyngeal swallow	Pharyngeal pooling
Thermal tactile stimulation	Delayed pharyngeal swallow	Pharyngeal pooling
Supraglottic swallow	Reduced TVF adduction	Aspiration during the swallow
	Delayed pharyngeal swallow	Aspiration before the swallow
Supersupraglottic swallow	Reduced laryngeal valving	Penetration or aspiration before or during the swallow

A-P = anterior-posterior, BOT = base of tongue, HLC = hyolaryngeal complex, TVF = true vocal folds, UES = upper esophageal sphincter.

Table 17–2. Symptom Approach for Application of Compensatory Strategies

The Symptoms of:	Secondary to Physiologic Abnormality of:	Compensation:
Anterior leakage	Poor orolingual control	Thickened liquid
Inadequate bolus preparation		Chopped or pureed diet
Discoordinated oral transfer		3-second prep
Oral residual		Cyclic ingestion
Pharyngeal pooling to the level of _____		Thickened liquid Volume regulation Chin tuck
	Delayed pharyngeal swallow	Thickened liquid Volume regulation 3-second prep Increased taste—sour bolus Thermal-tactile stimulation Chin tuck*
Nasal regurgitation	Poor pharyngeal motility	Thick consistencies
Inadequate epiglottic deflection	Decreased anterior hyoid movement	No identified compensatory strategy
	Intrinsic structural changes in supportive tissue	
Vallecular residual	Decreased base of tongue to posterior pharyngeal wall approximation	Cyclic ingestion Chin tuck Carbonation-physiology of residual not specified
	Inadequate epiglottic deflection	Cyclic ingestion Carbonation-physiology of residual not specified

224

Table 17–2. *continued*

The Symptoms of:	Secondary to Physiologic Abnormality of:	Compensation:
Inadequate opening of the UES	Decreased anterior hyoid movement	Head turn
	Intrinsic structural functional changes in cricopharyngeus	
Unilateral pharyngeal residue	Pharyngeal hemiparesis	Head turn to weaker side
Piriform sinus residual	Inadequate opening of the UES	Cyclic ingestion Carbonation-physiology of residual not specified Head turn
Penetration	Preswallow pharyngeal pooling	Thickened liquids Volume regulation 3-second prep Chin tuck* Increased taste—sour bolus Thermal-tactile stimulation
	Inadequate epiglottic deflection	No identified compensatory strategy
	Oral residual	Cyclic ingestion
	Pharyngeal residual	Cyclic ingestion Chin tuck Carbonation
	Reduced laryngeal valving	Supersupraglottic swallow
	Preswallow pharyngeal pooling	Same as for penetration Supraglottic or supersupraglottic swallow

continues

Table 17–2. *continued*

The Symptoms of:	Secondary to Physiologic Abnormality of:	Compensation:
Aspiration	Physiology not specified	Carbonation
	Reduced laryngeal valving	Supersupraglottic swallow
	Inadequate true vocal fold closure	Supraglottic swallow
	Oral residual	Same as for penetration
	Pharyngeal residual	Same as for penetration

*Precaution—use chin tuck only with pooling to valleculae. Use with pooling more inferior may increase airway invasion.

UES = upper esophageal sphincter.

POSTURAL CHANGES

Compensatory swallowing postures are designed to change pharyngeal dimensions and redirect bolus flow. Specific postures have been designed for specific motility disorders (see Tables 17-1 and 17-2). As with thickened liquids, a specific posture must be evaluated during an instrumental evaluation to determine effectiveness prior to implementation. Posture compensation should not be randomly applied but should be attempted for the specific dysmotility pattern for which it was designed. As with bolus modification, the use of a posture should be considered short term with rehabilitative management targeting the underlying pathophysiology.

Although posture generally is recommended over strict diet modification, many factors in addition to swallowing must be considered. Attention, memory, and awareness of deficit are critical for the patient to execute a posture adjustment. In a heterogeneous cohort of patients with aspiration, including stroke patients, Rasley et al. (1993) noted that postures were less effective in prevention of aspiration for patients with cognitive deficits. Moreover, honey-thick liquid was more effective than nectar-thick and chin tuck posture with thin liquids in preventing immediate aspiration on VFSS in patients with dementia and/or Parkinson's disease (Logemann et al., 2008).

The two most common postures used, chin tuck and head turn, are reviewed in this book. Although other postures and various combinations of these postures are available (see Logemann, 1998 for review), the chin tuck and head turn postures are the most clinically relevant in terms of management of the stroke patient.

Chin Tuck Posture

The chin tuck posture was designed to facilitate swallowing in patients with a delayed pharyngeal swallow or premature spillage with resulting preswallow pharyngeal pooling and aspiration (Logemann, 1983). The initial notion behind the use of this posture was that it would widen the valleculae. This, in turn, would yield a larger space for material to pool prior to pharyngeal swallow evocation, thereby decreasing aspiration. The initial research was completed to determine pharyngeal dimensions with the head in a neutral position and with the chin tucked (Welch, Logemann, Rademaker, & Kahrilas, 1993). Although results did not reveal a significant increase in vellecular width with the chin tuck posture, they did reveal narrowing of the laryngeal entrance and closer approximation of the laryngeal surface of the epiglottis with the posterior pharyngeal wall (PPW), which would yield improved airway protection. A subsequent study to determine the effects of chin tuck posture on aspiration was completed in a group of patients with neurogenic dysphagia and pre-swallow aspiration (Shanahan, Logemann, Rademaker, Pauloski, &

Kahrilas, 1993). Results revealed the chin tuck to be effective in preventing preswallow aspiration when pooling was limited to the valleculae. Aspiration persisted in patients with pooling to the piriform sinuses. It was suggested that aspiration persisted due to laryngeal elevation and shortening of the pharynx at onset of the pharyngeal swallow, which causeed hypopharyngeal material to enter the airway. Thus, the clinician may use this posture for patients with preswallow aspiration resulting from a delayed pharyngeal swallow or poor bolus control with premature spillage to the level of the valleculae, vallecular residual resulting from reduced base of tongue retraction, and for patients with airway invasion during the swallow due to reduced laryngeal closure.

With the chin tuck posture, the aim is for the patient to touch the chin to the neck. The spine should stay stable as the patient rotates his neck forward to look at his chest. The patient should assume this posture prior to oral transfer. Many stroke patients, however, have problems with bolus control or have cognitive deficits and cannot adequately coordinate timing of assuming the posture prior to bolus entry into the pharynx. In these patients, the use of straw delivery of the bolus with the straw positioned to where the patient must first assume the posture before ingestion may improve effectiveness of the posture.

Head Turn

A head turn posture, generally to the weaker side, was designed to clear unilateral pharyngeal residue in patients with pharyngeal hemiparesis. It was suggested that by closing off the weaker side, the bolus would be travel down the unaffected side of the pharynx (Kirchner, Scatliff, Dey, & Shedd, 1963; Logemann, 1983). This was demonstrated in healthy participants with the bolus traveling through the pharyngeal side opposite the head turn (Logemann et al., 1989). In addition, upper esophageal sphincter (UES) diameter increased and intrabolus pressure decreased in the healthy participants. In this same study, patients with lateral medullary stroke were evaluated with and without the head turn posture. Results revealed improved oropharyngeal swallowing efficiency and increased UES diameter with head turn; pressure was not studied. In a single descriptive case report using computed tomography, piriform sinus closure at the level of the hyoid with dilation of the hypopharynx opposite from the turned side was demonstrated (Tsukamoto, 2000).

For the clinician using videoendoscopy to evaluate swallowing, asymmetric piriform sinus residue may easily be identified. When postswallow residual is identified in the piriform sinus in the VFSS lateral view, a static anterior-posterior image should be obtained to identify if retention is bilateral or asymmetric. When asymmetric residue is noted, the patient should turn his or her head to the affected side. Although prior residual will not clear on the affected side with implementation of this posture, there should be improved bolus flow with minimal residual during subsequent swallows.

SENSORY ENHANCEMENT

Compensatory sensory techniques may involve temperature or taste. Thermal-tactile stimulation is reviewed under compensatory strategies. Research currently suggests only immediate effects of this strategy, thus supporting inclusion as a compensatory strategy.

Temperature

Numerous research studies have been undertaken to determine the effects of bolus temperature on swallowing. Most research has focused on cold temperature with studies generally concentrated on healthy geriatric participants. The majority of results suggest that temperature does not impact swallowing. In a series of studies, Shaker and colleagues found no effects of temperature on pharyngeal peristalsis (Shaker et al., 1993), duration of true vocal fold closure (Ren et al., 1993), or threshold volume required to evoke a pharyngeal swallow (Shaker et al., 1994) in healthy young and older adults. In a recent study in which a tasteless, odorless material was ingested by healthy young adults, results suggested that the warmer food at 50°C was subjectively judged to be easier to swallow than colder food (5°–35°C) (Miyaoka et al., 2006). No significant differences in durations of the oral and oropharyngeal phases were identified with the various temperatures; however, reduced suprahyoid amplitude as measured by surface electromyography (sEMG) was evident with 50°C as compared to 20°C. The authors concluded that the higher temperature of 50°C may facilitate swallowing, as they surmised that greater suprahyoid activity indicates increased effort required for laryngeal elevation. This notion seems counterintuitive as rehabilitation is frequently geared to increase distance, force, and speed of muscle movement.

Limited effects of temperature on bolus flow measure have been reported by Bisch, Logemann, Rademaker, Kahrilas, and Lazarus (1994). This study revealed no differences between cold and room temperature liquids on swallowing measures in the stroke patients. Longer pharyngeal response time and duration of laryngeal elevation was identified for the 1-ml volume in healthy participants.

Carbonation

The influence of carbonation on swallowing has been the focus of recent research studies. In healthy adults, no effects with carbonation were identified for timing and amplitude of contraction for the orbicularis oris, submental, and infrahyoid muscles using sEMG (Ding et al., 2003). Improvement in swallowing, however, has been identified in patients with dysphagia. The use of carbonation to facilitate swallowing was first reported by Jennings, Siroky, and Jackson (1992) in patients who underwent skull base tumor resection. Six of the 12 patients benefited from the use of a carbonated beverage to clear or reduce the amount of postswallow residual. Further evaluation of carbonation in a cohort of neurologically impaired patients revealed that carbonated liquids reduced airway invasion, and postswallow residual, and decreased pharyngeal transit time (PTT) as compared to noncarbonated thin liquids (Bulow, Olsson, & Ekberg, 2003). However, the interested reader should review the methodology of this study before assuming ready translation to clinical practice. Noncarbonated liquids were swallowed on cue whereas carbonated liquids were swallowed without verbal cue. Only participants who were able to sit upright and who could follow instructions were offered the opportunity to swallow the carbonated liquid.

Certain considerations must be made before employing carbonation as a compensatory strategy during VFSS. Unless mixed with barium, a carbonated liquid such as cola will not be visualized. Mixing the cola with barium will decrease and possibly neutralize the effects of the carbonation. If the clinician is interested in the ability of carbonation to clear pharyngeal residue, plain cola may be administered, and although it will not be visualized, the clearing of postswallow retention will be evident if this strategy is effective. If the clinician is interested in increasing swallowing speed or reducing airway invasion, a method described by Bulow et al. (2003) may be used. They added sodium bicarbonate to barium and thus were able to view bolus flow of the carbonated liquid. Of course, the effects of carbonation on airway invasion and postswallow residual are easily viewed with videoendoscopy.

Taste

The impact of taste on swallowing physiology and the potential of taste to facilitate disordered swallowing has become the focus of many research studies. The notion behind this line of research is two-fold. First, it has been suggested that increasing sensory input may facilitate disordered swallowing (Logemann, 1998). Second, taste sensitivity decreases with advancing age (Schiffman, 1993). Thus, findings from this line of research has increased clinical relevance for the stroke population as dysphagia is prominent in this group and the incidence of stroke increases with advancing age.

As reviewed in Chapter 3 (Table 3–1), taste may impact many aspects of swallowing in healthy adults including timing and amplitude of muscle contraction (Ding et al., 2003; Leow, Huckabee, Sharma, & Tooley, 2007), pressure (Palmer et al., 2005; Pelletier & Dhanaraj, 2006), number of swallows and volume per second (Chee et al., 2005), and oral preparation time (Leow et al., 2007). Studies have found that taste does not impact swallowing apnea duration (Butler, Postma, & Fischer, 2004; Hiss et al., 2004) or onset of the pharyngeal swallow when liquid is infused into the valleculae (Pouderoux, Logemann, & Kahrilas, 1996). Some of these studies have focused only on a sour bolus (Palmer et al., 2005; Pelletier & Dhanaraj, 2006), whereas others have evaluated tastes such as sweet, sour, bitter, and salty (Chee et al., 2005; Ding et al., 2003; Leow et al., 2007; Pouderoux & Kahrilas, 1995; Pouderoux et al., 1996).

Research on the effects of taste on swallowing in the neurogenic population has also demonstrated changes in swallowing physiology and supports the notion that heightened sensory stimulation may facilitate certain aspects of swallowing. In the first study to examine the effects of a sour bolus on swallowing pathophysiology, a cohort of patients with dysphagia as well as patients with other neurologic disorders were studied (Logemann et al., 1995). All patients were diagnosed with delayed onset of oral transfer and/or a delayed pharyngeal swallow on VFSS. Barium (1:1, barium to water) was compared against a sour bolus (1:1 barium to Real Lemon Juice). The stroke patients demonstrated a significant reduction in oral transfer onset, oral transfer time (OTT), stage transit duration (STD), and PTT; and oropharyngeal swallowing efficiency was significantly increased with the sour bolus. In the group with other neurogenic etiologies, the sour bolus resulted in faster onset of oral transfer, later onset of base of tongue (BOT) retraction, and shorter duration of BOT to PPW contact. Although the effects of the sour bolus on swallowing physiology were significant, the patients reported the taste to be unpleasant, thus negating its implementation as a functional compensatory strategy.

Recent research has attempted mixture suppression in an attempt to make a sour bolus more palatable yet also maintaining the positive physiologic effects demonstrated by Logemann et al. (1995). Mixture suppression involves the addition of a second taste (e.g., sweet) to the mixture to inhibit the impact of the first taste (e.g., sour). Pelletier and Lawless (2003) studied the impact of mixture suppression on 11 residents of a skilled nursing facility, 10 of whom had a neurogenic etiology (7 with dementia). All participants were previously diagnosed with dysphagia and were receiving thickened liquids. Participants swallowed water, high sour, and sour-sweet liquids. The high sour liquid was associated with decreased airway invasion as compared to water. Both the high sour liquid and the sour-sweet liquids were associated with an increase in spontaneous dry swallows. More work is required to determine the correct balance of mixtures to maintain improved swallowing function with high intensity sour while achieving palatability. Until then, the functional use of taste as a swallowing management strategy is limited.

Thermal-Tactile Stimulation

Thermal-tactile stimulation (TTS) is designed to heighten sensitivity in the central nervous system to increase the speed in which the pharyngeal swallow is evoked and was first described by Logemann (1983). Hence, TTS is recommended for patients with delayed onset of the pharyngeal swallow. The clinician is reminded from Chapter 3 that the concept of "delay" is evolving and that research has shown that the bolus may be in the pharynx prior to onset of the pharyngeal swallow with both single and sequential swallows in healthy adults (Chi-Fishman & Sonies, 2000; Daniels et al., 2004; Daniels & Foundas, 2001; Martin-Harris et al., 2007; Stephen et al., 2005). The presence of the bolus in the distal pharynx should be considered abnormal only when additional swallowing disorders are present.

Traditionally, TTS involves the vertical rubbing of the anterior faucial arches with a chilled laryngeal mirror (Logemann, 1998), although frozen ice sticks also have been used (Rosenbek et al., 1998). Ice sticks have been suggested due to the rapid temperature acceleration of a cold laryngeal mirror (Selinger, Prescott, & Hoffman, 1994). The back of the cold mirror, or ice stick, is initially placed at the base of the anterior arch, and brisk vertical up and down rubbing along the arch is completed five times. Both faucial arches are stimulated in this manner followed by the swallowing of a small amount of liquid or saliva if the patient cannot have oral intake. Three to four 5- to 10-minute daily treatment sessions have been recommended (Logemann, 1998).

Research on the effects of TTS in healthy adults is contradictory with some studies reporting no change in evocation of the pharyngeal swallow after TTS (Ali, Laundl, Wallace, deCarle, & Cook, 1996; Bove, Mansson, & Eliasson, 1998) and another study suggesting increased timing of the swallow response as well as the number of swallows following stimulation (Kaatzke-McDonald, Post, & Davis, 1996). Swallowing evocation may be at its peak in healthy adults with little room for improvement; therefore, perhaps study of participants with disordered swallowing may be best to determine the effectiveness of TTS. Lazzara, Lazarus, and Logemann (1986) were the first to report on the immediate effects of TTS on faster evocation of the pharyngeal swallow in neurologically impaired patients (one-half with stroke). TTS was completed in the radiology suite with immediate rescanning of the participant to determine improvement. Results revealed improvement in the majority of patients for at least one swallow. Four patients were further studied to probe impact of TTS on subsequent swallows. Results in this pilot study suggested that the influence of TTS may last for two to three swallows. Findings of positive immediate effects of TTS in shortening the time to onset of the pharyngeal swallow were supported by Rosenbek, Roecker, Wood, and Robbins (1996). Participants ranged from 1 month to more than 1 year poststroke. In a treatment trial to investigate more long-term effects of TTS, a single-subject ABAB (treatment-withdrawal) design was completed in seven stroke patients with a delayed pharyngeal swallow and airway invasion (Rosenbek et al., 1991). Each treatment period was for 1 week with participants receiving on average 18 trials in each of the five daily sessions. Results revealed reduced STD without change in penetration or aspiration in two participants, thus offering weak support for sustained effects of TTS. In the last of the series of studies on TTS, Rosenbek et al. (1998) studied treatment intensity ranging from 150 to 600 TTS trials distributed across 3 to 5 days. Results revealed that no one intensity level was more therapeutic than another.

Currently, results support only immediate effects of TTS, which would place it under a compensatory strategy. Until an appropriate and feasible treatment intensity is identified and applied in a research trial, the long-term rehabilitative effects of TTS remain elusive.

VOLITIONAL CONTROL OF ORAL TRANSFER

By volitionally delaying the onset of oral transfer, swallowing is changed from an automatic behavior to a more volitionally controlled action. This is the notion behind the 3-second prep as described by Kagel in the 1980s and reviewed by Huckabee and Pellitier (1999). In the 3-second prep, the patient silently counts to 3 prior to onset of oral transfer to facilitate organized execution of oral transfer and evocation of the pharyngeal swallow. This strategy does not have direct empirical evidence to support it, but the concept has been indirectly supported by other studies with preliminary favorable results. Although not a study of the 3-second prep, Ludlow et al. (2005) suggest that the self-initiated coordination of a button press with onset of swallowing may improve swallowing due to central volitional control. Moreover, Daniels et al. (2007) evaluated the effects of clinician-controlled verbal cue to swallow on bolus flow in healthy older adults. The participant was provided a verbal cue to swallow after placing the bolus in the oral cavity. Findings from this study as well as preliminary findings in patients with mild Alzheimer's disease (Daniels, Corey, Schulz, Foundas, & Rosenbek, 2007) reveal shorter OTT and STD with cue to swallow. Verbal cue affected bolus position at onset of timing measures thereby influencing duration. The bolus was positioned more posterior in the oral cavity at onset of oral transit and the leading edge of the bolus at onset of the pharyngeal swallow was more superior in the pharynx for cued as compared to noncued swallows. Anecdotal reports have suggested that verbal cue to swallow may decrease OTT and produce "apraxia of swallowing" in patients with a left hemispheric stroke (Logemann, 1998; Robbins & Levine, 1988; Robbins et al., 1993). Thus, results must be replicated in the stroke population to determine if the effects of cued swallow, either self-initiated or clinician-initiated, are beneficial or deleterious.

BREATH-HOLDING TECHNIQUES

The supraglottic and supersupraglottic swallow maneuvers are two techniques designed to facilitate airway protection (Logemann, 1998). Airway protection is at the level of the true vocal folds (TVF) for the supraglottic swallow and at the level of the laryngeal vestibule for the supersupraglottic swallow. They may be implemented to prevent aspiration (supraglottic swallow) and/or penetration (supersupraglottic swallow) before or during swallow. In addition to airway protection, these breath-holding maneuvers can impact temporal relationships and biomechanical events during swallowing. In a study of healthy adults, onset of hyoid, laryngeal, and BOT movement, laryngeal closure, and BOT-PPW contact occurred significantly later with either maneuver as compared to swallows without the maneuvers (Ohmae, Logemann, Kaiser, Hanson, & Kahrilas, 1996). In addition, onset of airway closure at the level of the arytenoids and the TVF was significantly earlier with either maneuver as compared to swallows without the maneuver; the duration of laryngeal closure and UES opening also significantly increased. In a case study of three patients with head and neck cancer treated with surgery and/or radiotherapy, BOT-PPW pressure and contact duration increased with the supersupraglottic swallow maneuver (Lazarus, Logemann, Song, Rademaker, & Kahrilas, 2002). Although impacting more than just laryngeal valving, the effects of these two breath-holding techniques have been shown to be immediate. No study has been completed to determine if repeated use produces long-term changes in swallowing physiology.

In the supraglottic swallow, the patient is instructed to hold his or her breath, swallow during breath-holding, and cough immediately after the swallow before inhalation. For the supersupraglottic swallow, the patient is instructed to hold his or her breath, bear down (this provides closure of the laryngeal vestibule), swallow while breath-holding and bearing down, and cough immediately after the swallow. It should be noted that for both maneuvers, patients are instructed to take a deep breath prior to holding their breath in the directions provided by Logemann (1998). The degree of laryngeal valving is influenced by the techniques, and instructions appear to be a critical component in attaining airway protection. A "hard" breath-hold has been shown more likely to achieve maximum laryngeal valving (TVF and false vocal fold adduction, arytenoid adduction and tilting) than an easy breath hold (Martin, Logemann, Shaker, & Dodds, 1993; Mendelsohn & Martin, 1993). Further research had suggested inhaling prior to the breath hold was least effective in attaining TVF adduction (Donzelli & Brady, 2004). The authors reported that participants abducted their TVF to take the deep breath and that, although they stopped breathing, they never adducted the TVF. To ensure that the patient is achieving maximum TVF adduction, the clinician can ask the patient to phonate "ah." If vocalization is evident, the TVF are not completely adducted. Videoendoscopy may also be used as visual feedback to achieve laryngeal valving with either breath-holding technique.

The "hard" breath hold is frequently effective in achieving laryngeal valving as it may create a Valsalva maneuver. The Valsalva maneuver has been associated with adverse events such as cardiac arrhythmia (Metzger & Therrien, 1990). As cardiovascular disease is associated with stroke, it is important to understand the impact of using breath-holding swallowing maneuvers in stroke patients. Chaudhuri et al. (2002) studied three groups of patients: (1) 11 patients with a recent stroke, dysphagia, coronary artery disease (CAD), (2) 4 patients with a recent stroke, dysphagia, no CAD, and (3) 8 orthopedic patients, no dysphagia, no CAD. Cardiac status was monitored for 4 hours. During this time period, subjects completed a swallowing treatment session involving performing either the supraglottic swallow or supersupraglottic swallow, a regular therapy session, and a meal. In the swallowing session, a minimum of eight swallows were completed using either technique. For the two groups with a stroke diagnosis, 87% of participants demonstrated arrhythmia during the swallowing session. The arrhythmia subsided after completion of the treatment and did not occur with other activities such as walking. In the orthopedic group, one participant exhibited bradycardia. Abnormal cardiac findings were equally evident with either maneuver. Although a Valsalva effect is created when lifting a heavy box or straining to have a bowel movement, it is brief and not repetitive; whereas, with swallowing using a breath-holding technique, the Valsalva effect may be slightly more sustained and repeated over the course of therapy or a meal. Thus, it is important for the clinician to review the medical history and discuss the treatment plan with medical staff prior to implementing breath-holding techniques in stroke patients.

BOLUS MODIFICATION

Bolus modification may involve thickening liquids or pureeing solids. The volume that a person swallows as well as the speed of bolus delivery may be controlled. In addition, the order in which boli of different consistencies are swallowed may be used to immediately improve swallowing. Many of these strategies are implemented due to disordered swallowing physiology; thus, effectiveness should be evaluated during the instrumental examination. On the other hand, others strategies are implemented secondary to the cognitive deficits often seen following stroke and may not require study during the instrumental evaluation.

Thickened Liquids

Increased consistency reduces bolus speed (Dantas et al., 1990). This decrease in speed should lead to improved bolus control thereby reducing premature spillage and the depth to which a bolus travels in the pharynx until the pharyngeal swallow is evoked. This may serve to explain the evidence of reduced aspiration on VFSS with thick liquids as compared to thin liquids (Kuhlemeier, Palmer, & Rosenberg, 2001). The understanding of the effects of consistency changes on swallowing physiology is based primarily on research comparing liquid and paste barium in healthy adults, although a few studies have focused on stroke patients and more recently, various liquid consistencies (Table 17–3).

Table 17–3. Consistency Effects on Swallowing

Study	Participants	Material	Results (thick as compared to thin)
Bisch et al. (1994)	10 healthy (M = 62 yrs) 10 stroke, mild dysphagia (M = 62 yrs) 8 stroke, moderate-severe dysphagia (M = 69 yrs)	Liquid barium Paste barium	↓ STD in both stroke groups ↓ BOT to PPW contact ↑ duration of UES opening
Bulow et al. (2003)	40 patients (M = 69 yrs) 19 with stroke	Solid (food mixed with high density barium) Thickened liquids (fruit puree mixed with high-density barium) Thin liquid (high-density barium) Carbonated thin liquid (high-density barium mixed with sodium bicarbonate)	↓ airway invasion ↓ airway invasion with carbonated thin liquid as compared to thin liquid ↑ PTT as compared to carbonated thin liquid ↑ postswallow residual as compared to thin liquids and carbonated thin liquids
Chi-Fishman & Sonies (2002)	13 healthy young (20–39 yrs) 11 healthy middle-aged (40–59 yrs) 7 healthy older (60–79 yrs)	Thin liquid 7 cp Nectar-thick liquid 243–260 cp Honey-thick liquid 724–759 cp Spoon-thick liquid 2760–2819 cp	↑ preswallow gesture duration ↑ TSD No additional temporal, amplitude, or velocity effects

Study	Participants	Consistencies	Results
Dantas et al. (1990)	10 healthy (M = 26 yrs)	Liquid barium 200 cp Paste barium 60,000 cp	↑ OTT ↑ PTT ↑ duration of UES opening ↑ duration of pharyngeal peristaltic pressure wave ↑ intrabolus pressure ↑ duration of hyoid displacement ↑ magnitude of hyoid and laryngeal movement
Dantas, Dodds, Massey, & Kern (1989)	9 healthy (M = 26 yrs)	Low-density liquid barium 200 cp High-density liquid barium 300 cp	↑ OTT ↑ PTT ↑ duration of UES opening Later onset of UES opening ↑ intrabolus pressure ↑ magnitude of anterior hyoid movement
Lazarus et al. (1993)	10 stroke (M = 62 yrs) 10 age-matched healthy	Liquid barium thinned with water Barium paste	Controls: ↑ duration of UES opening ↓ pharyngeal swallowing efficiency score* Both groups: ↑ BOT to PPW contact
Logemann et al. (2008)	351 dementia 228 PD 132 PD and dementia	Thin liquid barium 15 cp Nectar-thick liquid barium 300 cp Honey-thick liquid barium 3000 cp	↓ aspiration with honey-thick as compared to nectar-thick and chin tuck posture with thin liquids Honey-thick liquid least preferred by participants

continues

241

Table 17–3. *continued*

Study	Participants	Material	Results (thick as compared to thin)
Miller & Watkin (1996)	5 healthy (*M* = 26 yrs)	Water 0–10 cp Applesauce 400–8,000 cp Pudding >10,000 cp	↑ anterior lingual peak amplitude
Nicosia et al. (2000)	10 healthy middle aged (48–55 yrs) 10 healthy older (69–91 yrs)	Liquid, 3:1 water to barium Barium paste	↑ oral swallowing pressure ↑ time to reach peak swallowing pressure
Reimers-Neils et al. (1994)	5 healthy (25–42 yrs)	Liquids—fruit juice, tomato juice Thin paste—applesauce, pudding Thick paste—cheese spread, peanut butter	↑ EMG signal duration ↑ submental and infrahyoid EMG amplitude ↑ average and maximum EMG activity No difference between thin paste and liquids
Shaker et al. (1988)	5 healthy (*M* = 30 yrs)	Water Mashed potatoes	↑ tongue tip and dorsum pressure
Steele & Van Lieshout (2004)	4 healthy young (*M* = 27 yrs) 4 healthy older (*M* = 59 yrs)	Thin liquid 6–16 cp Nectar-thick liquid 466–470 cp Honey-thick liquid 1182–1774 cp	↓ sip size ↓ rate of sequential swallowing No significant differences in lingual behavior

↓ = decrease, ↑ = increase, BOT = base of tongue, cp = centipoise, EMG = electromyography, OTT = oral transit time, PD= Parkinson's disease, PPW = posterior pharyngeal wall, PTT = pharyngeal transit time, STD = stage transit duration, TSD = total swallow duration, UES = upper esophageal sphincter, M = mean.

*Pharyngeal swallowing efficiency score = 100% – [% pharyngeal residual + % aspirated] / PTT.

Although studies on the effectiveness of thickened liquids in preventing aspiration are lacking, clinicians frequently use thickened liquids in the management of their patients with dysphagia (Garcia, Chambers, & Molander, 2005). Only one study has evaluated the immediate effect of three compensatory strategies (nectar-thick liquid, honey-thick liquid, and chin tuck with thin liquids) in patients with VFSS-confirmed aspiration (Logemann et al., 2008). Patients were diagnosed with dementia and/or Parkinson's disease. Results indicated that honey-thick liquid was more effective than either nectar-thick or chin down posture in preventing thin liquid aspiration during the VFSS. However, an equally important finding was that one-half of the patients aspirated on all three compensatory interventions. How these results translate to the stroke population is unclear and requires further research; however, it does support the use of an instrumental examination to determine if a compensation technique is effective.

In deciding to recommend thickened liquids, clinicians must consider three key points:

1. *Patient satisfaction/Quality of life*: Patient dissatisfaction with food preparation, that is, thickened liquid, pureed diet, has been identified as highly related to patients' lack of compliance (Colodny, 2005). Moreover, dysphagic patients expressed preference for posture strategies over liquid alteration and preference for nectar-thick liquids over honey-thick liquids (Logemann et al., 2008).

2. *Risk/Benefit ratio*: Concerning the risks and benefits of thickened liquids, the clinician must consider aspiration, dehydration, and fatigue. Aspiration occurs less often with thickened liquids as compared to thin liquids (Kuhlemeier et al., 2001) with greater immediate elimination of aspiration using honey-thick liquids as compared to nectar-thick and chin tuck posture management (Logemann et al., 2008). However, no change in immediate aspiration status was evident in one-half of the patients studied.

Whereas aspiration is associated with the development of aspiration pneumonia in stroke patients (Holas, DePippo, & Reding, 1994; Johnson, McKenzie, & Sievers, 1993), other factors such as dependency for feeding and oral care, the number of decayed teeth, and tube feeding are more predictive of aspiration pneumonia (Langmore et al., 1998). Although an important clinical concern is prevention of aspiration, an additionally important concern is prevention of dehydration. Dehydration is not due to the thickening agent, which does not compromise free-water content or absorption. Rather, dehydration may ensue due to palatability, with patients drinking lesser amounts of the thickened liquid as compared to thin liquids. Whereas free-water may be obtained from additional food sources, ensuring adequate hydration is a prerequisite for patients receiving diet alteration. Last, thickened liquids increase intrabolus pressure (Dantas et al., 1990), leading to increased effort and strength to swallow (Miller & Watkin, 1996; Nicosia et al., 2000; Reimers-Neils, Logemann, & Larson, 1994) and possibly fatigue over the duration of a meal with an overall decrease in oral intake. Thus, strong collaboration between the speech pathologist and nutritionist is essential if thickened liquids are recommended.

3. *Correlation of mealtime and VFSS liquids*: Currently, thin and thick liquids ingested during mealtime and those used in the VFSS are not correlated in terms of rheologic properties (viscosity, density, yield stress). The interested reader is referred to Bourne (2002) for a review of rheology. Findings on lack of correlation apply when barium was used as the base and material was added to achieve the desired consistency (Cichero, Hay, Murdoch, & Halley, 1997) as well as to when the mealtime liquid (i.e., water, thickened liquid) served as the base and barium was added to create a radiopaque fluid (Cichero, Jackson, Halley, & Murdoch, 2000). Both strategies are used in the clinical setting. Since these studies were completed, standardized barium in thin liquid, nectar, and honey consistencies and commer-

cially available prethickened mealtime liquids are now available for clinical use. However, no published study has been completed to compare rheologic properties between these commercially available products. If the use of thickened liquids is critical to the prevention of liquid aspiration, concordance between mealtime and VFSS liquids would appear crucial. On the other hand, it must be acknowledged that there is an exponential amount of rheologic variation in the foods and liquids a person ingests. Every type of food and liquid cannot be evaluated in an instrumental evaluation. The wise clinician extrapolates findings from the limited number of consistencies administered during the instrumental evaluation and applies this information across the spectrum of what a person can safely swallow. Whether this notion can be applied to the thickened liquid argument is debatable.

As discussed earlier in this section, most compensatory strategies, including thickened liquids, must be evaluated for effectiveness during the instrumental evaluation (Logemann et al., 2008). Use of a thickened liquid should begin at the volume at which consistent aspiration of a thin liquid is observed. The remainder of the evaluation for liquids, including sequential swallowing, should proceed with thickened liquid consistency as the clinician must ensure that the compensatory strategy would be effective in normal mealtime situations of self-regulated liquid volumes. The clinician should start with a nectar consistency and only proceed to honey-thick liquid as indicated.

Due to reduced patient acceptance and the associated increased swallowing effort with potential for fatigue, the use of thickened liquids is frequently considered a last option in swallowing management. Generally, other compensatory strategies such as chin tuck, if proven effective in the instrumental evaluation, are recommended prior to implementing thickened liquids. However, the clinician must also consider the patient's cognitive status, which may be severely impaired in stroke patients. If the clinician is resolute that a patient's safety and oral intake is compromised without employment of a compensatory strategy for preswallow aspiration and if a patient's cognitive status precludes the use of compensatory postures, for example, the patient cannot consistently remember to use the posture, thickened liquids may be the only option at maintaining oral liquid intake. However, the goal should be to initiate rehabilitation to ameliorate pathophysiology and advance the diet as quickly as possible.

Modification of Food

A patient's ability to manipulate dense foods and solids can be evaluated with the CSE and VFSS. If mastication is poor, yielding inability to break down food or lingual strength is reduced and yields notable oral and oropharyngeal postswallow residual, diet alteration generally is considered. From the previous review of thickened liquids, the clinician will note that increased consistency requires increased muscular strength to propagate the bolus through the oral cavity and pharynx. Likewise, efficient mastication requires a functional set of teeth (or tough gums as is the case with some patients) and good lingual strength and movement. As with thickened liquids, diet modification is generally the last strategy implemented and if possible, initiated with the least restrictive diet. Concerning semisolids and solids, the order of least to most restrictive would be: (1) adding gravies to moisten more dense semisolids, (2) avoiding hard solids such as apples, (3) chopped foods, and (4) puree diet. Especially when more restrictive diets, such as puree, are recommended, the clinician must be concerned about decreased acceptance, which may lead to reduced intake and/or noncompliance.

When postswallow residual in the oral cavity and pharynx is the symptom observed, the use of cyclic ingestion would be a more optimal compensatory strategy compared to diet alteration. Cyclic ingestion involves altering ingestion of liquids and semisolid/masticated solid consistencies to facilitate clearing of postswallow residual. A dry swallow following every one to two swallows may also serve this purpose. In the instrumental evaluation, the clinician should note the patient's spontaneous initiation of a dry swallow to clear postswallow residual prior to asking the patient repeatedly to swallow or providing a liquid wash as this will provide information on sensation.

Volume and Rate of Delivery

The evaluation of swallowing generally is initiated with small liquid volumes to prevent aspiration of large quantities. If aspiration is consistent with a certain volume, compensatory intervention generally is initiated before increasing the volume. However, the reader may recall from earlier chapters that increased volume is associated with decreased OTT and (STD) in healthy adults (see Table 3–1) and provides increased sensory input. No study has been completed to determine if increased volume can have a therapeutic benefit for specific swallowing pathophysiology.

Current practice is to frequently regulate volume of liquid ingestion for a delayed pharyngeal swallow or reduced oral control if preswallow pooling with airway invasion is observed. Volume regulation may be completed on a global level with recommendation for small sips or it may be more exact by recommending a prescribed volume. Commercially available cups that allow regulation of the volume ingested are available. These cups have not been studied in terms of maintenance of volume over time, prevention of aspiration, or patient acceptance. In stroke patients who may be too cognitively impaired to self-regulate volume, volume regulation cups may be helpful.

Impulsive behavior, which is frequently evident in patients with right hemisphere or frontal stroke, may impact the preoral and oral phases in that the patient takes too large of a bite of a solid or continually stuffs food into the oral cavity without swallowing between each bite. This may lead to more concerns of asphyxia versus aspiration. With patients such as this, the underlying issue is cognition, not impaired swallowing physiology. For these patients, a team approach to patient management is critical. Mealtime supervision may be recommended, but this should not be considered treatment that is provided by the clinician. Rather, the dysphagia team must review and agree on eating/feeding strategies, and appropriate staff, such as the nursing assistant should provide supervision and daily monitoring of the meal. If swallowing pathophysiology is not identified in a patient such as this, then the clinician can concentrate solely on cognitive deficits, which in time should impact eating behavior.

Rate of presentation may include single versus sequential swallowing. Currently, it is unclear if sequential swallowing may improve certain dysmotility patterns evident with single swallows. By sequential swallowing, it is meant that a person continuously completes multiple swallows of a larger volume (e.g., 50–100 ml) as described by Chi-Fishman and Sonies (2000) and Daniels and colleagues (2004). Although these studies identified longer STD and pharyngeal transit time (PTT) as compared to single swallows, a cyclic elevation and partial lowering of the hyolaryngeal complex between swallows was identified for many participants. Chi-Fishman and Sonies (Chi-Fishman & Sonies, 2000) have suggested that as sequential swallowing has distinct biomechanical and sensorimotor properties such as bolus flow momentum, prolonged sensory stimulation, and heightened motor responsiveness, it may serve as a compensatory strategy. Research is indicated to identify if specific types of swallowing disorders are facilitated by sequential swallowing. If implemented for the wrong disorder, the risk of aspiration could be greater as the patient is self-administering large liquid volumes.

18 Rehabilitation of Oropharyngeal Dysphagia

The evolution of our clinical approaches to the management of dysphagia is bringing us to a point of exciting discoveries. Initially, as we struggled both in clinical practice and research to understand fundamental swallowing biomechanics, we developed a series of compensatory techniques that allowed for an immediate reduction in risks. These techniques are valuable for short-term risk management and will continue to hold an important place in the clinical armamentarium.

The rehabilitation of swallowing pathophysiology, although not new, is certainly now seeming to come into prominence. A cursory search of Medline reveals that from the years 1980 to 1989, out of 2,584 entries brought up using the search term "deglutition," only 6% were brought up again when the search term "rehabilitation" was added to the search. This increased to only 8% (of 4,368) from the years 1990 to 1999; and up to only 9% (of 2,776) from the shorter time span between 2000 to 2004. However, within the past 2 years, from 2005 to 2007, the percentage of references identified by including "rehabilitation" with "deglutition," compared to "deglutition" alone increased to a remarkable 23% of 1,660 references.

As we are developing greater sophistication in our understanding of dysphagia, we ultimately are developing greater specificity in patient management. No longer are we addressing all impairment in all patients with the same well-worn approaches. This greater specificity will ultimately lead to improved patient outcomes. A key example of this lies in the compensatory technique of thermal-tactile stimulation (TTS). First described by Logemann (1983) this application of a cold stimulus to the anterior faucial arches was targeted toward inhibiting preswallow pharyngeal pooling and thus the potential for aspiration prior to airway protection. TTS was based on a sound biologic probability: the anterior faucial arches are embedded with sensory receptors particularly responsive to cold and are innervated by the glossopharyngeal sensory nerve that is known to contribute to evocation of the pharyngeal swallow. However, subsequent research (Ali et al., 1996; Kaatzke-McDonald et al., 1996; Lazzara et al., 1986; Rosenbek et al., 1991; Rosenbek et al., 1996) has only weakly supported the effectiveness of TTS as a rehabilitation technique. These studies were based on the inclusion criteria of patients presenting with the symptom of pooling, rather than specifying a pathophysiologic etiology of sensory impairment. It would not be surprising then, that strong support was not identified for this sensory based technique as preswallow pooling can be the symptom of both a motor and a sensory impairment. With greater specificity in identifying sensory impairment, we may ultimately find that this type of approach can move from the compensatory realm of management into rehabilitation of a sensory-based swallowing impairment.

Emerging research in the rehabilitation of the dysphagic patient is making it increasingly clear that diagnostic precision is a mandate for rehabilitative effectiveness. Indeed, new information about both compensatory and rehabilitative techniques suggests substantial potential for both benefit and harm. The technique of effortful swallow has certainly seemed benign enough and has been applied regularly as both a compensation to facilitate bolus clearance during swallowing and, more recently, as a rehabilitative exercise to strengthen pharyngeal contraction. However, multiple studies have identified mixed outcomes for the effect of effortful swallow on pharyngeal pressure generation, and research by Bulow, Olsson, and Ekberg (1999, 2001, 2002) has offered the suggestion that this technique may inhibit anterior hyoid movement. Although replications of this work are needed, these data suggest the need for caution and careful evaluation before implementation of rehabilitation plans.

A review of our current rehabilitative strategies is outlined below, focusing heavily on techniques that are presumably well established (Table 18-1). In the subsequent chapter, exciting new developments that are still considered experimental and emerging into clinical work are detailed. Any discussion of rehabilitation should be, but rarely is, followed by a discussion of dose. How much rehabilitation is enough? Finally, as a rapidly expanding area of practice, a few thoughts are provided on areas that we perhaps need to develop in our efforts to increase rehabilitative specificity.

ORAL MOTOR EXERCISES

For as long as speech-language pathologists have been engaged in the provision of clinical services, there have been concerted therapeutic efforts to increase the strength and efficiency of orolingual structures. Initially these efforts were focused on improved speech articulatory performance, with an inevitable transfer of the developed exercises to the goal of improving oral phase swallowing and presumably tongue driving forces involved in pharyngeal phase swallowing. What is fairly astonishing however, given the prolonged use of these techniques, is the lack of sound research data to support these practices. In a historical publication on treatment of speech disorders, Van Riper (1954) commented that, "For centuries, speech correctionists have used diagrams, applicators, and instruments to ensure appropriate tongue, jaw, and lip placement. . . . If these devices and instruments have any real value, it seems to be that of vivifying the movements of the tongue and of providing a large number of varying tongue positions, from which the correct one may finally emerge" (pp. 236-238). Sadly, in the ensuing 50+ years, we have made little gains in quantifying treatment effects for oral motor therapy. We have many clinical descriptors of what to do, but have very few studies that document the clinical outcomes of these treatment approaches.

Table 18–1. Rehabilitative Strategies for Use with Specific Symptoms and Underlying Physiologic Abnormalities

The Symptoms of	Secondary to Physiologic Abnormality of	Rehabilitation Approach	Other Considerations
Anterior leakage	Poor orolingual control	Oral motor exercises: Tongue to palate pressure Tongue to tongue depressor pressure	Biofeedback device: IOPI or other oral pressure measurement device, mirror
Inadequate bolus preparation			
Inadequate bolus formation			
Oral residual			
Pharyngeal pooling to the level of _____	Delayed pharyngeal swallow	No known rehabilitation techniques at this time	
Nasal regurgitation	Poor pharyngeal motility	Effortful swallow Masako maneuver	Biofeedback device: sEMG of submental muscle group Precautions: attend to hyoid movement, may wish to add head lift maneuver as prophylactic

Inadequate epiglottic deflection	Decreased anterior hyoid movement	Head lift maneuver	Biofeedback device: sEMG of submental muscle group Precautions: attend to hyoid movement, may wish to add head lift maneuver as prophylactic
	Intrinsic structural changes in supportive tissue	No rehabilitation techniques at this time	
Vallecular residual	Decreased base of tongue to posterior pharyngeal wall approximation	Masako maneuver Effortful swallow Oral motor exercises	
	Inadequate epiglottic deflection*	See rehabilitation approaches for physiologic abnormalities resulting in inadequate epiglottic deflection above.	
Inadequate opening of the UES*	Decreased anterior hyoid movement*	Head lift maneuver	Biofeedback device: sEMG of submental muscle group Precautions: attend to hyoid movement, may wish to add head lift maneuver as prophylactic
	Intrinsic structural functional changes in cricopharyngeus	Mendelsohn maneuver	
Piriform sinus residual	Inadequate opening of the UES*	See rehabilitation approaches for physiologic abnormalities resulting in inadequate opening of the UES above.	

continues

253

The Symptoms of	Secondary to Physiologic Abnormality of	Rehabilitation Approach	Other Considerations
Penetration	Preswallow pharyngeal pooling*	Refer to rehabilitation approaches associated with physiologic abnormalities underlying penetration	
	Inadequate epiglottic deflection*		
	Inadequate supraglottic shortening/laryngeal elevation*		
	Oral residual*		
	Pharyngeal residual*		
Aspiration	Preswallow pharyngeal pooling*	Refer to rehabilitation approaches associated with physiologic abnormalities underlying aspiration	
	Inadequate true vocal fold closure	Vocal adduction exercises	
	Oral residual*	Refer to rehabilitation approaches associated with physiologic abnormalities underlying aspiration	
	Pharyngeal residual*		

Table 18–1. *continued*

*Occasionally a symptom will be caused by another symptom, which requires the clinician to problem-solve through to the initial presenting physiologic abnormality.

sEMG = surface electromyography; UES = upper esophageal sphincter.

Robbins and colleagues have initiated a research program designed to methodically address this gap in our knowledge. Using a hand-held, portable manometric device which measures lingual to palatal pressure, the Iowa Oral Pressure Instrument (IOPI), this research group initially investigated the influence of age on oral pressures (Robbins et al., 1995). Pressures were recorded at three lingual sites (tip, blade, dorsum) during a maximal isometric task and during saliva swallows in young and elder healthy participants. Results of this work suggest that functional swallowing pressures remain similar across age groups; however, functional reserve declines with age. Two implications are highlighted by the authors. First, elder individuals may have to work harder to produce functional pressures; second, age-related illness, such as stroke or even systemic infection, may put elder patients at higher risk of functional impairment. These findings were confirmed and elaborated in a study by Nicosia et al. (2000) that replicated methods in the prior study but added an analysis of temporal characteristics of pressure generation. Again, swallowing pressures did not differ between younger and elder participants, but elders generated decreased maximal isometric pressure. Additional temporal analysis of these data also suggests that elders require increased time to reach peak pressure. This supports the earlier supposition that elders have to work harder to reach functional swallowing pressures, and that they utilize what the researchers refer to as a pattern of "pressure building," in which multiple lingual gestures are recruited to reach peak pressure.

More recent studies by this research group have sought to evaluate the influence of rehabilitative efforts on generating increased functional reserve. In the first study of this kind, Robbins et al. (2005) designed a prospective study of 10 healthy elder participants (ages 70–89) who underwent an 8-week progressive lingual resistance exercise program. Using a videofluoroscopic swallow study (VFSS) to document functional change and measures of oral lingual pressure, researchers documented that all subjects significantly increased both isometric and swallowing pressures. Additionally, a subgroup of four participants who underwent magnetic resonance imaging of the tongue produced an increase in lingual volume averaging 5.1%. This study offers encouragement from a small treatment sample that oral-lingual exercises are effective in elderly individuals. Lazarus, Logemann, Haung, and Rademaker (2003) also sought to evaluate the influence of tongue strengthening exercises in healthy participants. However, instead of relying only on the IOPI, this group compared performance in 31 healthy young adults after participating for 1 month in one of three treatments groups: (1) no exercise, (2) standard tongue strength exercises using a tongue depressor, and (3) exercise using the IOPI. Data from this study suggest that either of the active exercise groups demonstrated substantially greater gains in tongue strength compared to the no exercise group but that type of exercise did not significantly influence outcome. Thus, at least in healthy participants, intervention to strengthen oral function does not appear to be dependent on instrumentation.

Only a single study has evaluated the influence of lingual exercise in patients with dysphagia subsequent to stroke (Robbins et al., 2007). Ten stroke patients were recruited to an 8-week intervention program of isometric lingual exercises using the IOPI as a biofeedback device. As in healthy elders, patients with stroke in this study increased maximum isometric pressures and increased swallowing pressures for some trials and some bolus conditions. Using VFSS as an outcome measures, oral transit time was decreased and pharyngeal response duration was increased. Postswallow pharyngeal residual was decreased for all textures. However, reductions of residual specifically in the oral cavity, cricopharyngeus, and piriform sinuses were not statistically significant. The Penetration-Aspiration Scale (Rosenbek et al., 1996) documented decreased aspiration. These physiologic changes were associated with reports of improved quality of life measured with the SWAL-QOL (McHorney et al., 2002) and increased tolerance of diet textures.

A single exercise of tongue to palate contact has been investigated in a series of studies; however, clinicians regularly employ a variety of other techniques for which no data are currently available. Although one research group has paved the way, significant research is left to be done to document the efficacy of oral lingual exercises on functional swallowing ability in stroke. As with all of the exercises to be discussed in subsequent sections, we require larger sample sizes, and treatment controls to document effects. Additionally, the influence of natural recovery needs to be extricated from experimental data. We have no evidence to suggest that the provision of oral lingual exercise can be contraindicated to functional swallowing and may be indeed be helpful. Thus, until further data emerge, this approach to rehabilitation may be included in a therapeutic regime.

EFFORTFUL SWALLOW

The effortful swallow was first introduced by Kahrilas et al. (Kahrilas, Lin, Logemann, Ergun, & Facchini, 1993; Kahrilas, Logemann, Krugler, & Flanagan, 1991; Kahrilas et al., 1992) as a compensatory technique. Very simply, the individual is instructed to swallow "with effort." Early work by these researchers suggested that increased effort in swallowing would result in immediate increased pressure on the bolus and thus decreased pharyngeal residual. Thus, this technique was routinely applied as a compensation for patients with pharyngeal motility disorders. Fortunately, we have acquired a fairly large body of evidence to guide our clinical practice and increase our specificity in using this technique.

The first of three research projects by Bulow and colleagues (1999), however, suggested a potential complication with this technique. They documented that effortful swallow resulted in decreased hyomandibular distance *before* the swallow, presumably as a type of preparatory set for increased effort. However, *during* the swallowing, this technique resulted in reduced laryngeal excursion and decreased overall anterior hyoid movement for airway protection and upper esophageal sphincter (UES) opening. This potential contraindication biomechanically makes sense and thus raises significant concerns. A relatively small group of floor of mouth muscles (anterior belly of digastric, mylohyoid, geniohyoid) pull the hyoid forward during swallowing; whereas the larger and longer posterior suprahyoids (posterior belly of digastric, stylohyoid) and the bulk of the middle pharyngeal constrictor pull the hyoid posteriorly. Execution of an effortful swallow does not allow increased effort within isolated muscles; rather, all muscles are presumably recruited with increased effort. Thus, the results of Bulow et al. can certainly be explained by posterior suprahyoid muscles overriding the small anterior suprahyoid muscles with a subsequent cumulative decrease in anterior hyoid movement.

Bulow et al. (2001) sought to expand their investigation of effortful swallow in patients with moderate to severe pharyngeal phase dysphagia. Based on this research, effortful swallow resulted in no change in the number of misdirected swallows, although depth of penetrated material into the larynx was reduced. In addition, despite the presumed effect of effortful swallow, they curiously documented no change in pharyngeal retention on VFSS. In an extension of this work, Bulow and colleagues (2002) evaluated intrabolus pressure in the distal pharynx and identified no significant increase in peak amplitude or duration of intrabolus pressure. No comment was made on hyoid movement in these two subsequent studies.

Certainly, if these studies withstand the scrutiny of replication, the findings may substantially change the way we apply rehabilitation techniques. For example, in the case of vallecular residual, if the symptom is caused by decreased base of tongue to posterior pharyngeal wall approximation, effortful swallow may be the treatment of choice. However, if the symptom is caused by decreased epiglottic deflection secondary to poor anterior hyoid movement, effortful swallow could potentially exacerbate the underlying physiologic abnormality and worsen the presentation of symptoms. Additionally, if a patient presents with impaired cricopharyngeal opening secondary to poor anterior hyoid movement, effortful swallow to increase pharyngeal motility through the distal pharynx may not only hinder hyoid movement but also may not be effective for its proposed intent.

Hind, Nicosia, Roecker, Carnes, and Robbins (2001) contributed different findings to the discussion on effortful swallow using VFSS and oral pressure measurement with the IOPI in healthy adults. This group documented increased oral pressure with effortful swallow and a trend toward decreased oral residual; however, they did not evaluate pharyngeal pressure. They also documented increased *duration* of maximal anterior hyoid excursion, laryngeal vestibule closure, and UES opening. Increased superior, but not anterior, hyoid movement was detected with this technique.

A further contribution was offered by Huckabee, Butler, Barclay, and Jit (2005) who evaluated submental surface electromyography (sEMG), and pressure at the proximal and distal pharynx and within the UES in 22 healthy participants. This study documented increased sEMG amplitude in submental muscles and, contrary to the findings of Bulow and colleagues (1999, 2001, 2002), increased pharyngeal manometric pressures with effortful swallows when compared to noneffortful swallows. Of particular relevance to the Bulow studies, this finding was more substantial in the lower pharynx as compared to the upper pharynx, suggesting that contributions of the pharyngeal constrictors are more responsible for pressure generation under effortful conditions than increased base of tongue retraction. Also of interest was the finding that although sEMG and pharyngeal pressure amplitude increased, there was no correlation between these two measures. Although recognizing that these two measures evaluate different mechanisms, the authors speculated that instructions for completing effortful swallow may influence the degree of pharyngeal pressure generation. Bulow and colleagues (1999), who identified no increase in pharyngeal pressure, instructed participants to "swallow very hard while squeezing the tongue in an upward-backward motion toward the soft palate" (p. 69). These instructions are similar to the instructions provided by Hind et al. (2001) who documented increased oral pressure. Other studies that have documented contradictory increased pharyngeal pressure have used instructions simply to "swallow hard" (Huckabee et al., 2005; Kahrilas et al., 1993; Kahrilas et al., 1991; Kahrilas et al., 1992). The question was raised if perhaps targeted increased orolingual pressure occurred at the expense of pharyngeal pressure.

This speculation gave rise to another study, which sought to evaluate the contribution of lingual movement in pharyngeal pressure generation. Huckabee and Steele (2006) evaluated not only submental sEMG and pharyngeal pressure, but also evaluated oral pressure generation in 20 healthy participants who completed noneffortful swallow as well as effortful swallow under two conditions: tongue emphasis and tongue inhibition. The authors hypothesized by emphasizing superior tongue to palate approximation, tongue to pharyngeal wall retraction would be inhibited, thus explaining the controversial finding of Bulow et al. (2001, 2002). Contrary to expectations, effortful swallow produced greater measurement at all five sensors (sEMG, two oral pressure, two pharyngeal pressure) with the tongue to palate emphasis condition producing greater measured amplitude and pressure than the tongue to palate inhibition condition. Thus, these data do not contribute to an explanation of discrepancies in pharyngeal pressure data across studies, but tend to support the finding that the effortful swallow increases pharyngeal pressure generation and that emphasizing tongue to palate approximation appears to increase the motor drive for pharyngeal pressure.

Other data exist that document temporal influences of effortful swallow on pharyngeal biomechanics. The first research on this topic was a study of 10 healthy participants presented by Olsson, Kjellin, and Ekberg (1996). The primary finding is this study was that duration of pressure at the tongue base was longer than that measured low in the pharynx during execution of this technique. This led the authors to suggest that an individual who is experiencing increased vallecular residue may best benefit from this technique, whereas an individual with piriform sinus residue may not and vice versa. In the previously discussed study by Hind et al. (2001), effortful swallow was found to elicit increased duration of pharyngeal response, maximum anterior hyoid excursion, laryngeal vestibule closure, UES opening, and total swallowing duration. These data suggest that effortful swallow prolongs most swallowing related events, either as a mechanism to increase strength or as a concomitant process.

Hiss and Huckabee (2005) confirmed the finding of longer duration of pharyngeal pressure with effortful swallowing in healthy participants but with the additional caveat that greater prolongation of the pressure wave was observed in the proximal pharynx compared to the distal pharynx. Additionally, this study identified that onsets of pharyngeal pressures and UES relaxation were delayed relative to the onset of submental sEMG contraction during performance of the effortful swallow and offered the suggestions that effortful swallow thus should be carefully considered in patients with coexisting delayed pharyngeal swallow. Steele and Huckabee (2007) clarified this information by peak of sEMG and pharyngeal pressure rather than onset. As before, longer overall durations of oral and pharyngeal pressure events were recorded during effortful swallowing when compared to noneffortful. However, shorter (rather than prolonged) latencies were documented from *peak* submental sEMG contraction to *peak* pressures during the effortful swallow. The combination of these findings supports the interpretation that the effortful swallow involves generation of higher velocity bolus driving forces that propel the bolus into and through the pharynx with greater efficiency, and that pressure is then sustained to facilitate more complete bolus clearance.

Until clarity is found, there are reasonable data to suggest that effortful swallow increases pharyngeal pressure, particularly in the distal pharynx, and increases duration of pressure in the upper pharynx. Data suggest increased pressure may be facilitated by emphasizing tongue to palate contact during execution of the maneuver. There are also reasonable preliminary data, paired with a logical biologic plausibility, that effortful swallow runs the risk of inhibiting anterior hyoid movement. A thoughtful rehabilitation program may pair this technique, with the head lift that is designed specifically to increase anterior hyoid movement. The resulting treatment approach would presumably accomplish a goal of increasing pharyngeal pressure generation, while concomitantly addressing anterior hyoid movement either prophylactically or as a therapeutic target. Finally, although effortful swallow may increase efficiency of bolus transport through the pharynx, a documented increased latency of onset may have implications for using the technique in patients with delayed pharyngeal swallow.

MENDELSOHN MANEUVER

As with the effortful swallow, the Mendelsohn maneuver was initially presented as a compensatory mechanism to facilitate bolus transfer through the UES. Execution of the technique requires an individual to initiate a pharyngeal swallow, and at the peak of hyolaryngeal excursion, maintain suprahyoid contraction before relaxing and completing the swallow. Prolonging suprahyoid contraction presumably prolongs UES opening to facilitate improved bolus flow. In more recent years, this technique has been applied as a rehabilitative maneuver, with the assumption that repetitive exercise results in overall improved cricopharyngeal compliance and more efficient bolus transport. No specific data are available to this effect, although some case series reports are summarized in a subsequent section on biofeedback modalities in which the Mendelsohn maneuver was a focus of treatment.

The first published report of this technique was proffered by Logemann and Kahrilas (1990). This case report documented the biomechanical effects of a series of swallowing maneuvers in a single patient with dysphagia subsequent to lateral medullary infarct. Based on this report, execution of a Mendelsohn maneuver improved swallowing efficiency greater than two-fold over other techniques. The following year, Kahrilas and colleagues (1991) published a manofluorographic investigation of this technique. In a sample of 10 healthy participants, they documented increased duration of anterior and superior excursion of the larynx and hyoid, thereby delaying closure of the UES. This would suggest an increase in duration of hyolaryngeal displacement, but not an increase in degree of anterior displacement of the hyolaryngeal complex. This is an important distinction. Miller and Watkin (1997) confirmed the finding of prolonged contraction using a real-time ultrasound study of lateral pharyngeal wall movement during execution of the Mendelsohn maneuver. This group documented increased duration of lateral pharyngeal wall movement compared to normal swallowing for this technique. In a more recent study by Boden, Hallgren, and Witt Hedstrom (2006), 10 healthy volunteers with no history of swallowing complaints were evaluated with manofluorography during execution of the Mendelsohn maneuver. With this maneuver, pharyngeal peak contraction and contraction duration were increased, suggesting not only prolonged contraction but also increased contraction of the pharyngeal muscles involved in swallowing.

All of the research on this technique, with the exception of the initial case report offered by Logemann and Kahrilas (1990) evaluates the influence of the Mendelsohn maneuver on the swallowing of healthy controls. Further research is needed to document the biomechanical effect in patients with neurologic disorders. Taken in light of the work on effortful swallow by Bulow et al. (1999, 2001, 2002), attention to hyoid movement during execution of this technique will be important. There are no data that implicate reduced degree of hyoid movement; however, this technique is known to produce increased strength of pharyngeal contraction. Until clear data identify that hyoid movement is not susceptible to inhibition from this technique, the prudent clinician will want to evaluate patients carefully before prescribing this technique. As with effortful swallow, rehabilitative specificity may emerge from these data.

A patient with prominent pyriform sinus residual, secondary to impaired hyoid movement would be better served with a technique focused on increasing anterior hyoid movement, such as head lift. However, a patient with adequate anterior hyoid movement but poor UES compliance as the source of residual may benefit more from the Mendelsohn maneuver.

Mastering the Mendelsohn maneuver will challenge both the patient and the clinician. The technique is not easy to accomplish. However, with persistence by both and implementation of biofeedback modalities to increase understanding, the technique offers substantial potential for improving swallowing biomechanics.

MASAKO MANEUVER (TONGUE-HOLD MANEUVER)

Our development of rehabilitation strategies is becoming increasingly intelligent in more recent years as our attention shifts to restoring swallowing function rather than compensating for impairment. To support our more global strengthening techniques of effortful swallow and Mendelsohn maneuver, clinical researchers have begun a more systematic analysis of impaired biomechanics with techniques designed specifically to address those impairments. The Masako maneuver, or tongue-hold maneuver, is the first of these techniques. The identification of this technique was based on work by Fujiu, Logemann, and Pauloski (1995), who documented that patients who have undergone base of tongue resection for cancer have consistently greater anterior movement of the posterior pharyngeal wall as a biomechanical compensation. Based on this finding, Fujiu and colleagues suggested a technique which mimics this disorder, thereby forcing the posterior pharyngeal wall to increase activation during swallowing. Individuals are instructed to "protrude the tongue maximally but comfortably, holding it between the central incisors" (p. 24).

In a clinical trial, Fujiu and Logemann (1996) documented that in 10 healthy participants, the technique resulted in significantly increased anterior bulging of the posterior pharyngeal wall but with no significant change in temporal features of swallowing biomechanics. The authors were careful to advise that use of the technique concomitantly inhibits base of tongue posterior retraction, thereby resulting in increased pharyngeal residual. Thus, the technique should be considered a targeted exercise for increasing posterior pharyngeal wall movement, rather than a compensatory technique.

Lazarus et al. (2002) evaluated the application of this technique in a small population of three patients with base of tongue resection. In this manofluorographic study, increased base of tongue to posterior pharyngeal wall contact pressures were recorded during maneuver conditions compared with those during nonmaneuver swallows. This increased hypopharyngeal pressure is remarkable given that base of tongue structures are resected and suggests substantially increased anterior movement of the posterior pharyngeal wall to approximate residual structures. Doltgen, Witte, Gumbley, and Huckabee. (Doeltgen, Witte, Gumbley, & Huckabee, 2007, submitted for publication) sought to further clarify pressure generation using this technique. Contrary to the findings seen in the patient population, an evaluation of 40 healthy individuals revealed that the tongue-hold maneuver produced no change in pressure generation at the level of the upper and mid-pharynx, while producing significantly lower pressure in the UES. When compared to healthy individuals, patients with base of tongue resection present changes in both structure and consequent function. It will be of substantial interest to the application of this technique in stroke patients with dysphagia to elucidate if increased pressure during execution of the technique is a consequence of anatomic change or functional change. To date, this research is not available.

In summary, the Masako maneuver is presented as a focused technique designed to increase contribution of the posterior pharyngeal wall during swallowing. Further research is needed to elucidate the effect of the technique on individuals with impaired swallowing but intact anatomy, as seen following stroke. The identification of techniques that are specific to a given pathophysiology allows for potentially improved patient outcomes; however, care should be taken that in isolating increased function in one aspect of swallowing, we do not inadvertently compromise other aspects in the delicate balance required for swallowing. Given that this technique is specifically designed to increase contribution of the pharyngeal constrictors, and the middle pharyngeal constrictors have attachments to the cornu of the hyoid, attention to hyoid movement will be important.

HEAD-LIFT EXERCISE

Another example of increased specificity in rehabilitative approaches is seen in the head-lift exercise. First identified by Shaker et al. (1997) this exercise consists of lying supine and completing a series of 'head lifts' three times per day for 6 weeks. Individuals are instructed to raise the head "high enough to observe the toes" and sustain this movement for 1 minute in the supine position. This is repeated three times. This is then followed by 30 repetitions of briefly raising and lowering the head.

Importantly, this exercise is not a swallowing-related task, thus other muscle groups are not the target of strengthening. The exercise is designed specifically for increasing UES opening through increased strength of the anterior suprahyoid muscle group. Two published EMG studies have documented this effect. An initial study by Jurell, Shaker, Mazur, Haig, and Wertsch (1996) documented EMG evidence of fatigue in the submental muscle group suggesting increased work with this exercise. This was followed by research by

Alfonso, Ferdjallah, Shaker, and Wertsch (1998) who documented increased EMG amplitude in the supra- and infrahyoid muscle groups with this technique.

The initial clinical study by Shaker and colleagues (1997) provided documentation of the effect of the technique in 31 healthy elderly participants. Two treatment groups were enrolled: one group completed a sham exercise, and the other completed the head-lift exercise for 6 weeks. Manofluorographic analysis revealed no change in any dimension of swallowing after the sham exercise; however, those completing the head-lift exercise demonstrated increased laryngeal excursion, increased width and duration of UES opening, and decreased intrabolus pressure within the UES. A crossover design then documented similar findings in those originally assigned to the alternate treatment group.

A subsequent study was completed to evaluate the effects of the exercise in individuals with chronic dysphagia, all of whom were tube fed. Shaker et al. (2002) published a clinical report of 27 patients with specific impairment of UES opening using the same research design. After 6 weeks of head-lift exercise, significant improvement was noted in UES opening, anterior laryngeal excursion, and postswallow aspiration. All participants were able to resume oral feeding. Finally, Easterling, Grande, Kern, Sears, and Shaker (2005) published a study which was designed to evaluate treatment compliance for a rehabilitation program incorporating the head-lift exercise. A group of 26 nondysphagic older adults were asked to perform the exercise and complete a questionnaire related to their performance. Four participants underwent pre- and post-treatment VFSS. The authors acknowledge that compliance is an issue; only slightly over half of those enrolled were able to complete the program. However, those who stayed in the program attained the treatment goals of increasing anterior hyoid and laryngeal excursion and UES opening.

To summarize, emergence of the head-lift exercise has offered significantly greater options for addressing swallowing pathophysiology than is commonly observed in dysphagia subsequent to stroke: that of decreased anterior hyoid movement. As this exercise is not done within the context of functional swallowing, concerns are not presented for adverse compensatory biomechanics. Additionally, this exercise does not require substantial cognitive power or motor control to complete, as is the case with the Mendelsohn maneuver. In many cases of dysphagia secondary to stroke, this technique may ultimately be the first-line rehabilitation approach given the importance of adequate hyoid movement on the cascade of pharyngeal biomechanics that follows.

19 Maximizing Rehabilitation Effectiveness

Much of our research which evaluates the effectiveness of rehabilitation strategies has initially, and sometimes exclusively, been conducted in healthy control participants. As a first step, this is critical, such that we can understand adaptability of biomechanics under optimal conditions before we seek to understand the influence of impairment of biomechanical flexibility. Clearly, in rehabilitation of the stroke patient, optimal conditions are rarely encountered. Stroke patients are frequently unwell, easily fatigued, cognitively compromised, and present with lesions that disrupt motor planning and neural transmission. This chapter addresses two issues that may influence rehabilitation effectiveness: biofeedback and treatment dose.

BIOFEEDBACK MODALITIES IN DYSPHAGIA REHABILITATION

Outcomes of swallowing rehabilitation may be limited by several factors:

■ We are dealing with a largely abstract concept.
Rehabilitation of impaired swallowing frequently requires neuromuscular adaptation of a pseudoreflexive process that most individuals typically perform without conscious thought or manipulation. In the event of dysphagia subsequent to stroke, clinicians ask individuals not only to

engage an impaired system but to modulate that system in a manner that is quite unlike anything they have ever done. Although execution of an effortful swallow may appear relatively simple, other techniques such as the Masako and Mendelsohn maneuvers will challenge even the patient with minor impairment and can sometimes present an overwhelming obstacle for those with cognitive impairment.

■ There are limited reliable means to assess if exercises are done correctly. Asking a patient to swallow with effort or sustain hyolaryngeal excursion may produce visible effort on the part of the patient, but it is unclear exactly where that effort lies. Swallowing produces very few externally observable cues on performance. Thus, it challenges the clinician to provide feedback to the patient for adaptation of behavior if the clinician has little insight into how that behavior is executed.

■ There is little objective measurement of change; thus, meaningful goal delineation is difficult at best. Research has unquestionably documented poor validity in the clinical assessment for evaluating swallowing biomechanics. This impacts our initial diagnostic formulation but also heavily influences our rehabilitation approaches. If we cannot see within the pharynx, how do we know pharyngeal improvement is occurring? Even if the patient presents with a known strong reflexive cough and therefore we can rely on decreased coughing as a measure of recovery, this represents a fairly large increment of change. How do we maintain motivation for treatment when external evidence of treatment is obscure? How do we document small increments of change?

■ Finally, as a consequence of the hurdles we face in rehabilitation, it is likely that treatment is discontinued prematurely due to frustration with the therapeutic process.

The swallowing clinician needs to be creative, inventive, and possess a bit of dogged determination to make identified rehabilitation techniques accessible to the neurologically impaired population. Mere instruction will rarely be sufficient. The emergence of surface electromyography (sEMG) as a biofeedback modality offers a valuable tool for facilitating this process. Biofeedback has been defined as:

> The technique of using equipment (usually electronic) to reveal to human beings some of their internal physiological events, normal and abnormal, in the form of visual and auditory signals in order to teach them to *manipulate these otherwise involuntary or unfelt events by manipulating the displayed signals*. (Basmajian & DeLuca, 1985, p. 132)

This final italicized point is an important one. In the event of cognitive impairment that hinders manipulation of swallow physiology, manipulation of a waveform may present a much easier, more accessible task. Kasman (1996, p. 4) extends on this definition by commenting that biofeedback modalities represent "instantaneous performance-contingent feedback . . . and provide an extension of the patients or clinicians senses." Because clinical measurement in swallowing presents such a challenge, our estimations of treatment response in the short term rely heavily on our "clinical sense." Although sEMG biofeedback cannot be considered diagnostic in nature, the additional quantitative information offered through observation of the waveform may be supportive enough to encourage patient and clinician alike to persevere with treatment when progress has not yet begun to manifest clinically.

Types of Biofeedback Modalities

Although the focus of this chapter is on sEMG biofeedback, biofeedback modalities for dysphagia rehabilitation may take many forms. Logemann and Kahrilas (1990) published a case report of a patient for whom the videofluoroscopic swallow study (VFSS) was used as a biofeedback modality to impress on a patient the concept of pharyngeal residual and clearance. Although clearly fluoroscopy has its limitations as biofeedback—the invasiveness and expense of the technique render it highly impractical—these authors provide a good lesson. Do not miss an opportunity when it presents itself to enhance insight into pathophysiology and recovery. Allowing the patient observation of the monitor during VFSS may add very little time and exposure to the study, but the on-line feedback of pharyngeal swallowing may provide a valuable baseline for extending patients' perception of swallowing behavior.

Other modalities have been reported. Denk and Kaider (1997) employed endoscopy as an ongoing biofeedback modality in a group of head and neck cancer patients. Those who received biofeedback recovered more rapidly than those in a control group without feedback. Additionally, in the earlier rehabilitation section discussing oral lingual exercises, the use of the Iowa Oral Performance Instrument was described as a biofeedback modality (Nicosia et al., 2000; Robbins et al., 2005; Robbins et al., 1995). Essentially, any tool that allows for a visual or auditory representation of some aspect of swallowing that can be immediately fed back to the patient to provide information about performance can be used as a biofeedback modality. Using this definition, ultrasound, oxygen saturation, endoscopy, manometry, and other clinical or diagnostic tools can be employed.

sEMG biofeedback is likely the most well recognized and documented feedback type for swallowing rehabilitation. This requires surface measurement of electrical activity in underlying musculature which is displayed as a time by amplitude waveform, which provides a visual representation of relative strength and timing of muscle contraction. Through on-line monitoring of muscle activity, this modality supplies an alternative feedback system of proprioception, thus attenuating the patient's or clinician's awareness of one aspect of swallowing behavior. By yielding a visible representation of even the smallest motor response, rehabilitative efforts are maximized, allowing the patient and clinician a means of confronting automatic physiologic behaviors and enhancing access to volitional motor control. Incorporated into swallowing treatment, the technique appears to be most useful for monitoring execution of rehabilitative techniques related to pharyngeal phase dysphagia; however, it may also be used to monitor activity associated with orolingual movement.

Nuts and Bolts

Electromyography is a method of measuring myoelectric impulses within a muscle during contraction. Clinical biofeedback applications require placement of surface electrodes on the skin surface overlying the target muscle or muscle group. Most commercially available sEMG biofeedback devices rectify and average the raw EMG data to produce a more responsive, comprehensible signal for patient use. Dual or multichannel devices will allow for measurement of multiple muscle sites. This may be helpful for observation and potential retraining of agonist/antagonist muscle groups or for use by the clinician to model targeted motor behavior. A detailed summary of measurement parameters that are commonly available on commercially available biofeedback devices has been published by Rubow (1984).

Surface electrode placement is a highly inferential process. As muscles within the head and neck are small and frequently overlapping, one can only assume the targeted muscle to be measured with surface electrodes. Despite this lack of specificity, the clinical feedback offered by this modality is the target rather than diagnostic information. Electrode placement for sEMG biofeedback is dependent on the clinical goals of treatment. A patient with specific impairment of supraglottic closure may be best served by placement of the electrodes on the lateral neck, overlying the upper strap muscles. Contraction of these muscles during swallowing contributes to supraglottic shortening. Patients with reduced anterior hyoid movement would benefit from electrode placement underneath the chin to measure the collective anterior suprahyoid muscle group. This placement also may be of value in addressing oral motor exercises as the electrodes will also detect intrinsic lingual muscle activity. Using this placement, the clinician will need to be aware of the depth of recording so as not to interpret increased lingual movement to represent increased floor of mouth contraction. Huckabee et al. (2005) and Huckabee and Steele (2006) have documented the influence of intrinsic lingual activity on submental measurement. If the goal of treatment is to increase anterior suprahyoid contraction, and exaggerated lingual to palatal approximation is used to increase sEMG amplitude, the target of treatment may be obscured by activity in the intrinsic lingual muscles (Huckabee et al., 2005). In this case the patient may need instruction not to engage lingual to palatal contact in an effort to increase measured sEMG amplitude. However, if the target of treatment is increased pharyngeal pressure during effortful type swallowing maneuvers, exaggerated tongue to palate contact that is evident in increased sEMG amplitude is known to correlate with increased pharyngeal pressure (Huckabee & Steele, 2006) and thus would be encouraged. The density of tissue in and around the neck region and the layered mantle of overlying muscle renders EMG measurement from the pharyngeal constrictor muscles impractical. Thus, direct feedback about the strength and timing of pharyngeal contraction is not available. However, as swallowing is a synergistic response with coordinated contraction of multiple muscle groups, the clinician may be able to infer information about the function of the pharynx from measurement at more external muscles.

Treatment Approach

It is important to realize that the incorporation of sEMG biofeedback into dysphagia rehabilitation programs is not a treatment unto itself. Biofeedback does not alter swallowing biomechanics. Swallowing maneuvers alter swallowing biomechanics; sEMG biofeedback offers a window into behavioral performance of these maneuvers. Thus, a treatment paradigm incorporating biofeedback as an adjunct will be quite similar to a treatment paradigm without, and would therefore incorporate periods of exercise, interspersed with periods of rest, and practice of compensatory mechanisms during oral intake. However, as sEMG monitors muscle activity, additional clinical (not diagnostic) information may be gleaned from analyzing the waveform that is quite difficult to acquire otherwise and therefore may shape the rehabilitative approach.

Within other areas of physical rehabilitation, neuromuscular deficits are often approached for treatment based on the underlying impairment. In the patient with spasticity, muscle relaxation and inhibition of tone may be the first approach, followed by gentle muscle strengthening. In the patient with apraxia, motor planning and performance are emphasized by breaking down tasks to address the pattern of the muscle response and improve the coordination of agonist/antagonist muscle groups. In the case of flaccidity, the approach is generally one of muscle strengthening. Our approach to rehabilitation of the dysphagic patient is yet quite unsophisticated. If you evaluate our rehabilitation techniques, they focus heavily on muscle strengthening, which may not always be the most appropriate paradigm. The use of biofeedback may provide some insights into the nature of the underlying motor task. This information can then be incorporated into the treatment paradigm. To facilitate this, treatment can be broken into four phases.

The initial phase of any treatment should include a clear focus on education and investment in the treatment plan. Certainly as with any treatment, the sharing of diagnostic information is critical, and in the patient with cognitive impairment from stroke, this may be facilitated by showing the patient his VFSS and comparing that with normal biomechanics. Although specific details can be deferred, the visualization of pathophysiology compared to normal can be quite striking and more easily comprehended than a verbal explanation, particularly for those with impaired comprehension. If introducing sEMG biofeedback, a full explanation of motor potentials and myo-electric activity also will likely exceed the interest or cognition of most patients. A very simple description will suffice: the device will be used to facilitate treatment by measuring the electrical activity of muscles used in swallowing and displaying that information on a computer screen so the patient can better learn swallowing maneuvers. It may be helpful to place electrodes first on the fore-arm, and then ask the patient to clinch his or her fist and observe the change in the feedback tracing. This method allows the patient to learn the technique of biofeedback using muscles that are less obscure and more easily observed. After the electrodes are placed to measure activity from the head and neck, the patient should be asked to simply open and close the mouth. A small movement will produce relatively small amplitude in the feedback tracing; a larger movement will result in greater deflection of the waveform. As jaw opening is easily observed and voluntarily controlled, this initial teaching step will further ensure that the basic application of biofeedback is reinforced before shifting the focus to swallowing. Relating degrees of movement to the relative effects on the feedback tracing will set a firm foundation for further treatment. Finally, the patient is asked to swallow and observe the effect of the swallow on the sEMG tracing. The clinician will want to encourage the patient to actively interpret the sEMG tracing and associate that with what he or she feels proprioceptively. For this purpose, the availability of a "freeze frame" option is essential. It is important, after each screen sweep, to hold that image and asked the patient to describe his motor events as related to the biofeedback tracing.

Once the patient has mastered the concept behind biofeedback-facilitated treatment and the electrodes are secured, valuable infor-mation may be gleaned from asking the patient to sit quietly and without volitional movement. Although there are not yet published data, clinical practice reveals that some patients will have consider-able difficulty with muscle relaxation. This raises a pertinent clinical question: Is there a potential subgroup of individuals with dysphagia who demonstrate features of spasticity? Our colleagues in physical medicine have long recognized that a spastic muscle is not likely to effectively perform a functional motor activity. The target of rehabilitation initially may be to inhibit the spastic response, thus freeing the muscle group to function under volitional control. sEMG is not a diagnostic tool and cannot be used to confirm spasticity as a clinical feature of dysphagia; however, it may serve as a clinical screening tool to aid the clinician in making appropriate referrals.

If the clinician determines through subsequent testing that increased muscle tone is indeed contributing to functionally impaired biomechanics, then this pathology can be addressed directly. A patient would be instructed first to sit quietly and observe the feedback tracing. Using this feedback to monitor the degree of tone in the resting muscle, the patient progressively works toward lowering the waveform amplitude and thus relaxing the targeted muscle. Once this task is achieved, differential contraction and relaxation of the targeted muscle group is practiced to carry over the relaxed state within the landscape of functional muscle contraction. Ultimately, intermittent volitional swallows are practiced with the patient instructed to demonstrate a relaxed state before and after swallowing execution.

Variation in patterns of muscular contraction, as visualized with sEMG waveforms, is common in normal swallowing. These variations are not, however, of great enough magnitude to impact the efficiency of deglutition. However, in some patient populations, particularly in patients with lateral medullary stroke, the organization, initiation, and execution of swallowing may be impaired and visible on the waveform. In this case, rehabilitative efforts may focus on reinforcement and mastery of a more efficient swallowing pattern. As referred to briefly in Chapter 20, interest in strength versus skill training is emerging (Chhadra & Sapienza, in press). In these patients, skill training may be more appropriate. Using the sEMG waveform as a direct visualization of muscle contraction, the patient is instructed to initiate swallowing with minimal anticipatory or struggling behavior. Their target is a clean peak of high amplitude and short duration. Repeated trials are used to shape motor behavior to achieve the target goal.

The Mendelsohn maneuver likely represents characteristics of both strength and skill training. As most clinicians will attest, this technique can be very difficult for patients to master; even in those patients without concomitant cognitive or language impairments. Use of sEMG biofeedback greatly enhances a patient's ability to complete this technique and thus reap the benefits. A patient is instructed to swallow and when the waveform elevates from baseline they are to hold that position for several seconds before allowing the waveform to return to baseline.

Finally, muscle strengthening is approached using traditional exercises of effortful swallow, and the more recent Masako maneuver. These appear to be highly effective if they are executed correctly and in the appropriate patient populations. As discussed in Chapter 18, the effortful swallowing involves simple swallowing "with effort." The Masako maneuver adapts this to maximize pharyngeal wall movement but executing the swallow with the tongue slightly protruded. Subjective estimates of strength or relative degree of laryngeal excursion during execution of these maneuvers are difficult to assess by observation or palpation. Using sEMG amplitude as a proxy measure of strength, the patient and clinician can gain valuable insight into motor performance.

Research Support for the Use of sEMG Biofeedback

Clinical sEMG biofeedback has been extensively evaluated in other realms of physical medicine and rehabilitation with numerous studies demonstrating clinical efficacy for a variety of neuromuscular disorders. Many of these studies have evaluated the use of sEMG in patients with intact cognition. However, a key study by Balliet, Levy, and Blood (1986) describes the use of sEMG as an adjunct to upper extremity retraining in cognitively impaired patients. In this study, five patients with chronic upper extremity paresis, all of whom had aphasia and notably impaired comprehension, regained functional upper extremity function after 50 sessions using EMG biofeedback of the weakened limb. This study documents the benefits of this technology in assisting patients who may otherwise not be treatment candidates based on the severity of cognitive/communication deficits. Indeed, dysphagic patients with unimpaired cognition may benefit from dysphagia rehabilitation without biofeedback; it is the patients with cognitive decline that will require the addition information from the external feedback. Although not an assessment of the application of biofeedback to dysphagia rehabilitation, the study carries significant implications as many dysphagic patients present with concomitant cognitive and/or communication deficits. These data, paired with research on motor learning theory, provide a foundation for its application in the realm of physical rehabilitation (Rubow, 1984; Wolf, 1994).

The discipline of speech-language pathology has yet to extensively evaluate this modality. The application of sEMG biofeedback in dysarthria rehabilitation, despite the neuromuscular nature of this type of disorder, has been grossly underevaluated. A string of case studies documents consistently both the short-term and long-term benefits of this treatment modality in facilitating primarily facial muscle control in patients with both acute and chronic deficits. As documented in some, but not all, of the studies, this increased control subsequently resulted in improved appearance and speech production skills through greater volitional use of primarily the labial articulators (Brown, Nahai, & Basmajian, 1991; Brudny, Hammerschlag, Cohen, & Ransohoff, 1988; Daniel-Whitney, 1989; Draizar, 1984; Jankel, 1978; Netsell & Cleeland, 1973). However, there are no experimentally controlled studies which compare this modality to more traditional treatment.

A similar string of case studies has begun to emerge regarding the use of sEMG biofeedback in swallowing treatment. The first such paper was presented by Draizar (1984) who outlined the use of biofeedback in the treatment of dysarthria and dysphagia; however, little detail is provided regarded specific treatment methods or evaluation of progress. A more detailed account was provided by Bryant (1991) who presented a description of the use of sEMG biofeedback in the treatment of a patient with oral pharyngeal carcinoma. This patient, a 40-year-old female with severe dysphagia secondary to resection and radiation was able to discontinue tube feedings and return to a near normal diet after 10 weeks of treatment. Relevant to stroke, Crary (1995) described the treatment course of 6 patients with chronic dysphagia secondary to brainstem infarct treated with sEMG biofeedback. Of these 6 patients, with a mean time since onset of 18.8 months (range: 5–54 months), all were able to return to oral feedings with discontinuation of tube feedings. Huckabee and Cannito (1999) extended this work by offering a report of 10 additional patients with dysphagia secondary to brainstem injury who participated in a 1-week accelerated swallowing treatment program with sEMG monitoring. Of these 10 patients, with a mean time postonset of 26 months, 8 returned to full oral feeding with removal of feeding tube on average of 5.3 months after treatment initiation. All maintained oral feeding with the exception of 2, both of whom suffered further neurologic injury unrelated to their swallowing disorder. Crary, Carnaby Mann, Groher, and Helseth (2004) completed an additional retrospective analysis of 45 patients, 25 of whom were dysphagic subsequent to stroke using a therapy approach with sEMG biofeedback. Of the stroke patients in this study, 92% demonstrated gains in functional oral intake with a return to full oral diet in 65% after an average of 12.32 sessions (range: 4–28 sessions).

These studies document positive outcomes in patients who are not within the acute phase of recovery. These are promising findings. What must be remembered, however, is that these outcome data suggest improvement subsequent to swallowing rehabilitation exercises. Although sEMG was used as an adjunct, no control groups were utilized to differentiate the effect of biofeedback over and above traditional treatment approaches.

DOSE

In the discussion of biofeedback modalities, several case series were presented as low-level evidence of the efficacy of swallowing rehabilitation (Crary, 1995; Huckabee & Cannito, 1999). Both of these programs were based on intensive provision of traditional neuromuscular exercises using biofeedback as a treatment adjunct. However, it is impossible to determine from these studies if the positive outcomes were due to the intensity of treatment or the use of exteroceptive feedback. Other studies which have demonstrated positive effects of neuromuscular treatments for dysphagia have also tended toward an intensive treatment approach.

In routine clinical practice, however, intensive rehabilitation practices do not appear to be the norm. An informal survey of 16 clinicians from 10 regional hospitals and rehabilitation centers in two countries was conducted by Maggie-Lee Huckabee. Clinicians were asked "On average, how often do you see your patients for dysphagia intervention?" These findings are summarized in Table 19–1. When consequently asked "How did you determine this schedule?" the

Table 19–1. An Informal Survey of Frequency of Dysphagia Intervention

Health Care Setting	Average Number Visits per Week and Duration of Sessions (range)
Acute hospital	Highly variable; as needed for diagnosis and compensation
Postacute rehabilitation	3.8 @ 32 min (3 @ 20 min to 5 @ 45 min)
Outpatient clinic	1.3 @ 43 min (1 @ 30 min to 2 @ 55 min)
Community therapy	0.06 @ 38 min (1 q 6 months @ 30 min to 1 @ 20 min)

overwhelming response from clinicians was that the treatment schedule was initially determined by administrative issues and resource availability and secondarily on what was thought to be best for the patient. No clinician in this limited sampling referred to the literature as a basis for their treatment frequency decisions.

Historically, in clinical training, the issue of treatment intensity is given little attention. A cursory review of several texts on the provision of clinical service in speech-language pathology reveals no mention of dose issues or treatment intensity. However, the issue of "dose" of service delivery in dysphagia management is critical. If a patient is deemed a treatment failure, perhaps this is actually a service delivery failure. Did the treatment not work, or was it not executed frequently enough to manifest clinical change? It is well understood that resource allocation may hinder the provision of intensive treatment. However, short bursts of intensive treatment may indeed produce more favorable outcomes and, therefore, decreased costs, as compared to protracted treatment offered at a much lower intensity. It becomes an issue of prioritization and scheduling. This issue translates to research activity as well. There is pressure to document efficacy of dysphagia management practices using randomized controlled trial studies. However, the evaluation of treatment efficacy is inherently encumbered by the evaluation of treatment intensity. One cannot assess efficacy without attending to dose. Although we have a string of studies, outlined below, that document positive effects of treatment, these studies were conducted at a set dose level; generally all were completed at a fairly intensive level of treatment. Adequate studies have yet to be published to compare intensities and determine if positive effects can be gained from a less intensive approach.

A Look to the Literature

Our colleagues in other areas of physical medicine and rehabilitation also have work to do in investigating dose effects. Remarkably few studies could be identified in a search of the literature. Sterr et al. (2002) evaluated two treatment intensities of constraint-induced movement therapy (CIMT). Fifteen adults with chronic hemiparesis secondary to stroke who were receiving CIMT therapy for 90% of waking hours were randomized to receive CIMT therapy with 6 hours of direct training or 3 hours of direct training per day for 14 days. Both groups demonstrated improved motor function, but the 6-hour training schedule was significantly more effective for improving motor function in this study population.

Coming closer to home, Denes, Perazzolog, and Piccione (1996) evaluated the influence of dose of treatment on language outcomes in 17 patients with global aphasia (>3 months postonset) randomized to intensive or traditional treatment. Intensive treatment was defined as 5 hours of treatment per week for 6 weeks; traditional treatment was defined as 2.5 hours per week for 6 months. Both treatment groups demonstrated improvement; however, the intensive group demonstrated significantly greater gains in a shorter period of time. However, the intensive group received a greater total number of sessions (130) compared to the traditional treatment group (60). Thus, the positive results are clouded by the inconsistency in design. A second series of studies was published by Hinckley and Craig (1998). This group evaluated naming skills in 40 individuals with aphasia secondary to stroke using an ABA treatment design. Their intensive treatment program consisted of 6 weeks of treatment at 23 hours per week. After establishing the effectiveness of this treatment protocol for improving naming skills when compared to no treatment, they then compared this intensive treatment approach to nonintensive therapy, defined as 6 weeks of treatment of 3 hours or less weekly at home. Significant improvements in naming ability were documented after the intensive treatment regimen. Nonsignificant improvements were achieved from the low-intensity treatment period, equivalent to no-treatment period. With reinitiation of the intensive treatment regimen, repeated significant improvement in naming skills was documented.

In the dysphagia literature we are amassing a slowly increasing body of literature to document outcomes of dysphagia intervention (Bartolome & Neumann, 1993; Carnaby, Hankey, & Pizzi, 2006; Crary, 1995; Huckabee & Cannito, 1999; Klor & Milianti, 1999; Neumann, 1993; Neumann, Bartolome, Buchholz, & Prosiegel, 1995; Robbins et al., 2007; Shaker et al., 2002; Shaker et al., 1997). Only two studies have compared treatment outcomes as a function of dose. Carnaby et al. (2006) evaluated three randomized levels of management in 306 acute stroke patients: (1) usual care as prescribed by the attending physician, (2) low-intensity intervention provided 3 times a week, and (3) high-intensity intervention provided at least daily. When comparing usual care and low-intensity intervention, high intensity therapy was associated with an increased proportion of patients who returned to a normal diet and recovered swallowing function by 6 months. Rosenbek et al. (1998) sought to evaluate the influence in the outcomes of treatment using thermal-tactile stimulation (TTS) This study included 45 male stroke patients who received TTS to the faucial arches using an ice stick. Each trial consisted of stroking one and then the other faucial arch 3 or more times each, then instructing the patient to "swallow hard." Participants were randomized to 1 of 4 treatment groups based on number of trials of stimulation per week across 3 to 5 days for 2 weeks: 150, 300, 450, or 600 trials. Based on this study, no single treatment intensity emerged as superior.

The application of neuromuscular electrical stimulation (NMES) as a treatment for dysphagia is discussed in some detail in Chapter 20. Much of the research on this emerging modality does not address treatment dose as a variable in outcomes. The exception is offered by the Manchester research group, who have systematically evaluated dose effects (Fraser et al., 2002; Power et al., 2004). An important point emerges from this collective work. In the case of NMES, dose can be defined by many treatment parameters: frequency, intensity, and duration of the electrical stimulus. Manipulation of these treatment parameters all influence treatment effect. Critically, the influence can be both positive and negative.

The Take-Home Point

Clinicians and researchers alike have considerable ground to cover to untangle the complex issues surrounding service delivery in dysphagia management. Much of our early outcome data suggest that intensive treatment can have positive outcomes on the biomechanics of swallowing. Limited data from other areas of physical medicine suggest that *more is better*. But we need to be cognizant that more may also be too much. Research on NMES suggests a potential negative influence of treatment at certain stimulation parameters. For neuromuscular strengthening this could potentially also manifest as muscle fatigue. Very clearly, more systematic randomized controlled trials of specific techniques executed through a range of intensities are needed.

Until further data are accrued and the picture becomes clearer, the practicing clinician should always question their provision of services. If outcomes are not favorable, is it the treatment, the patient, or the way in which the treatment was provided?

20 Emerging Modalities in Dysphagia Management

EXPIRATORY MUSCLE STRENGTH TRAINING

Effective function of the oral pharyngeal neuromuscular system is obviously critical for safe swallowing and has thus been the target of rehabilitation efforts. However, other subsystems support the swallowing process either directly or indirectly. A steady stream of research is emerging regarding the clinical application of expiratory muscle strength training (EMST) on swallowing biomechanics. This very promising approach has not yet emerged into widespread clinical use, but with a strong foundation of supportive data, this will likely take a prominent place in the repertoire of rehabilitation strategies for the dysphagic patient.

EMST was originally described in the respiratory medicine literature (Gosselink, 2002; Smeltzer, Lavietes, & Cook, 1996) but has been adapted for speech and swallowing rehabilitation purposes through the efforts of Sapienza and colleagues (Kim & Sapienza, 2005; Sapienza & Wheeler, 2006; Silverman et al., 2006). EMST utilizes a calibrated device consisting of a mouthpiece and a one-way, spring-loaded valve. Although variation exists in the literature, in general, the exercise consists of blowing into the device through the mouthpiece with sufficient effort to release the valve; the valve remains opened as long as air pressure continues. These training breaths are repeated in blocks of 5 to 10 minutes, several times a day, every day for a period of 4 to 8 weeks. The device is calibrated and adjustable, thus resistance can be increased as appropriate to achieve therapeutic goals.

Early work by Sapienza , Davenport, and Martin (2002) focused not on swallowing but on the novel goal of increasing pressure support in high school band students. High-intensity, low-repetition expiratory training was completed daily for 2 weeks using 4 sets of 6 breaths with the device set at 75% maximum expiratory pressure (MEP). Significantly increased expiratory pressure was reported within 2 weeks of initiating training. Given the confirmation of a positive training effect in this study, further research was conducted on healthy adults to gauge the 'training and detraining' effects relative to treatment dose. Thirty-two participants, divided into two duration-of-treatment groups, underwent EMST with accumulation of outcome measures pretreatment, immediately post-treatment, and again after 8 weeks without treatment. All participants demonstrated increased MEPs over baseline measures, regardless of treatment duration. Additionally, decline in performance was not dependent on training duration.

With indication of a treatment effect in healthy participants, several research works have addressed application of this technique in patients with neurologic disorders, although none as yet in the stroke population. A preliminary report by Silverman et al. (2006) documented treatment outcomes of 28 patients with moderate to severe Parkinson's disease during the "on" state of medication. Data from this pilot study suggest that respiratory muscle weakness may be amenable to EMST with the consequent potential for improved respiration, swallowing, cough, and speech production. An additional study of a single patient with Parkinson's disease was conducted by Saleem, Sapienza, and Okun (2005). A 20-week EMST program resulted in increased MEPs of 50% by the fourth week of training, with an eventual increase of 158% over the 20-week treatment protocol. After discontinuation of treatment, total MEP decreased 16%.

Two further studies have evaluated the influence of EMST on cough and speech production in individuals with multiple sclerosis, both demonstrating positive outcomes (Chiara, Martin, Davenport, & Bolser, 2006; Chiara, Martin, & Sapienza, 2007). Of particular relevance to airway protection was the finding of increased maximal voluntary cough in patients with moderate levels of disability.

With the goal of direct application of this modality to improving swallowing biomechanics, a very recent report investigated the activation of the submental muscle group as a function of EMST (Wheeler, Chiara, & Sapienza, 2007). Given the importance of this muscle group in anterior hyoid movement and subsequent effects on pharyngeal physiology, increased activation of these muscles would suggest a specific and direct influence of this treatment on swallowing biomechanics. The timing and amplitude of submental muscle activity was evaluated using surface EMG in 20 healthy participants. Participants performed a saliva swallow and a water swallow with expiratory pressure at 25% and 75% of MEP. As hypothesized, EMST increased activity in the submental muscle complex. Although formal trials of treatment effectiveness are yet to be completed, this physiologic outcome offers great promise that the therapeutic effects of EMST go beyond the respiratory support system.

EMST is an exciting development in rehabilitative research for swallowing impairment. With an emphasis on strengthening of the respiratory subsystem underlying swallowing, one would anticipate that further research will document improved capabilities for airway protection and clearance. With positive effects on floor of mouth muscles, future research may also support this use of this approach for other biomechanical deficits in pharyngeal swallowing. Which patient populations and under which conditions these improvements are evident are yet to be identified. In the interim, clinicians are well advised to keep an eye on the literature and eagerly anticipate the eventual benefits of this treatment in the management of dysphagia.

NEUROMUSCULAR ELECTRICAL STIMULATION[1]

As our focus in dysphagia management has shifted to rehabilitation, there is an emerging trend toward the utilization of neuromuscular electrical stimulation (NMES) as a therapeutic modality for swallowing impairment. The excitement generated by this technique has travelled quickly, and as a result, NMES has entered clinical practice well ahead of research to justify its application. This is not an uncommon pattern in clinical service delivery; however, the use of NMES has potential contraindications that should be considered.

NMES is defined as "the external control of innervated, but paretic or paralytic, muscles by electrical stimulation of the corresponding intact peripheral nerves" (Baker, McNeal, Benton, Bowman, & Waters, 1993, pp. 5-6). This is achieved through the carefully regulated administration of pulsed electrical current to nerves, myoneural junctions, or muscles (Ragnarsson, 1994), which results in changes in the ionic composition of the neural or muscular cell membrane and triggers transmission of a motor unit action potential with subsequent motor response. The clinical benefit arises from skeletal muscle contraction with subsequent effects on strength, reaction time, and stamina (Alon, 1991). The resulting contraction differs from physiologic muscle activity in the ordering of muscle fiber recruitment, the synchronicity of individual motor units, and the intensity of stimuli required to produce these changes. These are important distinctions when considering the complex patterned motor event of pharyngeal swallowing.

Not surprisingly, the literature addressing the use of NMES in physical rehabilitation is contradictory, with some reports of a posi-

---

[1]Significant portions of this section have been extracted from Huckabee, M. L., and Doeltgen, S. H. (2007). Emerging Modalities in Dysphagia Rehabilitation: Neuromuscular Electrical Stimulation. *New Zealand Medical Journal, 120*(1263), 1-9.

tive influence and other reports of minimal or no effect (Glanz, Klawansky, Stason, Berkey, & Chalmers, 1996). As with any treatment approach, one size does not fit all and the available literature supports this. Specific to swallowing rehabilitation, many clinical researchers and basic scientists are investigating the safety and efficacy of this technology. The quality of subsequent publications is variable and thus requires careful scrutiny of both methods and results before implementing this modality into clinical work. Although some of these data are reviewed below, the reader is directed to an intelligent review article offered by Steele, Thrasher, and Popovic (2007).

A Chronology of the NMES Literature in Swallowing

Park, O'Neill, and Martin (1997) published perhaps the first report of NMES applications in swallowing rehabilitation. This group investigated the effect of oral electrical stimulation on the physiologic abnormality of "delayed swallowing reflex" in four stroke patients with chronic dysphagia. Stimulation was applied to the posterior soft palate through a custom-designed palatal prosthesis with stimulation parameters set with a duration of 200 µsec, repeated at 1-second intervals and intensity at the patient's individual pain tolerance. Although two of four patients were identified to demonstrate decreased penetration/aspiration, NMES did not facilitate a more timely onset of swallowing, which was the primary target of treatment. Although many methodologic details were unjustified or unexplained, this initial work suggested a positive effect of this modality on at least some biomechanical features of swallowing.

The clinical effects of NMES on 110 stroke patients with dysphagia were investigated by Freed, Freed, Chatburn, and Christian (2001), who are responsible for development of the VitalStim™ device. Time postonset was not specified. Eighty-three patients were enrolled in an electrical stimulation (ES) group whereas 36 patients received what they considered to be a "standard" treatment, that of thermal-tactile stimulation (TTS). Randomization for treatment group assignment was not applied. Daily treatment for inpatients and 3 times weekly treatment for outpatients of 60 minutes in duration was administered by the primary investigator until the participants achieved a swallowing function score of at least 5 out of 6, or progress plateaued. Outcomes were based on a nonstandardized scale rating of pre- and post-treatment videofluoroscopic swallow studies (VFSS) that was completed by the primary investigator. Specific biomechanical changes were not evaluated. Ninety-eight percent of ES patients improved in some way, compared to 69% of TTS patients. Results of this study were promising at first glance; however, the design of this study limits the validity of the results. No justification or experimental control of stimulation parameters was undertaken or reported. TTS is problematic as a comparison treatment. This technique has not withstood the rigors of empirical research. Outcome measures were based on a nonvalidated rating scale and ratings were assigned only by the primary investigator, who also provided the treatment. Furthermore, an unspecified number of patients in the NMES group received concomitant dilatation of the upper esophageal sphincter, which is an accepted treatment in its own right. Unfortunately, these methodologic flaws erode the validity of the positive results and illustrate the need to interpret the available research with caution.

Leelamanit, Limsukul, and Geater (2002) evaluated the influence of synchronized electrical stimulation on the pathophysiologic feature of "reduced laryngeal elevation" in 23 patients with time postonset ranging from 3 to 12 months. Thyrohyoid muscle stimulation was provided through surface electrodes at a frequency of 60 Hz and an amplitude of 100 V, for 3 to 30 treatments of 4 hours per day until they demonstrated improved swallow. Again, the primary investigator rated treatment outcomes, which were based on a patient's ability to swallow more than 3 ml water without aspiration, adequate oral intake with weight gain, and improved laryngeal elevation during VFSS. Twenty patients demonstrated clinical improvement, whereas 3 patients had no improvement; 6 patients relapsed on follow-up at 2 to 9 months, but regained benefits with another round of treatment. This study has strength in its specific pathophysiologic target; however, no control group was utilized in this project and, as with the prior study, outcomes measures were by the primary investigator with no control for rater bias.

Burnett, Mann, Stoklosa, and Ludlow (2005) investigated self-triggered NMES using hooked-wire electrodes in the mylo- and thyrohyoid muscles in nine healthy adults. Stimulation was synchronized with swallowing behavior and delivered at a frequency of 30 Hz and at the highest comfortable intensity level. Objective measures of muscle activity were calculated to document treatment effects, rather than a nonvalidated subjective scale. No significant change in amplitude or duration of muscle activity was identified after self-triggered, synchronized electrical stimulation.

Subsequent to the questionably positive results reported by Freed et al. (2001), five very recent investigations have attempted to more critically evaluate NMES specifically using the VitalStim™ device. Suiter, Leder, and Ruark (2006) evaluated the influence of VitalStim™ treatment protocol on submental muscle activity in healthy participants using an AB/BA treatment design. Based on these data, 7 of 8 subjects exhibited no significant gains in myoelectric activity of the submental muscle group following 10 hours of NMES treatment; two subjects withdrew from the study due to mild skin irritations after treatment. The effects of stimulation on hyolaryngeal movement in healthy individuals at rest and during swallowing were investigated by Humbert et al. (2006). Ten different surface electrode placements were investigated using maximum tolerated stimulation. The National Institutes of Health-Swallowing Safety Scale (NIH-SSS) and specific biomechanical measures of the larynx and hyoid at rest and during swallowing were made by raters blind to the swallowing conditions of stimulation and no stimulation. Results of this study raise concerns for biomechanical safety of NMES. Significant hyolaryngeal descent occurred with stimulation at rest, and reduced hyolaryngeal elevation occurred during swallowing; both movements are antagonistic to functional swallowing. Stimulated swallows were also judged to be "less safe" than nonstimulated swallows.

These studies of individuals with unimpaired physiology have documented an absence of change or potential worsening of biomechanical function. It could be argued that similar effects may not be evident in patients with impaired physiology. In response, the effectiveness of the VitalStim™ protocol in a population of patients with chronic pharyngeal phase dysphagia was evaluated by Ludlow et al. (2007). Time postonset of dysphagia was 6 months or more. Blinded measurements were made of hyoid movement and subglottic air column position on VFSS during no-stimulation (no current induced); low-stimulation level (lowest intensity level, at which a participant felt a "tingling" sensation); and high-stimulation level (highest tolerable intensity without discomfort) conditions. Hyoid depression of up to 5 to 10 mm was observed during stimulation of the muscles at rest in 8 of 10 participants. Additionally, low levels of stimulation resulted in a slight improvement on the NIH-SSS but no improvement in aspiration or penetration. Higher levels of stimulation, which would facilitate muscle contraction, had no effect on aspiration or penetration. Because of interference with hyolaryngeal excursion, the authors conclude that "before such a tool is used in therapy, improved understanding of its' immediate effects should be gained in the presence of specific types of swallowing difficulties before it is applied widely . . . " (Ludlow et al., 2007, p. 9).

Conflicting results were identified in a study by Blumenfeld, Hahn, LePage, Leonard, and Belafsky (2006) who undertook at retrospective study of 40 consecutive patients who underwent traditional dysphagia therapy (a combination of therapeutic exercise, diet texture modifications, and compensatory maneuvers) compared to 40 prospective patients who underwent electrical stimulation therapy according to the VitalStim™ treatment paradigm. Patients were assigned a functional swallowing score, based on the nonvalidated scale used by Freed et al. (2001); no control was provided for rater bias. Not surprisingly given the research design, those patients who were evaluated retrospectively using standard treatment (for that time period) did not demonstrate gains in swallowing treatment to the degree of those prospectively studied patients who underwent ES. Twenty-two patients with swallowing disorders were evaluated by Kiger, Brown, and Watkins (2006) in another retrospective to prospective comparison of treatment. Participants were divided into two groups: the retrospective group received traditional dysphagia therapy whereas the prospective group received VitalStim™ therapy. VFSS or videoendoscopy was used to evaluate swallowing function pre- and post-treatment based on a 7-point ordinal rating scale that described the patients' biomechanical swallowing functions as well as their ability to swallow different food consistencies. The traditional treatment group improved more in the oral phase than the VitalStim™ group. No significant differences in post-treatment outcomes for the pharyngeal phase, diet consistency tolerated, and oral intake measures were identified between the two groups.

An interesting observation can be made through careful review of the current literature. Generally, studies using nonblinded subjective outcome measures based on nonvalidated rating scales, support clinical success using the VitalStim™ protocol. However, little or no positive effect and, indeed, concern for inhibition of hyoid movement was reported if blinded and more objective measures such as myoelectric activity, hyoid movement, or biomechanics were utilized as the basis for measuring outcomes.

Using a different approach, a research group in Manchester, United Kingdom, sought to systematically investigate the effects of NMES of the pharynx and the faucial pillars, respectively (Fraser et al., 2002; Power et al., 2004). Through a series of careful methodologic experiments, optimal stimulation parameters were identified that increased corticobulbar excitability based on evaluation of motor evoked potentials triggered from transcranial magnetic stimulation. These optimal parameters were interestingly specific to the site of stimulation. Importantly, certain stimulation parameters were found to inhibit neural transmission to the muscles associated with swallowing. This neural inhibition correlated with radiographically confirmed evidence of delayed swallowing in healthy research participants; in other words, stimulation created a pathophysiologic finding in unimpaired individuals (Power et al., 2004).

In summary, substantial excitement has been generated regarding the potential application of NMES in the treatment of swallowing impairment. Preliminary data are encouraging. However, clinical enthusiasm should be well balanced by a careful and intelligent evaluation of the presented data. Documentation of adverse effects urges the clinician to respect the potential risks associated with NMES and be a smart clinical consumer. In a chapter on NMSE, Alon (1991) comments that:

> The present disarray, and the natural tendency to accept nonscientific, subjective and commercially motivated claims . . . may threaten the substantive potential that electrical stimulation can offer as an objective clinical modality (p. 56).

This comment was offered in reference to NMES applications in physical therapy but should serve as a warning to swallowing clinical practitioners. In our endeavor to provide optimal and innovative rehabilitative services to our patients with swallowing impairment, our best intentions need to be balanced with judiciousness and a critical eye.

THE NEED FOR INTELLIGENT ENTHUSIASM

As our specificity in diagnosis improves and our depth of rehabilitative understanding deepens, we can eagerly anticipate new developments in swallowing rehabilitation. It is an exciting time in the profession. But as our existing data would indicate, it is also a time that we need to carefully consider emerging options and base our developing treatments on theory and outcome.

Exciting developments are emerging that involve adaptation of existing treatment and potential develop of new initiatives. As with EMST, The Lee Silverman Voice Treatment (LSVT) was originally described to address impairments of respiratory support and speech production in patients with Parkinson's disease. A series of efficacy studies have documented positive effects of this treatment (Ramig, Countryman, O'Brien, Hoehn, & Thompson, 1996; Ramig & Dromey, 1996; Ramig et al., 2001; Ramig, Sapir, Fox, & Countryman, 2001). Specific improvements have been documented for changes in facial expression (Spielman, Borod, & Ramig, 2003), speech intensity (Ramig, Countryman, Thompson, & Horii, 1995), vocal fold adduction (Smith, Ramig, Dromey, Perez, & Samandari, 1995), and subglottal air pressure (Ramig & Dromey, 1996). A single case report of a single patient with mild Parkinson's disease was published by El Sharkawi et al. (2002). Post-LSVT, the approximate amount of oral residue after 3 and 5-ml liquid swallows was significantly reduced, and an overall 51% reduction in the number of oral-tongue and tongue-base disorders was noted. Clearly future studies are required to determine if this effect extends to other patients with Parkinson's disease and other neurologic disorders such as stroke, but the findings are encouraging.

To guide us, several excellent review articles encourage us to think smartly about developing rehabilitation strategies and base our practices on rehabilitative theory. These authors have taken a very intelligent approach to reviewing literature from sports medicine, neurobiology, and muscle physiology to provide us with a diverse foundation of information on which to base our rehabilitative practices. A synopsis of this important information exceeds the scope of this text, but they should be considered critical readings for both clinicians and researchers alike. As such, these key references are provided below:

- Burkhead, L. M., Sapienza, C. M., & Rosenbek, J. C. (2007). Strength-training exercise in dysphagia rehabilitation: Principles, procedures, and directions for future research. *Dysphagia*, *22*, 251–265.

- Chhadra, C., & Sapienza, C. M. (in press). A review of neurogenic and myogenic adaptations associated with specific exercise. *Communicative Disorders Review*.

- Clark, H. M. (2003). Neuromuscular treatments for speech and swallowing: A tutorial. *American Journal of Speech-Language Pathology*, *12*, 400–415.

- Gabriel, D. A., Kamen, G., & Frost G. (2006) Neural adaptations to resistive exercise: Mechanisms and recommendations for training practices. *Sports Medicine*, *36*, 133–149.

- Kays, S., & Robbins, J. (2006). Effects of sensorimotor exercise on swallowing outcomes relative to age and age-related disease. *Seminars in Speech and Language*, *27*(4), 245–259.

- Sapienza, C. M., & Wheeler, K. (2006). Respiratory muscle strength training: Functional outcomes versus plasticity. *Seminars in Speech and Language*, *27*(4), 236–244.

- Solomon, N. P. (2006). What is orofacial fatigue and how does it affect function for swallowing and speech? *Seminars in Speech and Language*, *27*(4), 268–282.

- Stathopoulos, E., & Felson Duchan, J. (2006). History and principles of exercise-based therapy: How they inform our current treatment. *Seminars in Speech and Language*, *27*(4), 227–235.

21 Medical and Surgical Management

Randomized, controlled clinical trials have not been conducted to determine the effectiveness of medical or surgical interventions on the management of dysphagia following stroke. Although not exclusive to stroke, specific medical and surgical interventions have been proposed to target specific physiologic problems and are addressed in this chapter.

MEDICAL MANAGEMENT

Botulinum Toxin

Botulinum toxin (Botox) has been used since 2000 to treat upper esophageal dysfunction (UES) dysfunction. It is produced by the bacteria *Clostridium botulinum* and is the neurotoxin in botulism, which is a deadly, paralyzing disease that occurs when food contaminated with the toxin is swallowed. For therapeutic purposes, Botox is injected into target muscles to yield paralysis and atrophy. The duration of the effect of Botox is limited as nerve endings regenerate, thus requiring repeated reinjections (Ravich, 2001). Botox type A has been used to treat dysphagia due to UES dysfunction. Studies generally report improved swallowing on the instrumental examination and/or by patient report (Alberty, Oelerich, Ludwig, Hartmann, & Stoll, 2000; Haapaniemi, Laurikainen, Pulkkinen, & Marttila, 2001; Parameswaran & Soliman, 2002; Shaw & Searl, 2001), with results lasting from 1 to 14 months postinjection (Shaw & Searl, 2001). However, most of these studies are retrospective, completed in heterogeneous populations, and no study has incorporated a placebo control.

Dilation

Dilation may also be used to treat cricopharyngeal dysfunction; however, no study has specifically focused on this procedure in a group of dysphagic stroke patients. Dilation may be completed with a bougienage, a rigid dilator of a prescribed circumference, or a balloon, which is inflated to specific dimensions. Symptomatic response to cricopharyngeal disruption with either dilation or myotomy was studied in a heterogeneous group of subjects including two confirmed stroke patients (Ali et al., 1997). Results suggested that 58% of subjects who underwent dilation had a subjective improvement in swallowing at 6-weeks postprocedure. Long-term response was not assessed. Generally, response is short-term and repeated dilation is required. The clinician, however, must remember that it is rare for stroke patients to present with isolated UES dysfunction. As discussed in more detail in the following section, in the stroke population, the primary cause for reduced UES opening is attributable to decreased anterior HLC movement. Hence, Botox or dilation would not facilitate UES opening in patients for whom impaired anterior hyolaryngeal complex (HLC) movement was the underlying problem of decreased UES opening.

SURGICAL INTERVENTION

Cricopharyngeal Myotomy

Cricopharyngeal myotomy is the most common surgery performed to alleviate oropharyngeal dysphagia (Cook & Kahrilas, 1999); however, evidence supporting its use for dysphagia in stroke is limited. Although no controlled clinical trial has been completed to evaluate the effectiveness of cricopharyngeal myotomy in stroke patients with dysphagia, such a trial has been completed following surgery for head and neck cancer. Results revealed no significant differences in swallowing between those patients undergoing myotomy and those who did not (Jacobs et al., 1999). Thus far, studies in the neurogenic population, some of whom have included stroke patients in the participant cohort, frequently have been retrospective, have used subjective versus objective outcome measures, and have been limited by small sample sizes (e.g., Berg, Jacobs, Persky, & Cohen, 1985; Poirier et al., 1997). In their review of the efficacy of myotomy for neurogenic dysphagia, Cook and Karhilas (1999) report a 63% rate of improved response. The exact nature of UES dysfunction must be understood before proceeding with surgical or medical intervention in stroke patients with dysphagia. Generally following stroke, decreased anterior HLC traction is the cause of UES dysfunction, rather than failure of the muscle to relax (Logemann, 1998). In this case, myotomy or the medical interventions described previously would not improve the dysphagia. Specific criteria have been suggested before considering a patient with neurogenic dysphagia for myotomy: (a) normal voluntary swallowing, (b) adequate tongue movement, (c) intact laryngeal functioning and phonation, and (d) no dysarthria (Duranceau, 1997). These same criteria should also be applied when deciding on medical intervention for UES dysfunction. Manometric evaluation of the UES should facilitate identification of patients who will respond favorably to myotomy. It has been suggested that in patients with nonprogressive diseases, such as stroke or traumatic brain injury, a myotomy should not be completed until 6 months postinjury, as most patients recover function within that time frame (Logemann, 1998).

Laryngeal Procedures

Vocal fold medialization is the procedure generally performed to treat aspiration due to an incompetent larynx. As discussed in earlier chapters, the clinician will recall that unilateral true vocal fold paralysis is not uncommon in patients with a lateral medullary stroke. If recovery of function is anticipated (i.e., following stroke), augmentation of the vocal folds with an absorbable material such as collagen or fat is recommended (Ergun & Kahrilas, 1997). In a recent study of a heterogeneous population, including poststroke patients, who underwent videofluoroscopic swallow studies pre- and postvocal fold medialization, the incidence of airway invasion did not significantly decrease following surgery (Bhattacharyya, Kotz, & Shapiro, 2002).

A tracheotomy may be performed for stroke patients with chronic aspiration. Although it will not improve swallowing, it will facilitate pulmonary toileting. Tracheotomy generally is performed only on the most severe stroke patients. Laryngotracheal separation is a more radical attempt in preventing chronic aspiration, although allowing for oral intake. Whereas patients may return to oral diets, the ability to phonate is eliminated. If physiologic aspects of swallowing improve sufficiently, this procedure can be reversed, as the glottis is not affected (Eisele, 1991). Case reports have documented the successful use of this procedure with the neurogenic population; however, only limited specification of outcome measures was provided (Butcher, 1982; Krespi, Quatela, Sisson, & Som, 1984).

22 Lagniappe[1]

It is important that swallowing management be proven effective. To do this, large scale randomized controlled trials are warranted. Data from such studies can be used to support provision of services, staffing, and reimbursement from third-party payers for the evaluation and treatment of swallowing disorders. A clinical trial on swallowing intervention was recently completed in stroke patients with dysphagia and revealed positive results on the effects of treatment (Carnaby et al., 2006). In this study, 306 acute stroke patients with a clinical diagnosis of dysphagia were randomly assigned to one of three treatment groups: (1) usual care as prescribed by the physician ($n = 102$), (2) low-intensity treatment ($n = 102$), and (3) high-intensity treatment ($n = 102$). The usual care (control) group was managed by the physician in the routine manner and may have consisted of referral to speech pathology in which patients were primarily supervised for feedings and given precautions for safe swallowing. The low-intensity group received directed intervention composed of compensatory strategies and precautions for safe swallowing. The high-intensity group received direct swallowing

---

[1]Lagniappe (lan yap) is a Creole word derived from American Spanish meaning "a little something extra" and is a favorite expression and treat in New Orleans.

exercises. Treatment for the two experimental groups was based on results from the clinical swallowing examination and the videofluoroscopic swallow study.

Results revealed that the proportion of surviving patients who returned to a normal diet at 6 months was significantly greater for the high-intensity treatment group (70%) compared to the low-intensity treatment group (64%) which was greater than the usual care group (56%). Return to functional swallowing was significantly greater in the active treatment groups, and chest infection and complications related to dysphagia were significantly less in these two treatment groups compared to the control group. The number of sessions and duration of sessions were significantly greater for the experimental treatment groups compared to the control group. Not unexpectedly, the control group returned to a normal diet quicker than the treatment groups. It was noted that participants in the usual care group frequently received a regular diet prior to assessment.

Although not as rigorous as the randomized controlled clinical trial from Carnaby et al. (2006), other studies in the past decade have provided evidence of treatment effects of swallowing intervention using large cohorts of patients with nonprogressive neurologic disease including stroke (Bartolome, Prosiegel, & Yassouridis, 1997; Neumann, 1993; Neumann et al., 1995). In the Neumann et al. (1995) study, 58 consecutive patients were referred for swallowing therapy. Eleven patients were greater than 6 months following onset of deficits; the remaining 47 were less than 6 months. No patient was receiving exclusive oral intake with 86% receiving only tube feeding. Patients received either indirect (e.g., rehabilitative exercises, thermal-tactile stimulation) swallowing treatment or combined indirect and direct (e.g., compensatory postures and swallowing maneuvers) management. Treatment lasted a median of 15 weeks. Results revealed that 67% of patients were progressed to exclusive oral feeding at the end of treatment with only 14% receiving only tube feeding. Time from onset of deficit (greater than 6 months, less than 6 months) was not associated with outcome as both groups demonstrated a similar success rate in returning to oral intake. Patients greater than 6 months postdeficit tended to require a longer duration of treatment. These findings support earlier findings from Neumann (1993) and are supported by later findings from Bartolome et al. (1997). Of interest, Neumann (1993) identified decreased attention to be associated with negative outcomes. This was not confirmed by Neumann et al. (1995); however, attentional deficits were associated with longer treatment durations.

Additionally, in Chapter 19, several case series are reported, which suggest positive outcomes in treatment of patients averaging 1.5 years poststroke (Crary, 1995; Crary et al., 2004; Huckabee & Cannito, 1999). Thus, the influence of rehabilitative recovery is extricated from spontaneous recovery. From these findings, clinicians can confidently state that swallowing therapy is of benefit and that change in swallowing behavior cannot be accounted for exclusively by spontaneous recovery. Further research is need to replicate findings, determine response to specific types of treatment programs, and identify specific dosage requirements,

REASSESSMENT

Instrumental reassessment of swallowing must be considered on an individual basis in stroke patients and is influenced by changes in the patient's medical status, cognition, and response to swallowing treatment. Studies have suggested that significant improvement in swallowing occurs in the first month following stroke in those patients with supratentorial stroke (Barer, 1989; Logemann, 1998); however, continued dysphagia also has been documented at 6-months poststroke (Mann et al., 1999).

Certain external factors may help the clinician determine response to treatment. A gross estimate of onset of the laryngeal elevation and duration and distance of laryngeal movement may be achieved by palpating the larynx. Reduction in expectoration may indicate a more efficient swallow. Surface electromyography may facilitate objective quantification of treatment results. Before compensatory strategies are removed, however, instrumental re-evaluation is recommended. This will allow objective documentation of changes in biomechanical functioning as well as safety of swallowing with less restricted consistencies or without the use of postural compensation. The reassessment will also indicate if further treatment is warranted and guide the direction of continued rehabilitation.

If clinical improvement is not evident, outcome measures should be reviewed for appropriateness and modified if needed. Improvement cannot be properly determined if outcome measures are poorly selected. Outcomes measures should include both functional and objective swallowing measures. If outcome measures are appropriate but progress is not apparent, then modification of the treatment should be considered. For example, if the effortful swallow is used to target reduced base of tongue contact to the posterior pharyngeal wall and little progress is evident, the clinician may want to consider adding visual feedback such as surface electromyography (see Chapter 19). Additionally, as addressed in Chapter 19, an absence of treatment effect may indicate that the treatment dose was insufficient to produce the desired effect, and modifications in service delivery would be indicated.

If after considerable readjustment of the treatment plan and improvement in swallowing is still not evident, discontinuation of treatment must be considered. Reassessment of swallowing with an instrumental examination should be considered prior to termination of treatment to document lack of progress.

As the stroke patient is complex and behaviors in addition to swallowing are impaired, specific factors such as decreased cognition and attention may impede progress, particularly initially. In acute stroke patients, cognitive behaviors may need to be addressed before swallowing rehabilitation is undertaken. As cognition improves, the response to swallowing treatment may increase. Reassessment of swallowing should also be considered when a change in swallowing functioning is reported in those patients previously discharged from therapy. Re-evaluation by speech pathology may reveal changes in swallowing pathophysiology that are more amenable to rehabilitation. In addition, new treatment techniques may be available that may improve swallowing.

Optimal times when swallowing rehabilitation should be initiated or is most effective have not been established. It is frequently assumed that rehabilitation is best implemented in the acute phase poststroke; however, empiric research is not available to confirm this. Several case-series studies of rehabilitation of dysphagia have focused on treatment composed of the effortful swallow and Mendelsohn maneuver and have documented functional and physiologic improvement in patients well beyond the post-acute period (Crary, 1995; Crary et al., 2004; Huckabee & Cannito, 1999). The average time post-onset reported by Huckabee and Cannito was 26.9 months postonset (range: 8–84 months). Although the number of participants was limited ($N = 10$), time postonset was not a significant variable in recovery. One of the two patients with a time postonset of less than 1 year was the slowest to have tube feeding discontinued. As a result, reassessment and potential re-establishment of treatment should be considered when the clinician is reconsulted for previously treated patients.

LAST THOUGHTS

As our research increases and our clinical practice expands, the options for management of the patient with dysphagia increase. Greater diagnostic options will yield greater specificity in diagnosis, which consequently will yield improved patient outcomes. Our approaches to rehabilitation are broadening and novel methods are being developed and tested that will ultimately make rehabilitation accessible to all but the most cognitively impaired patient. It is, indeed, an exciting time to work in this area.

Expanding practice, however, carries weighty responsibilities. As we close this text on dysphagia in stroke, we would like to offer several issues for consideration:

1. *Diagnostic precision will be paramount:* In Chapter 14, the importance of the instrumental diagnostic assessment was emphasized, based on literature that documents poor sensitivity and specificity for the clinical assessment to detect pharyngeal swallowing impairment and aspiration. Although the videofluoroscopic swallow study(VFSS) is clearly the most comprehensive assessment for the patient with dysphagia subsequent to stroke, this type of assessment provides a biased view of swallowing, that of bolus flow changes secondary to biomechanical changes in a two dimensional plane. In Chapters 11 through 13, we discussed other adjunct options for instrumental assessment that may be required to clarify when the VFSS does not reveal underlying pathophysiology. The clinician should not hesitate to rely on the multidisciplinary team to expand the diagnostic repertoire when needed. It is understood that not all clinicians are trained or have privileges to complete some of these adjunctive procedures. This does not imply that they are unavailable to you, only that you will need to establish strong collaborations with colleagues in otolaryngology and gastroenterology. The broad range of neuromuscular and neurosensory pathophysiologies and the complex interrelationships between biomechanical forces in the pharynx demand a clear diagnosis before management begins in order to prescribe a treatment approach that is efficacious and not harmful.

2. *We can do harm:* As a profession, we have been clinging to an assumption that we could try anything for any problem . . . "it might not help, but it won't hurt." Newer data from the liter-

ature are beginning to dismantle this assumption and will likely continue to do so. Old approaches are more carefully evaluated such that we fully understand both positive and negative ramifications of a particular adaptation of swallowing biomechanics. Clinical practice is dynamic and challenges the clinician to keep up with the literature so that as this information emerges, clinical practice can be adapted. As new rehabilitation approaches emerge, particularly those that involve invasive procedures, it is important that we exercise caution and intelligence in incorporating these approaches into our clinical work. If a technique is powerful enough to positively affect swallowing biomechanics, it is also likely powerful enough to adversely affect it as well. However, a precaution does not justify restriction. As an example, take the issue of aspiration. Early practice in dysphagia management (for the profession as a whole and an emerging clinician in particular) generally involved inhibition of oral intake at the first signs of aspiration with the assumption that inhibiting aspiration would inhibit the development of pneumonia. We now know that the link between the two is not as strong as originally presumed. Langmore et al. (1998) has carefully evaluated risks factors for development of pneumonia and "dysphagia was concluded to be an important risk for aspiration pneumonia, but generally not sufficient to cause pneumonia unless other risk factors are present as well" (p. 69). Restriction in itself may yield adverse outcomes. Research outlined in Chapter 16 identifies continued risks of aspiration pneumonia with the presence of a nasogastric tube. Thus, inhibiting prandial aspiration may not address the problem of pneumonia. Additionally, although not yet fully explored, one could speculate that the sensory input offered through oral ingestion is critical for recovery of swallowing impairment and that withholding it could impair recovery at the very least and exacerbate an existing problem at the worst. Dysphagia management appears to respond best with intensive management (see data presented in Chapters 18 and

19 and earlier in this chapter). However, it requires careful, intelligent approaches to developing treatment plans that are based on the literature and that maximize outcomes without taking unnecessary risks.

Our definition of management is changing: As was discussed in Chapter 18, we appear to be expanding our focus more heavily into rehabilitation research. Bolstered by the emergence of data that support these efforts, clinicians can strengthen their confidence in the application of rehabilitation programs. Rehabilitation will finally surpass compensation. It would never be considered acceptable for a physician to treat a urinary tract infection by advising bed rest and aspirin. Antibiotics would be expected. Likewise, except in cases of severe cognitive impairment where rehabilitation is not accessible to the patient, recommending a diet change and chin tuck is not an acceptable approach for swallowing impairment. Moreover, monitoring a patient is not management. Rehabilitation is expected. Intensive efforts are vital for success, and our research has documented preliminary evidence of substantial improvement even in patients with chronic and severe swallowing disability. We have not yet identified clear parameters for rehabilitation candidacy. Until these data emerge, every stroke patient should be considered a rehabilitation candidate until he or she proves not to be. Bottom line— once the clinician decides the patient will not benefit from treatment, he or she will not benefit from treatment. Until that decision is made, there is potential. The responsibility for rehabilitation should not be taken lightly given the social and health ramifications of nonoral status. At the 2007 meeting of the Dysphagia Research Society, a presentation was given by Deborah Batjer, a very determined woman who recovered swallowing function after 2.5 years of nonoral feeding secondary to neurologic injury. She commented, "As you already know, dysphagia is a package deal. It is not just the dysfunctional synchronization of nerves and muscles. It also involves a complex matrix of emotions." In her talk, she also provided great insights into the possibility of recovery. "I will never forget the clinician's words after she saw my dismal test results. Without offering any promise of success (and, more importantly, of not predicting failure), she simply said, 'Let's try.' This was all I needed to hear; a hopeful message with effort to back it up."

References

Addington, W. R., Stephens, R. E., & Gilliland, K. A. (1999). Assessing the laryngeal cough reflex and the risk of developing pneumonia after stroke: An interhospital comparison. *Stroke, 30*(6), 1203-1207.

Addington, W. R., Stephens, R. E., & Goulding, R. E. (1999). Anesthesia for the superior laryngeal nerves and tartaric acid-induced cough. *Archives of Physical Medicine and Rehabilitation, 80*(12), 1584-1586.

Adnerhill, I., Ekberg, O., & Groher, M. E. (1989). Determining normal bolus size for thin liquids. *Dysphagia, 4*(1), 1-3.

Aithal, G. P., Nylander, D., Dwarakanath, A. D., & Tanner, A. R. (1999). Subclinical esophageal peristaltic dysfunction during the early phase following a stroke. *Digestive Diseases and Sciences, 44*(2), 274-278.

Alberts, M. J., Horner, J., Gray, L., & Brazer, S. R. (1992). Aspiration after stroke: Lesion analysis by brain MRI. *Dysphagia, 7*(3), 170-173.

Alberty, J., Oelerich, M., Ludwig, K., Hartmann, S., & Stoll, W. (2000). Efficacy of botulinum toxin A for treatment of upper esophageal sphincter dysfunction. *Laryngoscope, 110*(7), 1151-1156.

Alfonso, M., Ferdjallah, M., Shaker, R., & Wertsch, J. J. (1998). Electrophysiologic validation of deglutitive UES opening head lift exercise [Abstract]. *Gastroenterology, 114*(4), G2942.

Ali, G. N., Laundl, T. M., Wallace, K. L., deCarle, D. J., & Cook, I. J. (1996). Influence of cold stimulation on the normal pharyngeal swallow response. *Dysphagia, 11*(1), 2-8.

Ali, G. N., Wallace, K. L., Laundl, T. M., Hunt, D. R., deCarle, D. J., & Cook, I. J. (1997). Predictors of outcome following cricopharyngeal disruption for pharyngeal dysphagia. *Dysphagia, 12*(3), 133-139.

Alon, G. (1991). Principles of electrical stimulation. In R. M. Nelson & D. P. Currier (Eds.), *Clinical electrotherapy* (2nd ed., pp. 35-101). Norwalk, CT: Appleton & Lange.

American Speech-Language-Hearing Association. (1992). *Instrumental diagnostic procedures for swallowing* [guidelines, knowledge, and skills, position statement]. Retrieved September 24, 2007 from ASHA professional Web site: http://www.asha.org/docs/html/GLKSPS1992-00092.html

Amri, M., & Car, A. (1988). Projections from the medullary swallowing center to the hypoglossal motor nucleus: A neuroanatomical and electrophysiological study in sheep. *Brain Research*, *441*(1-2), 119-126.

Amri, M., Car, A., & Jean, A. (1984). Medullary control of the pontine swallowing neurones in sheep. *Experimental Brain Research*, *55*(1), 105-110.

Amri, M., Car, A., & Roman, C. (1990). Axonal branching of medullary swallowing neurons projecting on the trigeminal and hypoglossal motor nuclei: Demonstration by electrophysiological and fluorescent double labeling techniques. *Experimental Brain Research*, *81*(2), 384-390.

Anis, M. K., Abid, S., Jafri, W., Abbas, Z., Shah, H. A., Hamid, S., et al. (2006). Acceptability and outcomes of the percutaneous endoscopic gastrostomy (PEG) tube placement-patients' and care givers' perspectives. *BMC Gastroenterology*, *6*, 37.

Aviv, J. E. (1997). Effects of aging on sensitivity of the pharyngeal and supraglottic areas. *American Journal of Medicine*, *103*(5A), 74S-76S.

Aviv, J. E., Martin, J. H., Jones, M. E., Wee, T. A., Diamond, B., Keen, M. S., et al. (1994). Age-related changes in pharyngeal and supraglottic sensation. *Annals of Otology, Rhinology, and Laryngology*, *103*(10), 749-752.

Aviv, J. E., Martin, J. H., Kim, T., Sacco, R. L., Thomson, J. E., Diamond, B., et al. (1999). Laryngopharyngeal sensory discrimination testing and the laryngeal adductor reflex. *Annals of Otology, Rhinology, and Laryngology*, *108*(8), 725-730.

Aviv, J. E., Martin, J. H., Sacco, R. L., Zagar, D., Diamond, B., Keen, M. S., et al. (1996). Supraglottic and pharyngeal sensory abnormalities in stroke patients with dysphagia. *Annals of Otology, Rhinology, and Laryngology*, *105*(2), 92-97.

Baker, L. L., McNeal, D. R., Benton, L. A., Bowman, B. R., & Waters, R. L. (1993). *Neuromuscular electrical stimulation: A practical guide.* Downey, CA: Los Amigos Research and Education Institute, Inc.

Balliet, R., Levy, B., & Blood, K. M. (1986). Upper extremity sensory feedback therapy in chronic cerebrovascular accident patients with impaired expressive aphasia and auditory comprehension. *Archives of Physical Medicine and Rehabilitation*, *67*(5), 304-310.

Barer, D. H. (1989). The natural history and functional consequences of dysphagia after hemispheric stroke. *Journal of Neurology, Neurosurgery, and Psychiatry*, *52*(2), 236-241.

Bartolome, G., & Neumann, S. (1993). Swallowing therapy in patients with neurological disorders causing cricopharyngeal dysfunction. *Dysphagia*, *8*(2), 146-149.

Bartolome, G., Prosiegel, M., & Yassouridis, A. (1997). Long-term functional outcome in patients with neurogenic dysphagia. *NeuroRehabilitation*, *9*, 195-204.

Basmajian, J. V., & DeLuca, C. J. (1985). *Muscles alive: Their functions revealed by electromyography* (5th ed.). Baltimore: Williams and Wilkins.

Bath, P. M., Bath, F. J., & Smithard, D. G. (2000). Interventions for dysphagia in acute stroke. *Cochran Database System Review*.

Beckstead, R. M., Morse, J. R., & Norgren, R. (1980). The nucleus of the solitary tract in the monkey: Projections to the thalamus and brain stem nuclei. *Journal of Comparative Neurology*, *190*(2), 259-282.

Benjamin, R. M., & Burton, H. (1968). Projection of taste nerve afferents to anterior opercular-insular cortex in squirrel monkey (Saimiri sciureus). *Brain Research*, *7*(2), 221-231.

Berg, H. M., Jacobs, J. B., Persky, M. S., & Cohen, N. L. (1985). Cricopharyngeal myotomy: A review of surgical results in patients with cricopharyngeal achalasia of neurogenic origin. *Laryngoscope*, *95*(11), 1337-1340.

Bhattacharyya, N., Kotz, T., & Shapiro, J. (2002). Dysphagia and aspiration with unilateral vocal cord immobility: Incidence, characterization, and response to surgical treatment. *Annals of Otology, Rhinology, and Laryngology*, *111*(8), 672-679.

Bickerman, H. A., & Barach, A. L. (1954). The experimental production of cough in human subjects induced by citric acid aerosols; Preliminary studies on the evaluation of antitussive agents. *American Journal of the Medical Sciences*, *228*(2), 156-163.

Bickerman, H. A., Cohen, B. M., & German, E. (1956). The cough response of normal human subjects stimulated experimentally by citric acid aerosol: Alterations produced by antitussive agents. I. Methology. *American Journal of the Medical Sciences*, *232*(1), 57-66.

Bisch, E. M., Logemann, J. A., Rademaker, A. W., Kahrilas, P. J., & Lazarus, C. L. (1994). Pharyngeal effects of bolus volume, viscosity, and temperature in patients with dysphagia resulting from neurologic impairment and in normal subjects. *Journal of Speech and Hearing Research*, *37*(5), 1041–1059.

Blumenfeld, L., Hahn, Y., Lepage, A., Leonard, R., & Belafsky, P. C. (2006). Transcutaneous electrical stimulation versus traditional dysphagia therapy: A nonconcurrent cohort study. *Otolaryngology-Head and Neck Surgery*, *135*(5), 754–757.

Boden, K., Hallgren, A., & Witt Hedstrom, H. (2006). Effects of three different swallow maneuvers analyzed by videomanometry. *Acta Radiologica*, *47*(7), 628–633.

Borr, C., Hielscher-Fastabend, M., & Lucking, A. (2007). Reliability and validity of cervical auscultation. *Dysphagia*, *22*(3), 225–234.

Bourne, M. (2002). *Food texture and viscosity: Concept and measurement* (2nd ed.). New York: Academic Press.

Bove, M., Mansson, I., & Eliasson, I. (1998). Thermal oral-pharyngeal stimulation and elicitation of swallowing. *Acta Oto-Laryngologica*, *118*(5), 728–731.

Broderick, J., Brott, T., Kothari, R., Miller, R., Khoury, J., Pancioli, A., et al. (1998). The Greater Cincinnati/Northern Kentucky Stroke Study: Preliminary first-ever and total incidence rates of stroke among blacks. *Stroke*, *29*(2), 415–421.

Broussard, D. L., & Altschuler, S. M. (2000). Central integration of swallow and airway-protective reflexes. *American Journal of Medicine*, *108*(Suppl. 4a), 62S–67S.

Brown, D. M., Nahai, F., & Basmajian, J. V. (1991). Electromyographic biofeedback in the reeducation of facial palsy. *Americal Journal of Physical Medicine*, *57*, 183–190.

Brudny, J., Hammerschlag, P. E., Cohen, N. L., & Ransohoff, J. (1988). Electromyographic rehabilitation of facial function and introduction of a facial paralysis grading scale for hypoglossal-facial nerve anastomosis. *Laryngoscope*, *98*(4), 405–410.

Bryant, M. (1991). Biofeedback in the treatment of a selected dysphagic patient. *Dysphagia*, *6*(3), 140–144.

Bulow, M., Olsson, R., & Ekberg, O. (1999). Videomanometric analysis of supraglottic swallow, effortful swallow, and chin tuck in healthy volunteers. *Dysphagia*, *14*(2), 67–72.

Bulow, M., Olsson, R., & Ekberg, O. (2001). Videomanometric analysis of supraglottic swallow, effortful swallow, and chin tuck in patients with pharyngeal dysfunction. *Dysphagia, 16*(3), 190-195.

Bulow, M., Olsson, R., & Ekberg, O. (2002). Supraglottic swallow, effortful swallow, and chin tuck did not alter hypopharyngeal intrabolus pressure in patients with pharyngeal dysfunction. *Dysphagia, 17*(3), 197-201.

Bulow, M., Olsson, R., & Ekberg, O. (2003). Videoradiographic analysis of how carbonated thin liquids and thickened liquids affect the physiology of swallowing in subjects with aspiration on thin liquids. *Acta Radiologica, 44*(4), 366-372.

Burkhead, L. M., Sapienza, C. M., & Rosenbek, J. C. (2007). Strength-training exercise in dysphagia rehabilitation: Principles, procedures, and directions for future research. *Dysphagia, 22*(3), 251-265.

Burnett, T. A., Mann, E. A., Stoklosa, J. B., & Ludlow, C. L. (2005). Self-triggered functional electrical stimulation during swallowing. *Journal of Neurophysiology, 94*(6), 4011-4018.

Butcher, R. B., 2nd. (1982). Treatment of chronic aspiration as a complication of cerebrovascular accident. *Laryngoscope, 92*(6 Pt. 1), 681-685.

Butler, S. G. (Ed.). (2006). *The SLP's clinical use of pharyngeal and upper esopahgeal sphincter manometry*.Lincoln Park, NJ: KayPentax.

Butler, S. G., Postma, G. N., & Fischer, E. (2004). Effects of viscosity, taste, and bolus volume on swallowing apnea duration of normal adults. *Otolaryngology-Head and Neck Surgery, 131*(6), 860-863.

Butler, S. G., Stuart, A., Pressman, H., Poage, G., & Roche, W. J. (2007). Preliminary investigation of swallowing apnea duration and swallow/respiratory phase relationships in individuals with cerebral vascular accident. *Dysphagia, 22*(3), 215-224.

Callahan, C. M., Haag, K. M., Buchanan, N. N., & Nisi, R. (1999). Decision-making for percutaneous endoscopic gastrostomy among older adults in a community setting. *Journal of the American Geriatrics Society, 47*(9), 1105-1109.

Campion, M. B., Haynos, J., & Palmer, J. B. (2007). An individualized approach to the videofluoroscopic swallowing study. *Perspectives on Swallowing and Swallowing Disorders, 16*(1), 7-11.

Car, A. (1970). Cortical control of the bulbar swallowing center [in French]. *Journal of Physiology (Paris), 62*(4), 361-386.

Car, A. (1973). Cortical control of deglutition. 2. Medullary impact of corti-cofugal swallowing pathways [in French]. *Journal of Physiology (Paris)*, *66*(5), 553–575.

Car, A., & Amri, M. (1982). Pontine deglutition neurons in sheep. I. Activity and localization [in French]. *Experimental Brain Research*, *48*(3), 345–354.

Car, A., Jean, A., & Roman, C. (1975). A pontine primary relay for ascending projections of the superior laryngeal nerve. *Experimental Brain Research*, *22*(2), 197–210.

Carl, L. R., & Johnson, P. R. (2006). *Drugs and dysphagia: How medications can affect eating and swallowing*. Austin, TX: Pro-Ed.

Carnaby, G., Hankey, G. J., & Pizzi, J. (2006). Behavioural intervention for dysphagia in acute stroke: A randomised controlled trial. *Lancet Neurology*, *5*(1), 31–37.

Carpenter, M. B. (1978). *Core text of neuroanatomy* (1st ed.). Baltimore: Williams and Wilkins.

Carter, K., Anderson, C., Hacket, M., Feigin, V., Barber, P. A., Broad, J. B., et al. (2006). Trends in ethnic disparities in stroke incidence in Auckland, New Zealand, during 1981 to 2003. *Stroke*, *37*(1), 56–62.

Castell, J. A., Dalton, C. B., & Castell, D. O. (1990). Pharyngeal and upper esophageal sphincter manometry in humans. *American Journal of Physiology*, *258*(2 Pt. 1), G173–G178.

Cerenko, D., McConnel, F. M., & Jackson, R. T. (1989). Quantitative assessment of pharyngeal bolus driving forces. *Otolaryngology-Head and Neck Surgery*, *100*(1), 57–63.

Chang, A. B., Phelan, P. D., Roberts, R. G., & Robertson, C. F. (1996). Capsaicin cough receptor sensitivity test in children. *European Respiratory Journal*, *9*(11), 2220–2223.

Chang, A. B., Phelan, P. D., & Robertson, C. F. (1997). Cough receptor sensitivity in children with acute and non-acute asthma. *Thorax*, *52*(9), 770–774.

Chaudhuri, G., Hildner, C. D., Brady, S., Hutchins, B., Aliga, N., & Abadilla, E. (2002). Cardiovascular effects of the supraglottic and super-supraglottic swallowing maneuvers in stroke patients with dysphagia. *Dysphagia*, *17*(1), 19–23.

Chee, C., Arshad, S., Singh, S., Mistry, S., & Hamdy, S. (2005). The influence of chemical gustatory stimuli and oral anaesthesia on healthy human pharyngeal swallowing. *Chemical Senses*, *30*(5), 393–400.

Chen, M. Y., Ott, D. J., Peele, V. N., & Gelfand, D. W. (1990). Oropharynx in patients with cerebrovascular disease: Evaluation with videofluoroscopy. *Radiology, 176*(3), 641-643.

Chhadra, C., & Sapienza, C. M. (in press). A review of neurogenic and myogenic adaptions associated with specific exercise. *Communicative Disorders Review.*

Chhetri, D. K., & Berke, G. S. (1997). Ansa cervicalis nerve: Review of the topographic anatomy and morphology. *Laryngoscope, 107*(10), 1366-1372.

Chi-Fishman, G., & Sonies, B. C. (2000). Motor strategy in rapid sequential swallowing: New insights. *Journal of Speech, Language, and Hearing Research, 43*(6), 1481-1492.

Chi-Fishman, G., & Sonies, B. C. (2002). Kinematic strategies for hyoid movement in rapid sequential swallowing. *Journal of Speech, Language, and Hearing Research, 45*(3), 457-468.

Chiara, T., Martin, A. D., Davenport, P. W., & Bolser, D. C. (2006). Expiratory muscle strength training in persons with multiple sclerosis having mild to moderate disability: Effect on maximal expiratory pressure, pulmonary function, and maximal voluntary cough. *Archives of Physical Medicine and Rehabilitation, 87*(4), 468-473.

Chiara, T., Martin, D., & Sapienza, C. (2007). Expiratory muscle strength training: speech production outcomes in patients with multiple sclerosis. *Neurorehabilitation and Neural Repair, 21*(3), 239-249.

Chua, K. S., & Kong, K. H. (1996). Functional outcome in brain stem stroke patients after rehabilitation. *Archives of Physical Medicine and Rehabilitation, 77*(2), 194-197.

Cichero, J. A., Hay, G., Murdoch, B. E., & Halley, P. J. (1997). Videofluoroscopic fluids versus mealtime fluids: Differences in viscosity and density made clear. *Journal of Medical Speech Language Pathology, 5,* 203-215.

Cichero, J. A., Jackson, O., Halley, P. J., & Murdoch, B. E. (2000). How thick is thick? Multicenter study of the rheological and material property characteristics of mealtime fluids and videofluoroscopy fluids. *Dysphagia, 15*(4), 188-200.

Cichero, J. A., & Murdoch, B. E. (2002). Detection of swallowing sounds: Methodology revisited. *Dysphagia, 17*(1), 40-49.

Ciocon, J. O., Silverstone, F. A., Graver, L. M., & Foley, C. J. (1988). Tube feedings in elderly patients. Indications, benefits, and complications. *Archives of Internal Medicine, 148*(2), 429-433.

Clark, H. M. (2003). Neuromuscular treatments for speech and swallowing: A tutorial. *American Journal of Speech-Language Pathology, 12*(4), 400-415.

Clave, P., de Kraa, M., Arreola, V., Girvent, M., Farre, R., Palomera, E., et al. (2006). The effect of bolus viscosity on swallowing function in neurogenic dysphagia. *Alimentary Pharmacology and Therapeutics, 24*(9), 1385-1394.

Collins, M. J., & Bakheit, A. M. (1997). Does pulse oximetry reliably detect aspiration in dysphagic stroke patients? *Stroke, 28*(9), 1773-1775.

Colodny, N. (2000). Comparison of dysphagics and nondysphagics on pulse oximetry during oral feeding. *Dysphagia, 15*(2), 68-73.

Colodny, N. (2002). Interjudge and intrajudge reliabilities in fiberoptic endoscopic evaluation of swallowing (FEES) using the Penetration-Aspiration Scale: A replication study. *Dysphagia, 17*(4), 308-315.

Colodny, N. (2005). Dysphagic independent feeders' justifications for noncompliance with recommendations by a speech-language pathologist. *American Journal of Speech-Language Pathology, 14*(1), 61-70.

Cook, I. J. (1993). Cricopharyngeal function and dysfunction. *Dysphagia, 8*(3), 244-251.

Cook, I. J., Dodds, W. J., Dantas, R. O., Kern, M. K., Massey, B. T., Shaker, R., et al. (1989). Timing of videofluoroscopic, manometric events, and bolus transit during the oral and pharyngeal phases of swallowing. *Dysphagia, 4*(1), 8-15.

Cook, I. J., & Kahrilas, P. J. (1999). AGA technical review on management of oropharyngeal dysphagia. *Gastroenterology, 116*(2), 455-478.

Cook, I. J., Weltman, M. D., Wallace, K., Shaw, D. W., McKay, E., Smart, R. C., et al. (1994). Influence of aging on oral-pharyngeal bolus transit and clearance during swallowing: scintigraphic study. *American Journal of Physiology, 266*(6 Pt. 1), G972-G977.

Crary, M. A. (1995). A direct intervention program for chronic neurogenic dysphagia secondary to brainstem stroke. *Dysphagia, 10*(1), 6-18.

Crary, M. A., Carnaby Mann, G. D., Groher, M. E., & Helseth, E. (2004). Functional benefits of dysphagia therapy using adjunctive sEMG biofeedback. *Dysphagia, 19*(3), 160-164.

Curtis, D. J., Braham, S. L., Karr, S., Holborow, G. S., & Worman, D. (1988). Identification of unopposed intact muscle pair actions affecting swallowing: Potential for rehabilitation. *Dysphagia, 3*(2), 57-64.

Daggett, A., Logemann, J., Rademaker, A., & Pauloski, B. (2006). Laryngeal penetration during deglutition in normal subjects of various ages. *Dysphagia, 21*(4), 270-274.

Daniel-Whitney, B. (1989). Severe spastic-ataxic dysarthria in a child with traumatic brain injury: Questions for management. In K. Yorkston & D.

Beukelman (Eds.), *Recent advances in clinical dysarthria* (pp. 129-137). Boston: College-Hill.

Daniels, S. K. (2000). Swallowing apraxia: A disorder of the praxis system? *Dysphagia, 15*(3), 159-166.

Daniels, S. K., Brailey, K., & Foundas, A. L. (1999). Lingual discoordination and dysphagia following acute stroke: Analyses of lesion localization. *Dysphagia, 14*(2), 85-92.

Daniels, S. K., Brailey, K., Priestly, D. H., Herrington, L. R., Weisberg, L. A., & Foundas, A. L. (1998). Aspiration in patients with acute stroke. *Archives of Physical Medicine and Rehabilitation, 79*(1), 14-19.

Daniels, S. K., Corey, D. M., Hadskey, L. D., Legendre, C., Priestly, D. H., Rosenbek, J. C., et al. (2004). Mechanism of sequential swallowing during straw drinking in healthy young and older adults. *Journal of Speech, Language, and Hearing Research, 47*(1), 33-45.

Daniels, S. K., Corey, D. M., Schulz, P. E., Foundas, A. L., & Rosenbek, J. C. (2007). Effects of evaluation variables on swallowing performance in mild Alzheimer's disease [Abstract]. *Dysphagia, 22*, 386.

Daniels, S. K., & Foundas, A. L. (1997). The role of the insular cortex in dysphagia. *Dysphagia, 12*(3), 146-156.

Daniels, S. K., & Foundas, A. L. (1999). Lesion localization in acute stroke patients with risk of aspiration. *Journal of Neuroimaging, 9*(2), 91-98.

Daniels, S. K., & Foundas, A. L. (2001). Swallowing physiology of sequential straw drinking. *Dysphagia, 16*(3), 176-182.

Daniels, S. K., Foundas, A. L., Iglesia, G. C., & Sullivan, M. A. (1996). Lesion site in unilateral stroke patients with dysphagia. *Journal of Stroke and Cerebrovascular Disease, 6*, 30-34.

Daniels, S. K., McAdam, C. P., Brailey, K., & Foundas, A. L. (1997). Clinical assessment of swallowing and prediction of dysphagia severity. *American Journal of Speech-Language Pathology, 6*(4), 7-24.

Daniels, S. K., Schroeder, M. F., DeGeorge, P. C., Corey, D. M., & Rosenbek, J. C. (2007). Effects of verbal cue on bolus flow during swallowing. *American Journal of Speech-Language Pathology, 16*(2), 140-147.

Daniels, S. K., Schroeder, M. F., McClain, M., Corey, D. M., Rosenbek, J. C., & Foundas, A. L. (2006). Dysphagia in stroke: Development of a standard method to examine swallowing recovery. *Journal of Rehabilitation, Research, and Development, 43*(3), 347-356.

Dantas, R. O., Dodds, W. J., Massey, B. T., & Kern, M. K. (1989). The effect of high- vs low-density barium preparations on the quantitative fea-tures of swallowing. *AJR American Journal of Roentgenology, 153*(6), 1191-1195.

Dantas, R. O., Kern, M. K., Massey, B. T., Dodds, W. J., Kahrilas, P. J., Brasseur, et al. (1990). Effect of swallowed bolus variables on oral and pharyngeal phases of swallowing. *American Journal of Physiology, 258*(5 Pt. 1), G675-G6781.

Davalos, A., Ricart, W., Gonzalez-Huix, F., Soler, S., Marrugat, J., Molins, A., et al. (1996). Effect of malnutrition after acute stroke on clinical out-come. *Stroke, 27*(6), 1028-1032.

Davies, A. E., Kidd, D., Stone, S. P., & MacMahon, J. (1995). Pharyngeal sen-sation and gag reflex in healthy subjects. *Lancet, 345*(8948), 487-488.

Denes, G., Perazzolog, C., & Piccione, F. (1996). Intensive versus regular speech therapy in global aphasia: A controlled study. *Aphasiology, 10*(4), 385-394.

Denk, D. M., & Kaider, A. (1997). Videoendoscopic biofeedback: a simple method to improve the efficacy of swallowing rehabilitation of patients after head and neck surgery. *ORL Journal of Otorhinolaryngology and Its Related Specalities, 59*(2), 100-105.

Dennis, M., Lewis, S., Cranswick, G., & Forbes, J. (2006). FOOD: A multicen-tre randomised trial evaluating feeding policies in patients admitted to hospital with a recent stroke. *Health Technology Assessessment, 10*(2), iii-iv, ix-x, 1-120.

DePippo, K. L., Holas, M. A., & Reding, M. J. (1992). Validation of the 3-oz water swallow test for aspiration following stroke. *Archives of Neurol-ogy, 49*(12), 1259-1261.

DePippo, K. L., Holas, M. A., & Reding, M. J. (1994). The Burke dysphagia screening test: Validation of its use in patients with stroke. *Archives of Physical Medicine and Rehabilitation, 75*(12), 1284-1286.

Dick, T. E., Oku, Y., Romaniuk, J. R., & Cherniack, N. S. (1993). Interaction between central pattern generators for breathing and swallowing in the cat. *Journal of Physiology, 465*, 715-730.

Dicpinigaitis, P. V. (2003). Cough reflex sensitivity in cigarette smokers. *Chest, 123*(3), 685-688.

Dicpinigaitis, P. V., & Rauf, K. (1998). The influence of gender on cough reflex sensitivity. *Chest, 113*(5), 1319-1321.

Ding, R., Logemann, J. A., Larson, C. R., & Rademaker, A. W. (2003). The effects of taste and consistency on swallow physiology in younger and older healthy individuals: A surface electromyographic study. *Journal of Speech, Language, and Hearing Research, 46*(4), 977–989.

Dodds, W. J., Hogan, W. J., Reid, D. P., Stewart, E. T., & Arndorfer, R. C. (1973). A comparison between primary esophageal peristalsis following wet and dry swallows. *Journal of Applied Physiology, 35*(6), 851–857.

Dodds, W. J., Man, K. M., Cook, I. J., Kahrilas, P. J., Stewart, E. T., & Kern, M. K. (1988). Influence of bolus volume on swallow-induced hyoid movement in normal subjects. *AJR American Journal of Roentgenology, 150*(6), 1307–1309.

Doeltgen, S. H., Witte, U., Gumbley, F., & Huckabee, M. L. (2007). Pharyngeal pressure generation during tonguehold maneuver [Abstract]. *Dysphagia, 22*, 374.

Doeltgen, S. H., Witte, U., Gumbley, F., & Huckabee, M. L. (submitted for publication). Evaluation of manometric measures during tongue hold swallows.

Donzelli, J., & Brady, S. (2004). The effects of breath-holding on vocal fold adduction: implications for safe swallowing. *Archives of Otolaryngology-Head and Neck Surgery, 130*(2), 208–210.

Doty, R. W. (1968). Neural organization of deglutition. In C. F. Code (Ed.), *Handbook of physiology: Alimentary canal: Motility* (Vol. Sec. 6, Vol. 4, pp. 1861–1902). Washington, DC: American Physiology Society.

Doty, R. W., & Bosma, J. F. (1956). An electromyographic analysis of reflex deglutition. *Journal of Neurophysiology, 19*(1), 44–60.

Doty, R. W., Richmond, W. H., & Storey, A. T. (1967). Effect of medullary lesions on coordination of deglutition. *Experimental Neurology, 17*(1), 91–106.

Dozier, T. S., Brodsky, M. B., Michel, Y., Walters, B. C., Jr., & Martin-Harris, B. (2006). Coordination of swallowing and respiration in normal sequential cup swallows. *Laryngoscope, 116*(8), 1489–1493.

Draizar, A. (1984). Clinical EMG feedback in motor speech disorders. *Archives of Physical Medicine and Rehabilitation, 65*(8), 481–484.

Dua, K. S., Ren, J., Bardan, E., Xie, P., & Shaker, R. (1997). Coordination of deglutitive glottal function and pharyngeal bolus transit during normal eating. *Gastroenterology, 112*(1), 73–83.

Duffy, J. R. (2005). *Motor speech disorders* (2nd ed.). St. Louis, MO: Mosby.

Duranceau, A. (1997). Cricopharyngeal myotomy in the management of neurogenic and muscular dysphagia. *Neuromuscular Disorders*, 7 (Suppl. 1), S85–S89.

Dziewas, R., Ritter, M., Schilling, M., Konrad, C., Oelenberg, S., Nabavi, D. G., et al. (2004). Pneumonia in acute stroke patients fed by nasogastric tube. *Journal of Neurology, Neurosurgery, and Psychiatry*, 75(6), 852–856.

Dziewas, R., Soros, P., Ishii, R., Chau, W., Henningsen, H., Ringelstein, E. B., et al. (2003). Neuroimaging evidence for cortical involvement in the preparation and in the act of swallowing. *Neuroimage*, 20(1), 135–144.

Easterling, C., Grande, B., Kern, M., Sears, K., & Shaker, R. (2005). Attaining and maintaining isometric and isokinetic goals of the Shaker exercise. *Dysphagia*, 20(2), 133–138.

Eisele, D. W. (1991). Surgical approaches to aspiration. *Dysphagia*, 6(2), 71–78.

El Sharkawi, A., Ramig, L., Logemann, J. A., Pauloski, B. R., Rademaker, A. W., Smith, C. H., et al. (2002). Swallowing and voice effects of Lee Silverman Voice Treatment (LSVT): A pilot study. *Journal of Neurology, Neurosurgery, and Psychiatry*, 72(1), 31–36.

Ergun, G. A., & Kahrilas, P. J. (1997). Medical and surgical treatment interventions in deglutitive dysfunction. In A. L. Perlman & K. Schulze-Delreiu (Eds.), *Deglutition and its disorders* (pp. 463–490). San Diego, CA: Singular.

Ferrari, M., Olivieri, M., Sembenini, C., Benini, L., Zuccali, V., Bardelli, E., et al. (1995). Tussive effect of capsaicin in patients with gastroesophageal reflux without cough. *American Journal of Respiratory and Critical Care Medine*, 151(2 Pt. 1), 557–561.

Finestone, H. M., Greene-Finestone, L. S., Wilson, E. S., & Teasell, R. W. (1996). Prolonged length of stay and reduced functional improvement rate in malnourished stroke rehabilitation patients. *Archives of Physical Medicine and Rehabilitation*, 77(4), 340–345.

Foundas, A. L., Macauley, B. L., Raymer, A. M., Maher, L. M., Heilman, K. M., & Gonzalez Rothi, L. J. (1995). Ecological implications of limb apraxia: Evidence from mealtime behavior. *Journal of the International Neuropsychological Society*, 1(1), 62–66.

Fraser, C., Power, M., Hamdy, S., Rothwell, J., Hobday, D., Hollander, I., et al. (2002). Driving plasticity in human adult motor cortex is associated with improved motor function after brain injury. *Neuron*, 34(5), 831–840.

Freed, M. L., Freed, L., Chatburn, R. L., & Christian, M. (2001). Electrical stimulation for swallowing disorders caused by stroke. *Respiratory Care*, *46*(5), 466–474.

Fujiu, M., & Logemann, J. A. (1996). Effect of a tongue-holding maneuver on posterior pharyngeal wall movement during deglutition. *American Journal of Speech-Language Pathology*, *5*(1), 23–30.

Fujiu, M., Logemann, J. A., & Pauloski, B. (1995). Increased post-operative posterior pharyngeal wall movement in patients with anterior oral cancer: Preliminary findings and possible implications for treatment. *American Journal of Speech-Language Pathology*, *4*(1), 24–30.

Gabriel, D. A., Kamen, G., & Frost, G. (2006). Neural adaptations to resistive exercise: Mechanisms and recommendations for training practices. *Sports Medicine*, *36*(2), 133–149.

Garcia, J. M., Chambers, E. T., & Molander, M. (2005). Thickened liquids: practice patterns of speech-language pathologists. *American Journal of Speech-Language Pathology*, *14*(1), 4–13.

Gariballa, S. E., Parker, S. G., Taub, N., & Castleden, M. (1998). Nutritional status of hospitalized acute stroke patients. *British Journal of Nutrition*, *79*(6), 481–487.

Garon, B. R., Engle, M., & Ormiston, C. (1995). Reliability of the 3-oz water swallow test utilizing cough reflex as sole indicator of aspiration. *Journal of Neurologic Rehabilitation*, *9*, 139–143.

Garon, B. R., Engle, M., & Ormiston, C. (1997). A randomized control study to determine the effects of unlimited oral intake of water in patients with identified aspiration. *Journal of Neurologic Rehabilitation*, *11*, 139–148.

Glanz, M., Klawansky, S., Stason, W., Berkey, C., & Chalmers, T. C. (1996). Functional electrostimulation in poststroke rehabilitation: A meta-analysis of the randomized controlled trials. *Archives of Physical Medicine and Rehabilitation*, *77*(6), 549–553.

Gordon, C., Hewer, R. L., & Wade, D. T. (1987). Dysphagia in acute stroke. *British Medical Journal (Clinical Research Ed)*, *295*(6595), 411–414.

Gosselink, R. (2002). Respiratory rehabilitation: Improvement of short- and long-term outcome. *European Respiratory Journal*, *20*(1), 4–5.

Gottlieb, D., Kipnis, M., Sister, E., Vardi, Y., & Brill, S. (1996). Validation of the 50 ml drinking test for evaluation of post-stroke dysphagia. *Disability and Rehabilitation*, *18*(10), 529–532.

Gumbley, F., Huckabee, M. L., Doeltgen, S. H., Witte, U., & Moran, C. (in press). Effects of bolus volume on pharyngeal contact pressure during normal swallowing. *Dysphagia*.

Haapaniemi, J. J., Laurikainen, E. A., Pulkkinen, J., & Marttila, R. J. (2001). Botulinum toxin in the treatment of cricopharyngeal dysphagia. *Dysphagia*, *16*(3), 171-175.

Hadjikoutis, S., Pickersgill, T. P., Dawson, K., & Wiles, C. M. (2000). Abnormal patterns of breathing during swallowing in neurological disorders. *Brain*, *123 (Pt. 9)*, 1863-1873.

Hamdy, S., Aziz, Q., Rothwell, J. C., Crone, R., Hughes, D., Tallis, R. C., et al. (1997). Explaining oropharyngeal dysphagia after unilateral hemispheric stroke. *Lancet*, *350*(9079), 686-692.

Hamdy, S., Aziz, Q., Rothwell, J. C., Power, M., Singh, K. D., Nicholson, D. A., et al. (1998). Recovery of swallowing after dysphagic stroke relates to functional reorganization in the intact motor cortex. *Gastroenterology*, *115*(5), 1104-1112.

Hamdy, S., Aziz, Q., Rothwell, J. C., Singh, K. D., Barlow, J., Hughes, D. G., et al. (1996). The cortical topography of human swallowing musculature in health and disease. *Nature Medicine*, *2*(11), 1217-1224.

Hamdy, S., Mikulis, D. J., Crawley, A., Xue, S., Lau, H., Henry, S., et al. (1999). Cortical activation during human volitional swallowing: An event-related fMRI study. *American Journal of Physiology*, *277*(1 Pt. 1), G219-G225.

Hamdy, S., Rothwell, J. C., Brooks, D. J., Bailey, D., Aziz, Q., & Thompson, D. G. (1999). Identification of the cerebral loci processing human swallowing with H2(15)O PET activation. *Journal of Neurophysiology*, *81*(4), 1917-1926.

Hamidon, B. B., Abdullah, S. A., Zawawi, M. F., Sukumar, N., Aminuddin, A., & Raymond, A. A. (2006). A prospective comparison of percutaneous endoscopic gastrostomy and nasogastric tube feeding in patients with acute dysphagic stroke. *Medical Journal of Malaysia*, *61*(1), 59-66.

Hamlet, S. L., Nelson, R. J., & Patterson, R. L. (1990). Interpreting the sounds of swallowing: Fluid flow through the cricopharyngeus. *Annals of Otology, Rhinology, and Laryngology*, *99*(9 Pt. 1), 749-752.

Hanna-Pladdy, B., Heilman, K. M., & Foundas, A. L. (2003). Ecological implications of ideomotor apraxia: Evidence from physical activities of daily living. *Neurology*, *60*(3), 487-490.

Hasan, M., Meara, R. J., Bhowmick, B. K., & Woodhouse, K. (1995). Percutaneous endoscopic gastrostomy in geriatric patients: Attitudes of health care professionals. *Gerontology, 41*(6), 326-331.

Heilman, K. M., Watson, R. T., & Valenstein, E. (2003). Neglect and related disorders. In K. M. Heilman & E. Valenstein (Eds.), *Clinical neuropsychology* (4th ed., pp. 296-346). New York: Oxford University Press.

Hiiemae, K. M., & Palmer, J. B. (1999). Food transport and bolus formation during complete feeding sequences on foods of different initial consistency. *Dysphagia, 14*(1), 31-42.

Hinckley, J. J., & Craig, H. K. (1998). Influence of rate of treatment on the naming ability of adults with chronic aphasia. *Aphasiology, 12*(11), 989-1006.

Hind, J. A., Nicosia, M. A., Roecker, E. B., Carnes, M. L., & Robbins, J. (2001). Comparison of effortful and noneffortful swallows in healthy middle-aged and older adults. *Archives of Physical Medicine and Rehabilitation, 82*(12), 1661-1665.

Hinds, N. P., & Wiles, C. M. (1998). Assessment of swallowing and referral to speech and language therapists in acute stroke. *Quarterly Journal of Medicine, 91*(12), 829-835.

Hirst, L. J., Ford, G. A., Gibson, G. J., & Wilson, J. A. (2002). Swallow-induced alterations in breathing in normal older people. *Dysphagia, 17*(2), 152-161.

Hiss, S. G., & Huckabee, M. L. (2005). Timing of pharyngeal and upper esophageal sphincter pressures as a function of normal and effortful swallowing in young healthy adults. *Dysphagia, 20*(2), 149-156.

Hiss, S. G., Strauss, M., Treole, K., Stuart, A., & Boutilier, S. (2003). Swallowing apnea as a function of airway closure. *Dysphagia, 18*(4), 293-300.

Hiss, S. G., Strauss, M., Treole, K., Stuart, A., & Boutilier, S. (2004). Effects of age, gender, bolus volume, bolus viscosity, and gustation on swallowing apnea onset relative to lingual bolus propulsion onset in normal adults. *Journal of Speech, Language, and Hearing Research, 47*(3), 572-583.

Hiss, S. G., Treole, K., & Stuart, A. (2001). Effects of age, gender, bolus volume, and trial on swallowing apnea duration and swallow/respiratory phase relationships of normal adults. *Dysphagia, 16*(2), 128-135.

Holas, M. A., DePippo, K. L., & Reding, M. J. (1994). Aspiration and relative risk of medical complications following stroke. *Archives of Neurology, 51*(10), 1051-1053.

Horner, J., Brazer, S. R., & Massey, E. W. (1993). Aspiration in bilateral stroke patients: A validation study. *Neurology*, *43*(2), 430–433.

Horner, J., Massey, E. W., & Brazer, S. R. (1990). Aspiration in bilateral stroke patients. *Neurology*, *40*(11), 1686–1688.

Horner, J., Massey, E. W., Riski, J. E., Lathrop, D. L., & Chase, K. N. (1988). Aspiration following stroke: Clinical correlates and outcome. *Neurology*, *38*(9), 1359–1362.

Huckabee, M. L., Butler, S. G., Barclay, M., & Jit, S. (2005). Submental surface electromyographic measurement and pharyngeal pressures during normal and effortful swallowing. *Archives of Physical Medicine and Rehabilitation*, *86*(11), 2144–2149.

Huckabee, M. L., & Cannito, M. P. (1999). Outcomes of swallowing rehabilitation in chronic brainstem dysphagia: A retrospective evaluation. *Dysphagia*, *14*(2), 93–109.

Huckabee, M. L., Deecke, L., Cannito, M. P., Gould, H. J., & Mayr, W. (2003). Cortical control mechanisms in volitional swallowing: The Bereitschaftspotential. *Brain Topography*, *16*(1), 3–17.

Huckabee, M. L., & Doeltgen, S. H. (2007). Emerging modalities in dysphagia rehabilitation: Neuromuscular electrical stimulation. *New Zealand Medical Journal*, *120*(1263), 1–9.

Huckabee, M. L., & Pelletier, C. A. (1999). *Management of adult neurogenic dysphagia.* San Diego, CA: Singular.

Huckabee, M. L., & Steele, C. M. (2006). An analysis of lingual contribution to submental surface electromyographic measures and pharyngeal pressure during effortful swallow. *Archives of Physical Medicine and Rehabilitation*, *87*(8), 1067–1072.

Huggins, P. S., Tuomi, S. K., & Young, C. (1999). Effects of nasogastric tubes on the young, normal swallowing mechanism. *Dysphagia*, *14*(3), 157–161.

Hughes, T. A., & Wiles, C. M. (1996). Clinical measurement of swallowing in health and in neurogenic dysphagia. *Quarterly Journal of Medicine*, *89*(2), 109–116.

Humbert, I. A., Poletto, C. J., Saxon, K. G., Kearney, P. R., Crujido, L., Wright-Harp, W., et al. (2006). The effect of surface electrical stimulation on hyolaryngeal movement in normal individuals at rest and during swallowing. *Journal of Applied Physiology*, *101*(6), 1657–1663.

Iizuka, M., & Reding, M. (2005). Use of percutaneous endoscopic gastrostomy feeding tubes and functional recovery in stroke rehabilitation: A case-matched controlled study. *Archives of Physical Medicine and Rehabilitation, 86*(5), 1049–1052.

Irie, H., & Lu, C. C. (1995). Dynamic evaluation of swallowing in patients with cerebrovascular accident. *Clinical Imaging, 19*(4), 240–243.

Jacob, P., Kahrilas, P. J., Logemann, J. A., Shah, V., & Ha, T. (1989). Upper esophageal sphincter opening and modulation during swallowing. *Gastroenterology, 97*(6), 1469–1478.

Jacobs, J. R., Logemann, J., Pajak, T. F., Pauloski, B. R., Collins, S., Casiano, R. R., et al. (1999). Failure of cricopharyngeal myotomy to improve dysphagia following head and neck cancer surgery. *Archives of Otolaryngology-Head and Neck Surgery, 125*(9), 942–946.

James, A., Kapur, K., & Hawthorne, A. B. (1998). Long-term outcome of percutaneous endoscopic gastrostomy feeding in patients with dysphagic stroke. *Age and Ageing, 27*(6), 671–676.

Jankel, W. R. (1978). Bell palsy: Muscle reeducation by electromyograph feedback. *Archives of Physical Medicine and Rehabilitation, 59*(5), 240–242.

Jean, A. (1984a). Brainstem organization of the swallowing network. *Brain, Behavior, and Evolution, 25*(2–3), 109–116.

Jean, A. (1984b). Control of the central swallowing program by inputs from the peripheral receptors. A review. *Journal of Autonomic Nervous System, 10*(3–4), 225–233.

Jean, A. (1990). Brainstem control of swallowing: Localization and organization of the central pattern generator for swallowing. In A. Taylor (Ed.), *Neurophysiology of the jaws and teeth.* London: MacMillan Press.

Jean, A., Amri, M., & Calas, A. (1983). Connections between the ventral medullary swallowing area and the trigeminal motor nucleus of the sheep studied by tracing techniques. *Journal of the Autonomic Nervous System, 7*(2), 87–96.

Jean, A., & Car, A. (1979). Inputs to the swallowing medullary neurons from the peripheral afferent fibers and the swallowing cortical area. *Brain Research, 178*(2–3), 567–572.

Jennings, K. S., Siroky, D., & Jackson, C. G. (1992). Swallowing problems after excision of tumors of the skull base: Diagnosis and management in 12 patients. *Dysphagia, 7*(1), 40–44.

Johnson, E. R., McKenzie, S. W., & Sievers, A. (1993). Aspiration pneumonia in stroke. *Archives of Physical Medicine and Rehabilitation, 74*(9), 973–976.

Jurell, K. C., Shaker, R., Mazur, A., Haig, A. J., & Wertsch, J. J. (1996). Spectral analysis to evaluate hyoid muscles involvement in neck exercise [Abstract]. *Muscle Nerve, 19*, 1224.

Kaatzke-McDonald, M. N., Post, E., & Davis, P. J. (1996). The effects of cold, touch, and chemical stimulation of the anterior faucial pillar on human swallowing. *Dysphagia, 11*(3), 198-206.

Kahrilas, P. J., Dodds, W. J., Dent, J., Logemann, J. A., & Shaker, R. (1988). Upper esophageal sphincter function during deglutition. *Gastroenterology, 95*(1), 52-62.

Kahrilas, P. J., Lin, S., Chen, J., & Logemann, J. A. (1996). Oropharyngeal accommodation to swallow volume. *Gastroenterology, 111*(2), 297-306.

Kahrilas, P. J., Lin, S., Logemann, J. A., Ergun, G. A., & Facchini, F. (1993). Deglutitive tongue action: Volume accommodation and bolus propulsion. *Gastroenterology, 104*(1), 152-162.

Kahrilas, P. J., Logemann, J. A., Krugler, C., & Flanagan, E. (1991). Volitional augmentation of upper esophageal sphincter opening during swallowing. *American Journal of Physiology, 260*(3 Pt. 1), G450-G456.

Kahrilas, P. J., Logemann, J. A., Lin, S., & Ergun, G. A. (1992). Pharyngeal clearance during swallowing: A combined manometric and videofluoroscopic study. *Gastroenterology, 103*(1), 128-136.

Kasman, G. (1996). Motor learning with EMG biofeedback: An information processing perspective for rehabilitation. *Biofeedback, 59*, 240-242.

Kastelik, J. A., Thompson, R. H., Aziz, I., Ojoo, J. C., Redington, A. E., & Morice, A. H. (2002). Sex-related differences in cough reflex sensitivity in patients with chronic cough. *American Journal of Respiration and Critical Care Medicine, 166*(7), 961-964.

Kelly, A. M., Drinnan, M. J., & Leslie, P. (2007). Assessing penetration and aspiration: How do videofluoroscopy and fiberoptic endoscopic evaluation of swallowing compare? *Laryngoscope, 117*(10), 1723-1727.

Kelly, A. M., Leslie, P., Beale, T., Payten, C., & Drinnan, M. J. (2006). Fibreoptic endoscopic evaluation of swallowing and videofluoroscopy: Does examination type influence perception of pharyngeal residue severity? *Clinical Otolaryngology, 31*(5), 425-432.

Kern, M., Bardan, E., Arndorfer, R., Hofmann, C., Ren, J., & Shaker, R. (1999). Comparison of upper esophageal sphincter opening in healthy asymptomatic young and elderly volunteers. *Annals of Otology, Rhinology and Laryngology, 108*(10), 982-989.

Kern, M. K., Jaradeh, S., Arndorfer, R. C., & Shaker, R. (2001). Cerebral cortical representation of reflexive and volitional swallowing in humans. *American Journal of Physiology-Gastrointestinal and Liver Physiology*, *280*(3), G354–G360.

Kessler, J. P., & Jean, A. (1985). Identification of the medullary swallowing regions in the rat. *Experimental Brain Research*, *57*(2), 256–263.

Kidd, D., Lawson, J., Nesbitt, R., & MacMahon, J. (1993). Aspiration in acute stroke: A clinical study with videofluoroscopy. *Quarterly Journal of Medicine*, *86*(12), 825–829.

Kiger, M., Brown, C. S., & Watkins, L. (2006). Dysphagia management: An analysis of patient outcomes using VitalStim therapy compared to traditional swallow therapy. *Dysphagia*, *21*(4), 243–253.

Kim, H., Chung, C. S., Lee, K. H., & Robbins, J. (2000). Aspiration subsequent to a pure medullary infarction: Lesion sites, clinical variables, and outcome. *Archives of Neurology*, *57*(4), 478–483.

Kim, J., & Sapienza, C. M. (2005). Implications of expiratory muscle strength training for rehabilitation of the elderly: Tutorial. *Journal of Rehabilitation Resarch and Development*, *42*(2), 211–224.

Kirchner, J. A., Scatliff, J. H., Dey, F. L., & Shedd, D. P. (1963). The pharynx after laryngectomy. Changes in its structure and function. *Laryngoscope*, *73*, 18–33.

Klahn, M. S., & Perlman, A. L. (1999). Temporal and durational patterns associating respiration and swallowing. *Dysphagia*, *14*(3), 131–138.

Kleindorfer, D., Broderick, J., Khoury, J., Flaherty, M., Woo, D., Alwell, K., et al. (2006). The unchanging incidence and case-fatality of stroke in the 1990s: A population-based study. *Stroke*, *37*(10), 2473–2478.

Klor, B. M., & Milianti, F. J. (1999). Rehabilitation of neurogenic dysphagia with percutaneous endoscopic gastrostomy. *Dysphagia*, *14*(3), 162–164.

Kobayashi, H., Hoshino, M., Okayama, K., Sekizawa, K., & Sasaki, H. (1994). Swallowing and cough reflexes after onset of stroke. *Chest*, *105*(5), 1623.

Krespi, Y. P., Quatela, V. C., Sisson, G. A., & Som, M. L. (1984). Modified tracheoesophageal diversion for chronic aspiration. *Laryngoscope*, *94*(10), 1298–1301.

Kuhlemeier, K. V., Palmer, J. B., & Rosenberg, D. (2001). Effect of liquid bolus consistency and delivery method on aspiration and pharyngeal retention in dysphagia patients. *Dysphagia*, *16*(2), 119–122.

Kuhlemeier, K. V., Yates, P., & Palmer, J. B. (1998). Intra- and interrater variation in the evaluation of videofluorographic swallowing studies. *Dysphagia*, *13*(3), 142-147.

Kuypers, H. G. (1958a). Corticobular connexions to the pons and lower brain-stem in man: An anatomical study. *Brain*, *81*(3), 364-388.

Kuypers, H. G. (1958b). Some projections from the peri-central cortex to the pons and lower brain stem in monkey and chimpanzee. *Journal of Comparative Neurology*, *110*(2), 221-255.

Langmore, S. E., & Aviv, J. E. (2001). Endoscopic procedures to evaluate oropharyngeal swallowing. In S. E. Langmore (Ed.), *Endoscopic evaluation and treatment of swallowing disorders* (pp. 73-100). New York: Thieme.

Langmore, S. E., Terpenning, M. S., Schork, A., Chen, Y., Murray, J. T., Lopatin, D., et al. (1998). Predictors of aspiration pneumonia: How important is dysphagia? *Dysphagia*, *13*(2), 69-81.

Lazarus, C., Logemann, J. A., Huang, C. F., & Rademaker, A. W. (2003). Effects of two types of tongue strengthening exercises in young normals. *Folia Phoniatrica et Logopaedica*, *55*(4), 199-205.

Lazarus, C., Logemann, J. A., Rademaker, A. W., Kahrilas, P. J., Pajak, T., Lazar, R., et al. (1993). Effects of bolus volume, viscosity, and repeated swallows in nonstroke subjects and stroke patients. *Archives of Physical Medicine and Rehabilitation*, *74*(10), 1066-1070.

Lazarus, C., Logemann, J. A., Song, C. W., Rademaker, A. W., & Kahrilas, P. J. (2002). Effects of voluntary maneuvers on tongue base function for swallowing. *Folia Phoniatrica et Logopaedica*, *54*(4), 171-176.

Lazzara, G., Lazarus, C., & Logemann, J. A. (1986). Impact of thermal stimulation on the triggering of the swallowing reflex. *Dysphagia*, *1*, 73-77.

Leder, S. B. (1996). Gag reflex and dysphagia. *Head and Neck*, *18*(2), 138-141.

Leder, S. B. (1997). Videofluoroscopic evaluation of aspiration with visual examination of the gag reflex and velar movement. *Dysphagia*, *12*(1), 21-23.

Leder, S. B. (2000). Use of arterial oxygen saturation, heart rate, and blood pressure as indirect objective physiologic markers to predict aspiration. *Dysphagia*, *15*(4), 201-205.

Leder, S. B., Acton, L. M., Lisitano, H. L., & Murray, J. T. (2005). Fiberoptic endoscopic evaluation of swallowing (FEES) with and without blue-dyed food. *Dysphagia*, *20*(2), 157-162.

Leder, S. B., & Espinosa, J. F. (2002). Aspiration risk after acute stroke: comparison of clinical examination and fiberoptic endoscopic evaluation of swallowing. *Dysphagia, 17*(3), 214–218.

Leder, S. B., Ross, D. A., Briskin, K. B., & Sasaki, C. T. (1997). A prospective, double-blind, randomized study on the use of a topical anesthetic, vasoconstrictor, and placebo during transnasal flexible fiberoptic endoscopy. *Journal of Speech, Language, and Hearing Research, 40*(6), 1352–1357.

Leelamanit, V., Limsakul, C., & Geater, A. (2002). Synchronized electrical stimulation in treating pharyngeal dysphagia. *Laryngoscope, 112*(12), 2204–2210.

Leopold, N. A., & Kagel, M. C. (1997). Dysphagia—Ingestion or deglutition? A proposed paradigm. *Dysphagia, 12*(4), 202–206.

Leow, L. P., Huckabee, M. L., Sharma, S., & Tooley, T. P. (2007). The influence of taste on swallowing apnea, oral preparation time, and duration and amplitude of submental muscle contraction. *Chemical Senses, 32*(2), 119–128.

Leslie, P., Drinnan, M. J., Finn, P., Ford, G. A., & Wilson, J. A. (2004). Reliability and validity of cervical auscultation: A controlled comparison using videofluoroscopy. *Dysphagia, 19*(4), 231–240.

Leslie, P., Drinnan, M. J., Ford, G. A., & Wilson, J. A. (2002). Swallow respiration patterns in dysphagic patients following acute stroke. *Dysphagia, 17*(3), 202–207.

Lin, Y. N., Chen, S. Y., Wang, T. G., Chang, Y. C., Chie, W. C., & Lien, I. N. (2005). Findings of videofluoroscopic swallowing studies are associated with tube feeding dependency at discharge in stroke patients with dysphagia. *Dysphagia, 20*(1), 23–31.

Linden, P., Kuhlemeier, K. V., & Patterson, C. (1993). The probability of correctly predicting subglottic penetration from clinical observations. *Dysphagia, 8*(3), 170–179.

Linden, P., & Siebens, A. A. (1983). Dysphagia: Predicting laryngeal penetration. *Archives of Physical Medicine and Rehabilitation, 64*(6), 281–284.

Link, D. T., Willging, J. P., Miller, C. K., Cotton, R. T., & Rudolph, C. D. (2000). Pediatric laryngopharyngeal sensory testing during flexible endoscopic evaluation of swallowing: Feasible and correlative. *Annals of Otology, Rhinology, and Laryngology, 109*(10 Pt. 1), 899–905.

Logemann, J. A. (1983). *Evaulation and treatment of swallowing disorders* (1st ed.). San Diego, CA: College-Hill.

Logemann, J. A. (1998). *Evaluation and treatment of swallowing disorders* (2nd ed.). Austin, TX: Pro-Ed.

Logemann, J. A., Gensler, G., Robbins, J., Lindblad, A., Brandt, D., Hind, J. A., et al. (2008). A randomized study of three interventions for aspiration of thin liquids in patients with dementia and Parkinson's disease. *Journal of Speech, Language, and Hearing Research, 51*, 173–183.

Logemann, J. A., & Kahrilas, P. J. (1990). Relearning to swallow after stroke-Application of maneuvers and indirect biofeedback: A case study. *Neurology, 40*(7), 1136–1138.

Logemann, J. A., Kahrilas, P. J., Cheng, J., Pauloski, B. R., Gibbons, P. J., Rademaker, A. W., et al. (1992). Closure mechanisms of laryngeal vestibule during swallow. *American Journal of Physiology, 262*(2 Pt. 1), G338–G344.

Logemann, J. A., Kahrilas, P. J., Kobara, M., & Vakil, N. B. (1989). The benefit of head rotation on pharyngoesophageal dysphagia. *Archives of Physical Medicine and Rehabilitation, 70*(10), 767–771.

Logemann, J. A., Pauloski, B. R., Colangelo, L., Lazarus, C., Fujiu, M., & Kahrilas, P. J. (1995). Effects of a sour bolus on oropharyngeal swallowing measures in patients with neurogenic dysphagia. *Journal of Speech and Hearing Research, 38*(3), 556–563.

Logemann, J. A., Pauloski, B. R., Rademaker, A. W., Colangelo, L. A., Kahrilas, P. J., & Smith, C. H. (2000). Temporal and biomechanical characteristics of oropharyngeal swallow in younger and older men. *Journal of Speech, Language, and Hearing Research, 43*(5), 1264–1274.

Logemann, J. A., Shanahan, T., Rademaker, A. W., Kahrilas, P. J., Lazar, R., & Halper, A. (1993). Oropharyngeal swallowing after stroke in the left basal ganglion/internal capsule. *Dysphagia, 8*(3), 230–234.

Logemann, J. A., Veis, S., & Colangelo, L. (1999). A screening procedure for oropharyngeal dysphagia. *Dysphagia, 14*(1), 44–51.

Lucas, C. E., Yu, P., Vlahos, A., & Ledgerwood, A. M. (1999). Lower esophageal sphincter dysfunction often precludes safe gastric feeding in stroke patients. *Archives of Surgery, 134*(1), 55–58.

Ludlow, C. L., Humbert, I., Poletto, C. J., Saxon, K. G., Kearney, P. R., Crujido, L., et al. (2005). *The use of coordination training for the onset of intramuscular stimulation in dysphagia.* Paper presented at the 10th annual conference of the International FES Society, Montreal, Quebec, Canada.

Ludlow, C. L., Humbert, I., Saxon, K., Poletto, C., Sonies, B., & Crujido, L. (2007). Effects of surface electrical stimulation both at rest and during swallowing in chronic pharyngeal dysphagia. *Dysphagia, 22*(1), 1–10.

Mamun, K., & Lim, J. (2005). Role of nasogastric tube in preventing aspiration pneumonia in patients with dysphagia. *Singapore Medical Journal, 46*(11), 627–631.

Mann, G. (2002). *MASA: The Mann Assessment of Swallowing Ability.* Clifton Park, NY: Thomson Delmar Learning.

Mann, G., & Hankey, G. J. (2001). Initial clinical and demographic predictors of swallowing impairment following acute stroke. *Dysphagia, 16*(3), 208–215.

Mann, G., Hankey, G. J., & Cameron, D. (1999). Swallowing function after stroke: Prognosis and prognostic factors at 6 months. *Stroke, 30*(4), 744–748.

Mann, G., Hankey, G. J., & Cameron, D. (2000). Swallowing disorders following acute stroke: Prevalence and diagnostic accuracy. *Cerebrovascular Disorders, 10*(5), 380–386.

Martin-Harris, B., Brodsky, M. B., Michel, Y., Ford, C. L., Walters, B., & Heffner, J. (2005). Breathing and swallowing dynamics across the adult lifespan. *Archives of Otolaryngology-Head and Neck Surgery, 131*(9), 762–770.

Martin-Harris, B., Brodsky, M. B., Michel, Y., Lee, F. S., & Walters, B. (2007). Delayed initiation of the pharyngeal swallow: Normal variability in adult swallows. *Journal of Speech, Language, and Hearing Research, 50*(3), 585–594.

Martin-Harris, B., & Easterling, C. S. (2006). *Esophageal swallowing physiology and disorders* [Electronic presentation]. Rockville, MD: American Speech-Language-Hearing Association.

Martin, B. J., Logemann, J. A., Shaker, R., & Dodds, W. J. (1993). Normal laryngeal valving patterns during three breath-hold maneuvers: A pilot investigation. *Dysphagia, 8*(1), 11–20.

Martin, B. J., Logemann, J. A., Shaker, R., & Dodds, W. J. (1994). Coordination between respiration and swallowing: Respiratory phase relationships and temporal integration. *Journal of Applied Physiology, 76*(2), 714–723.

Martin, R. E., Goodyear, B. G., Gati, J. S., & Menon, R. S. (2001). Cerebral cortical representation of automatic and volitional swallowing in humans. *Journal of Neurophysiology, 85*(2), 938–950.

Martino, R., Foley, N., Bhogal, S., Diamant, N., Speechley, M., & Teasell, R. (2005). Dysphagia after stroke: Incidence, diagnosis, and pulmonary complications. *Stroke, 36*(12), 2756-2763.

Martino, R., Terrault, N., Ezerzer, F., Mikulis, D., & Diamant, N. E. (2001). Dysphagia in a patient with lateral medullary syndrome: Insight into the central control of swallowing. *Gastroenterology, 121*(2), 420-426.

McConnel, F. M. (1988). Analysis of pressure generation and bolus transit during pharyngeal swallowing. *Laryngoscope, 98*(1), 71-78.

McCullough, G. H., Rosenbek, J. C., Wertz, R. T., McCoy, S., Mann, G., & McCullough, K. (2005). Utility of clinical swallowing examination measures for detecting aspiration post-stroke. *Journal of Speech, Language, and Hearing Research, 48*(6), 1280-1293.

McCullough, G. H., Wertz, R. T., & Rosenbek, J. C. (2001). Sensitivity and specificity of clinical/bedside examination signs for detecting aspiration in adults subsequent to stroke. *Journal of Communication Disorders, 34*(1-2), 55-72.

McCullough, G. H., Wertz, R. T., Rosenbek, J. C., Mills, R. H., Ross, K. B., & Ashford, J. R. (2000). Inter- and intrajudge reliability of a clinical examination of swallowing in adults. *Dysphagia, 15*(2), 58-67.

McCullough, G. H., Wertz, R. T., Rosenbek, J. C., Mills, R. H., Webb, W. G., & Ross, K. B. (2001). Inter- and intrajudge reliability for videofluoroscopic swallowing evaluation measures. *Dysphagia, 16*(2), 110-118.

McHorney, C. A., Martin-Harris, B., Robbins, J., & Rosenbek, J. (2006). Clinical validity of the SWAL-QOL and SWAL-CARE outcome tools with respect to bolus flow measures. *Dysphagia, 21*(3), 141-148.

McHorney, C. A., Robbins, J., Lomax, K., Rosenbek, J. C., Chignell, K., Kramer, A. E., et al. (2002). The SWAL-QOL and SWAL-CARE outcomes tool for oropharyngeal dysphagia in adults: III. Documentation of reliability and validity. *Dysphagia, 17*(2), 97-114.

Mendelsohn, M. S., & Martin, R. E. (1993). Airway protection during breath-holding. *Annals of Otology, Rhinology, and Laryngology, 102*(12), 941-944.

Meng, N. H., Wang, T. G., & Lien, I. N. (2000). Dysphagia in patients with brainstem stroke: Incidence and outcome. *American Journal of Physical Medicine and Rehabilitation, 79*(2), 170-175.

Mesulam, M. M., & Mufson, E. J. (1985). The insula of Reil in man and monkey: architectonics, connectivity, and function. In A. Peters & E. G. Jones

(Eds.), *Cerebral cortex, Volume 4, Association and auditory cortices* (pp. 179–226). New York: Plenum.

Metzger, B. L., & Therrien, B. (1990). Effect of position on cardiovascular response during the Valsalva maneuver. *Nursing Research*, *39*(4), 198–202.

Midgren, B., Hansson, L., Karlsson, J. A., Simonsson, B. G., & Persson, C. G. (1992). Capsaicin-induced cough in humans. *American Review of Respiratory Disease*, *146*(2), 347–351.

Miller, A. J. (1972). Characteristics of the swallowing reflex induced by peripheral nerve and brain stem stimulation. *Experimental Neurology*, *34*(2), 210–222.

Miller, A. J. (1999). *The neuroscientific principles of swallowing and dysphagia*. San Diego, CA: Singular.

Miller, A. J., Bieger, D., & Conklin, J. L. (1997). Functional controls of deglutition. In A. L. Perlman & K. Schulze-Delreiu (Eds.), *Deglutition and its disorders* (pp. 43–98). San Diego, CA: Singular.

Miller, A. J., & Bowman, J. P. (1977). Precentral cortical modulation of mastication and swallowing. *Journal of Dental Research*, *56*(10), 1154.

Miller, F. R., & Sherrington, C. S. (1916). Some observations on the buccopharyngeal stage of reflex deglutition in the cat. *Quarterly Journal of Experimental Physiology*, *9*, 147–186.

Miller, J. L., & Watkin, K. L. (1996). The influence of bolus volume and viscosity on anterior lingual force during the oral stage of swallowing. *Dysphagia*, *11*(2), 117–124.

Miller, J. L., & Watkin, K. L. (1997). Lateral pharyngeal wall motion during swallowing using real time ultrasound. *Dysphagia*, *12*(3), 125–132.

Miyaoka, Y., Haishima, K., Takagi, M., Haishima, H., Asari, J., & Yamada, Y. (2006). Influences of thermal and gustatory characteristics on sensory and motor aspects of swallowing. *Dysphagia*, *21*(1), 38–48.

Morice, A. H., Kastelik, J. A., & Thompson, R. (2001). Cough challenge in the assessment of cough reflex. *British Journal of Clinical Pharmacology*, *52*(4), 365–375.

Mosier, K., & Bereznaya, I. (2001). Parallel cortical networks for volitional control of swallowing in humans. *Experimental Brain Research*, *140*(3), 280–289.

Mufson, E. J., & Mesulam, M. M. (1984). Thalamic connections of the insula in the rhesus monkey and comments on the paralimbic connectivity of the medial pulvinar nucleus. *Journal of Comparative Neurology*, *227*(1), 109–120.

Mullan, H., Roubenoff, R. A., & Roubenoff, R. (1992). Risk of pulmonary aspiration among patients receiving enteral nutrition support. *JPEN Journal of Parenteral and Enteral Nutrition*, *16*(2), 160–164.

Murray, J. (1999). *Manual of dysphagia assessment in adults*. San Diego, CA: Singular.

Murray, J., Langmore, S. E., Ginsberg, S., & Dostie, A. (1996). The significance of accumulated oropharyngeal secretions and swallowing frequency in predicting aspiration. *Dysphagia*, *11*(2), 99–103.

Nakajoh, K., Nakagawa, T., Sekizawa, K., Matsui, T., Arai, H., & Sasaki, H. (2000). Relation between incidence of pneumonia and protective reflexes in post-stroke patients with oral or tube feeding. *Journal of Internal Medicine*, *247*(1), 39–42.

Netsell, R., & Cleeland, C. S. (1973). Modification of lip hypertonia in dysarthria using EMG feedback. *Journal of Speech and Hearing Disorders*, *38*(1), 131–140.

Neumann, S. (1993). Swallowing therapy with neurologic patients: Results of direct and indirect therapy methods in 66 patients suffering from neurological disorders. *Dysphagia*, *8*(2), 150–153.

Neumann, S., Bartolome, G., Buchholz, D., & Prosiegel, M. (1995). Swallowing therapy of neurologic patients: Correlation of outcome with pretreatment variables and therapeutic methods. *Dysphagia*, *10*(1), 1–5.

Nicosia, M. A., Hind, J. A., Roecker, E. B., Carnes, M., Doyle, J., Dengel, G. A., et al. (2000). Age effects on the temporal evolution of isometric and swallowing pressure. *Journals of Gerontology Series: Biological Sciences and Medical Sciences*, *55*(11), M634–M640.

Nilsson, H., Ekberg, O., Bulow, M., & Hindfelt, B. (1997). Assessment of respiration during video fluoroscopy of dysphagic patients. *Academic Radiology*, *4*(7), 503–507.

Nishino, T., & Hiraga, K. (1991). Coordination of swallowing and respiration in unconscious subjects. *Journal of Applied Physiology*, *70*(3), 988–993.

Norton, B., Homer-Ward, M., Donnelly, M. T., Long, R. G., & Holmes, G. K. (1996). A randomised prospective comparison of percutaneous endoscopic gastrostomy and nasogastric tube feeding after acute dysphagic stroke. *British Medical Journal*, *312*(7022), 13–16.

Odderson, I. R., Keaton, J. C., & McKenna, B. S. (1995). Swallow management in patients on an acute stroke pathway: Quality is cost effective. *Archives of Physical Medicine and Rehabilitation, 76*(12), 1130-1133.

Ohmae, Y., Logemann, J. A., Kaiser, P., Hanson, D. G., & Kahrilas, P. J. (1995). Timing of glottic closure during normal swallow. *Head and Neck, 17*(5), 394-402.

Ohmae, Y., Logemann, J. A., Kaiser, P., Hanson, D. G., & Kahrilas, P. J. (1996). Effects of two breath-holding maneuvers on oropharyngeal swallow. *Annals of Otology, Rhinology, and Laryngology, 105*(2), 123-131.

Olsson, R., Kjellin, O., & Ekberg, O. (1996). Videomanometric aspects of pharyngeal constrictor activity. *Dysphagia, 11*(2), 83-86.

Olsson, R., Nilsson, H., & Ekberg, O. (1995). Simultaneous videoradiography and pharyngeal solid state manometry (videomanometry) in 25 nondysphagic volunteers. *Dysphagia, 10*(1), 36-41.

Palmer, J. B., & Hiiemae, K. M. (2003). Eating and breathing: Interactions between respiration and feeding on solid food. *Dysphagia, 18*(3), 169-178.

Palmer, J. B., Rudin, N. J., Lara, G., & Crompton, A. W. (1992). Coordination of mastication and swallowing. *Dysphagia, 7*(4), 187-200.

Palmer, P. M., McCulloch, T. M., Jaffe, D., & Neel, A. T. (2005). Effects of a sour bolus on the intramuscular electromyographic (EMG) activity of muscles in the submental region. *Dysphagia, 20*(3), 210-217.

Panther, K. (2005). The Frazier free water protocol. *Perspectives on Swallowing and Swallowing Disorders, 14*(1), 4-9.

Parameswaran, M. S., & Soliman, A. M. (2002). Endoscopic botulinum toxin injection for cricopharyngeal dysphagia. *Annals of Otology, Rhinology, and Laryngology, 111*(10), 871-874.

Park, C. L., O'Neill, P. A., & Martin, D. F. (1997). A pilot exploratory study of oral electrical stimulation on swallow function following stroke: An innovative technique. *Dysphagia, 12*(3), 161-166.

Park, R. H., Allison, M. C., Lang, J., Spence, E., Morris, A. J., Danesh, B. J., et al. (1992). Randomised comparison of percutaneous endoscopic gastrostomy and nasogastric tube feeding in patients with persisting neurological dysphagia. *British Medical Journal, 304*(6839), 1406-1409.

Parker, C., Power, M., Hamdy, S., Bowen, A., Tyrrell, P., & Thompson, D. G. (2004). Awareness of dysphagia by patients following stroke predicts swallowing performance. *Dysphagia, 19*(1), 28-35.

Passingham, R. (1993). *The frontal lobes and voluntary action.* Oxford: Oxford University Press.

Pelletier, C. A., & Dhanaraj, G. E. (2006). The effect of taste and palatability on lingual swallowing pressure. *Dysphagia, 21*(2), 121-128.

Pelletier, C. A., & Lawless, H. T. (2003). Effect of citric acid and citric acid-sucrose mixtures on swallowing in neurogenic oropharyngeal dysphagia. *Dysphagia, 18*(4), 231-241.

Perlman, A. L., Booth, B. M., & Grayhack, J. P. (1994). Videofluoroscopic predictors of aspiration in patients with oropharyngeal dysphagia. *Dysphagia, 9*(2), 90-95.

Perlman, A. L., He, X., Barkmeier, J., & Van Leer, E. (2005). Bolus location associated with videofluoroscopic and respirodeglutometric events. *Journal of Speech, Language, and Hearing Research, 48*(1), 21-33.

Perlman, A. L., Schultz, J. G., & VanDaele, D. J. (1993). Effects of age, gender, bolus volume, and bolus viscosity on oropharyngeal pressure during swallowing. *Journal of Applied Physiology, 75*(1), 33-37.

Poirier, N. C., Bonavina, L., Taillefer, R., Nosadini, A., Peracchia, A., & Duranceau, A. (1997). Cricopharyngeal myotomy for neurogenic oropharyngeal dysphagia. *Journal of Thoracic and Cardiovascular Surgery, 113*(2), 233-240; discussion 240-231.

Pouderoux, P., & Kahrilas, P. J. (1995). Deglutitive tongue force modulation by volition, volume, and viscosity in humans. *Gastroenterology, 108*(5), 1418-1426.

Pouderoux, P., Logemann, J. A., & Kahrilas, P. J. (1996). Pharyngeal swallowing elicited by fluid infusion: Role of volition and vallecular containment. *American Journal of Physiology, 270*(2 Pt. 1), G347-G354.

Pounsford, J. C., & Saunders, K. B. (1985). Diurnal variation and adaptation of the cough response to citric acid in normal subjects. *Thorax, 40*(9), 657-661.

Power, M., Fraser, C., Hobson, A., Rothwell, J. C., Mistry, S., Nicholson, D. A., et al. (2004). Changes in pharyngeal corticobulbar excitability and swallowing behavior after oral stimulation. *American Journal of Physiology-Gastrointestinal and Liver Physiology, 286*(1), G45-G50.

Preiksaitis, H. G., & Mills, C. A. (1996). Coordination of breathing and swallowing: Effects of bolus consistency and presentation in normal adults. *Journal of Applied Physiology, 81*(4), 1707-1714.

Rademaker, A. W., Pauloski, B. R., Colangelo, L. A., & Logemann, J. A. (1998). Age and volume effects on liquid swallowing function in normal women. *Journal of Speech, Language, and Hearing Research, 41*(2), 275-284.

Ragnarsson, K. T. (1994). The physiologic aspects and clinical application of functional electrical stimulation in rehabilitation. In J. A. Downey, S. J. Myers, E. G. Gonzalez, & J. S. Lieberman (Eds.), *The physiological basis of rehabilitation medicine* (2nd ed., pp. 573-597). Boston: Butterworth-Heinemann.

Ramig, L. O., Countryman, S., O'Brien, C., Hoehn, M., & Thompson, L. (1996). Intensive speech treatment for patients with Parkinson's disease: Short- and long-term comparison of two techniques. *Neurology, 47*(6), 1496-1504.

Ramig, L. O., Countryman, S., Thompson, L. L., & Horii, Y. (1995). Comparison of two forms of intensive speech treatment for Parkinson disease. *Journal of Speech and Hearing Research, 38*(6), 1232-1251.

Ramig, L. O., & Dromey, C. (1996). Aerodynamic mechanisms underlying treatment-related changes in vocal intensity in patients with Parkinson disease. *Journal of Speech and Hearing Research, 39*(4), 798-807.

Ramig, L. O., Sapir, S., Countryman, S., Pawlas, A. A., O'Brien, C., Hoehn, M., & Thompson, L. L. (2001). Intensive voice treatment (LSVT) for patients with Parkinson's disease: A 2-year follow-up. *Journal of Neurology, Neurosurgery and Psychiatry, 71*(4), 493-498.

Ramig, L. O., Sapir, S., Fox, C., & Countryman, S. (2001). Changes in vocal loudness following intensive voice treatment (LSVT) in individuals with Parkinson's disease: A comparison with untreated patients and normal age-matched controls. *Movement Disorders, 16*(1), 79-83.

Ramsey, D., Smithard, D., Donaldson, N., & Kalra, L. (2005). Is the gag reflex useful in the management of swallowing problems in acute stroke? *Dysphagia, 20*(2), 105-107.

Rasley, A., Logemann, J. A., Kahrilas, P. J., Rademaker, A. W., Pauloski, B. R., & Dodds, W. J. (1993). Prevention of barium aspiration during videofluoroscopic swallowing studies: Value of change in posture. *AJR American Journal of Roentgenology, 160*(5), 1005-1009.

Ravich, W. J. (2001). Botulinum toxin for UES dysfunction: therapy or poison? *Dysphagia, 16*(3), 168-170.

Reimers-Neils, L., Logemann, J., & Larson, C. (1994). Viscosity effects on EMG activity in normal swallow. *Dysphagia, 9*(2), 101-106.

Ren, J., Shaker, R., Zamir, Z., Dodds, W. J., Hogan, W. J., & Hoffmann, R. G. (1993). Effect of age and bolus variables on the coordination of the glottis and upper esophageal sphincter during swallowing. *American Journal of Gastroenterology, 88*(5), 665-669.

Richter, J. E., & Castell, J. A. (1989). Esophageal manometry. In D. W. Gelfand & J. E. Richter (Eds.), *Dysphagia: Diagnosis and treatment* (pp. 83–114). New York: IgatsuShoin.

Robbins, J., Coyle, J., Rosenbek, J., Roecker, E., & Wood, J. (1999). Differentiation of normal and abnormal airway protection during swallowing using the penetration-aspiration scale. *Dysphagia, 14*(4), 228–232.

Robbins, J., Gangnon, R. E., Theis, S. M., Kays, S. A., Hewitt, A. L., & Hind, J. A. (2005). The effects of lingual exercise on swallowing in older adults. *Journal of the American Geriatrics Society, 53*(9), 1483–1489.

Robbins, J., Hamilton, J. W., Lof, G. L., & Kempster, G. B. (1992). Oropharyngeal swallowing in normal adults of different ages. *Gastroenterology, 103*(3), 823–829.

Robbins, J., Kays, S. A., Gangnon, R. E., Hind, J. A., Hewitt, A. L., Gentry, L. R., & Taylor, A. J. (2007). The effects of lingual exercise in stroke patients with dysphagia. *Archives of Physical Medicine and Rehabilitation, 88*(2), 150–158.

Robbins, J., & Levine, R. L. (1988). Swallowing after unilateral stroke of the cerebral cortex: Preliminary experience. *Dysphagia, 3*(1), 11–17.

Robbins, J., & Levine, R. (1993). Swallowing after lateral medullary syndrome plus. *Clinics in Communication Disorders, 3*(4), 45–55.

Robbins, J., Levine, R., Wood, J., Roecker, E. B., & Luschei, E. (1995). Age effects on lingual pressure generation as a risk factor for dysphagia. *Journals of Gerontology Series: A Biological Sciences and Medical Sciences, 50*(5), M257–M262.

Robbins, J., Levine, R. L., Maser, A., Rosenbek, J. C., & Kempster, G. B. (1993). Swallowing after unilateral stroke of the cerebral cortex. *Archives of Physical Medicine and Rehabilitation, 74*(12), 1295–1300.

Roland, P. E., Larsen, B., Lassen, N. A., & Skinhoj, E. (1980). Supplementary motor area and other cortical areas in organization of voluntary movements in man. *Journal of Neurophysiology, 43*(1), 118–136.

Roman, C. (1986). Neural control of deglutition and esophageal motility in mammals [in French]. *Journal of Physiology (Paris), 81*(2), 118–131.

Rosenbek, J. C., Robbins, J., Fishback, B., & Levine, R. L. (1991). Effects of thermal application on dysphagia after stroke. *Journal of Speech and Hearing Research, 34*(6), 1257–1268.

Rosenbek, J. C., Robbins, J., Willford, W. O., Kirk, G., Schiltz, A., Sowell, T. W., et al. (1998). Comparing treatment intensities of tactile-thermal application. *Dysphagia, 13*(1), 1-9.

Rosenbek, J. C., Robbins, J. A., Roecker, E. B., Coyle, J. L., & Wood, J. L. (1996). A Penetration-Aspiration Scale. *Dysphagia, 11*(2), 93-98.

Rosenbek, J. C., Roecker, E. B., Wood, J. L., & Robbins, J. (1996). Thermal application reduces the duration of stage transition in dysphagia after stroke. *Dysphagia, 11*(4), 225-233.

Rossignol, S., & Dubuc, R. (1994). Spinal pattern generation. *Current Opinions in Neurobiology, 4*(6), 894-902.

Rothwell, P. M., Coull, A. J., Giles, M. F., Howard, S. C., Silver, L. E., Bull, L. M., et al. (2004). Change in stroke incidence, mortality, case-fatality, severity, and risk factors in Oxfordshire, UK from 1981 to 2004 (Oxford Vascular Study). *Lancet, 363*(9425), 1925-1933.

Rubow, R. (1984). Reinforcement and compliance on training and transfer in biofeedback-based rehabilitation of motor speech disorders. In M. R. McNeil, J. C. Rosenbek, & A. E. Aronson (Eds.), *The dysarthrias: Physiology, acoustics, perception, and managment* (pp. 207-229). San Diego, CA: College-Hill Press.

Sacco, R. L., Boden-Albala, B., Gan, R., Chen, X., Kargman, D. E., Shea, S., et al. (1998). Stroke incidence among white, black, and Hispanic residents of an urban community: The Northern Manhattan Stroke Study. *American Journal of Epidemiology, 147*(3), 259-268.

Saito, Y., Ezure, K., Tanaka, I., & Osawa, M. (2003). Activity of neurons in ventrolateral respiratory groups during swallowing in decerebrate rats. *Brain Development, 25*(5), 338-345.

Sala, R., Munto, M. J., de la Calle, J., Preciado, I., Miralles, T., Cortes, A., et al. (1998). [Swallowing changes in cerebrovascular accidents: Incidence, natural history, and repercussions on the nutritional status, morbidity, and mortality]. *Revista de Neurologia, 27*(159), 759-766.

Salassa, J. R., DeVault, K. R., & McConnel, F. M. (1998). Proposed catheter standards for pharyngeal manofluorography (videomanometry). *Dysphagia, 13*(2), 105-110.

Saleem, A. F., Sapienza, C. M., & Okun, M. S. (2005). Respiratory muscle strength training: treatment and response duration in a patient with early idiopathic Parkinson's disease. *NeuroRehabilitation, 20*(4), 323-333.

Sapienza, C. M., Davenport, P. W., & Martin, A. D. (2002). Expiratory muscle training increases pressure support in high school band students. *Journal of Voice, 16*(4), 495–501.

Sapienza, C. M., & Wheeler, K. (2006). Respiratory muscle strength training: Functional outcomes versus plasticity. *Seminars in Speech and Language, 27*(4), 236–244.

Schelp, A. O., Cola, P. C., Gatto, A. R., Silva, R. G., & Carvalho, L. R. (2004). [Incidence of oropharyngeal dysphagia associated with stroke in a regional hospital in Sao Paulo State - Brazil]. *Arquivos de Neuro-Psiquiatria, 62*(2B), 503–506.

Schiffman, S. S. (1993). Perception of taste and smell in elderly persons. *Critical Reviews in Food Science and Nutrition, 33*(1), 17–26.

Schroeder, M. F., Daniels, S. K., McClain, M., Corey, D. M., & Foundas, A. L. (2006). Clinical and cognitive predictors of swallowing recovery in stroke. *Journal of Rehabilitation, Research, and Development, 43*(3), 301–310.

Schulz, M. L. (1994). *The somatotopic arrangement of motor fibers in the periventricular white matter and internal capsule in the Rhesus monkey.* Dissertation. Boston University, Boston.

Schulze-Delrieu, K., & Miller, R. (1997). Clinical assessment of dysphagia. In A. L. Perlman & K. Schulze-Delreiu (Eds.), *Deglutition and its disorders* (pp. 125–152). San Diego, CA: Singular.

Scott, A., Perry, A., & Bench, J. (1998). A study of interrater reliability when using videofluoroscopy as an assessment of swallowing. *Dysphagia, 13*(4), 223–227.

Selinger, M., Prescott, T. E., & Hoffman, I. (1994). Temperature acceleration in cold oral stimulation. *Dysphagia, 9*(2), 83–87.

Selley, W. G., Flack, F. C., Ellis, R. E., & Brooks, W. A. (1989a). Respiratory patterns associated with swallowing: Part 1. The normal adult pattern and changes with age. *Age and Ageing, 18*(3), 168–172.

Selley, W. G., Flack, F. C., Ellis, R. E., & Brooks, W. A. (1989b). Respiratory patterns associated with swallowing: Part 2. Neurologically impaired dysphagic patients. *Age and Ageing, 18*(3), 173–176.

Shaker, R., Cook, I. J., Dodds, W. J., & Hogan, W. J. (1988). Pressure-flow dynamics of the oral phase of swallowing. *Dysphagia, 3*(2), 79–84.

Shaker, R., Dodds, W. J., Dantas, R. O., Hogan, W. J., & Arndorfer, R. C. (1990). Coordination of deglutitive glottic closure with oropharyngeal swallowing. *Gastroenterology, 98*(6), 1478–1484.

Shaker, R., Easterling, C., Kern, M., Nitschke, T., Massey, B., Daniels, S., et al. (2002). Rehabilitation of swallowing by exercise in tube-fed patients with pharyngeal dysphagia secondary to abnormal UES opening. *Gastroenterology, 122*(5), 1314–1321.

Shaker, R., Kern, M., Bardan, E., Taylor, A., Stewart, E. T., Hoffmann, R. G., et al. (1997). Augmentation of deglutitive upper esophageal sphincter opening in the elderly by exercise. *American Journal of Physiology, 272*(6 Pt. 1), G1518–G1522.

Shaker, R., Ren, J., Bardan, E., Easterling, C., Dua, K., Xie, P., et al. (2003). Pharyngoglottal closure reflex: Characterization in healthy young, elderly and dysphagic patients with predeglutitive aspiration. *Gerontology, 49*(1), 12–20.

Shaker, R., Ren, J., Podvrsan, B., Dodds, W. J., Hogan, W. J., Kern, M., et al. (1993). Effect of aging and bolus variables on pharyngeal and upper esophageal sphincter motor function. *American Journal of Physiology, 264*(3 Pt. 1), G427–G432.

Shaker, R., Ren, J., Zamir, Z., Sarna, A., Liu, J., & Sui, Z. (1994). Effect of aging, position, and temperature on the threshold volume triggering pharyngeal swallows. *Gastroenterology, 107*(2), 396–402.

Shanahan, T. K., Logemann, J. A., Rademaker, A. W., Pauloski, B. R., & Kahrilas, P. J. (1993). Chin-down posture effect on aspiration in dysphagic patients. *Archives of Physical Medicine and Rehabilitation, 74*(7), 736–739.

Sharma, J. C., Fletcher, S., Vassallo, M., & Ross, I. (2001). What influences outcome of stroke-Pyrexia or dysphagia? *International Journal of Clinical Practice, 55*(1), 17–20.

Shaw, D. W., Cook, I. J., Gabb, M., Holloway, R. H., Simula, M. E., Panagopoulos, V., et al. (1995). Influence of normal aging on oral-pharyngeal and upper esophageal sphincter function during swallowing. *American Journal of Physiology, 268*(3 Pt. 1), G389–G396.

Shaw, G. Y., & Searl, J. P. (2001). Botulinum toxin treatment for cricopharyngeal dysfunction. *Dysphagia, 16*(3), 161–167.

Shiba, K., Satoh, I., Kobayashi, N., & Hayashi, F. (1999). Multifunctional laryngeal motoneurons: An intracellular study in the cat. *Journal of Neuroscience, 19*(7), 2717–2727.

Silverman, E. P., Sapienza, C. M., Saleem, A., Carmichael, C., Davenport, P. W., Hoffman-Ruddy, B., et al. (2006). Tutorial on maximum inspiratory and expiratory mouth pressures in individuals with idiopathic Parkinson disease (IPD) and the preliminary results of an expiratory muscle strength training program. *NeuroRehabilitation, 21*(1), 71-79.

Sinha, U. K., James, A., & Hasan, M. (2001). Audit of percutaneous endoscopic gastrostomy (PEG): A questionnaire survey of hospital consultants. *Archives of Gerontology and Geriatrics, 32*(2), 113-118.

Smeltzer, S. C., Lavietes, M. H., & Cook, S. D. (1996). Expiratory training in multiple sclerosis. *Archives of Physical Medicine and Rehabilitation, 77*(9), 909-912.

Smith Hammond, C. A., Goldstein, L. B., Zajac, D. J., Gray, L., Davenport, P. W., & Bolser, D. C. (2001). Assessment of aspiration risk in stroke patients with quantification of voluntary cough. *Neurology, 56*(4), 502-506.

Smith, M. E., Ramig, L. O., Dromey, C., Perez, K. S., & Samandari, R. (1995). Intensive voice treatment in Parkinson disease: laryngostroboscopic findings. *Journal of Voice, 9*(4), 453-459.

Smithard, D. G., O'Neill, P. A., England, R. E., Park, C. L., Wyatt, R., Martin, D. F., et al. (1997). The natural history of dysphagia following a stroke. *Dysphagia, 12*(4), 188-193.

Smithard, D. G., O'Neill, P. A., Parks, C., & Morris, J. (1996). Complications and outcome after acute stroke. Does dysphagia matter? *Stroke, 27*(7), 1200-1204.

Solomon, N. P. (2006). What is orofacial fatigue and how does it affect function for swallowing and speech? *Seminars in Speech and Language, 27*(4), 268-282.

Spielman, J. L., Borod, J. C., & Ramig, L. O. (2003). The effects of intensive voice treatment on facial expressiveness in Parkinson disease: Preliminary data. *Cognitive and Behavioral Neurology, 16*(3), 177-188.

Splaingard, M. L., Hutchins, B., Sulton, L. D., & Chaudhuri, G. (1988). Aspiration in rehabilitation patients: videofluoroscopy vs bedside clinical assessment. *Archives of Physical Medicine and Rehabilitation, 69*(8), 637-640.

Stathopoulos, E., & Felson Duchan, J. (2006). History and principles of exercise-based therapy: How they inform our current treatment. *Seminars in Speech and Language, 27*(4), 227-235.

Steele, C. M., & Huckabee, M. L. (2007). The influence of orolingual pressure on the timing of pharyngeal pressure events. *Dysphagia, 22*(1), 30-36.

Steele, C. M., Thrasher, A. T., & Popovic, M. R. (2007). Electric stimulation approaches to the restoration and rehabilitation of swallowing: A review. *Neurological Research, 29*(1), 9-15.

Steele, C. M., & Van Lieshout, P. H. (2004). Influence of bolus consistency on lingual behaviors in sequential swallowing. *Dysphagia, 19*(3), 192-206.

Stephen, J. R., Taves, D. H., Smith, R. C., & Martin, R. E. (2005). Bolus location at the initiation of the pharyngeal stage of swallowing in healthy older adults. *Dysphagia, 20*(4), 266-272.

Sterr, A., Elbert, T., Berthold, I., Kolbel, S., Rockstroh, B., & Taub, E. (2002). Longer versus shorter daily constraint-induced movement therapy of chronic hemiparesis: An exploratory study. *Archives of Physical Medicine and Rehabilitation, 83*(10), 1374-1377.

Stoeckli, S. J., Huisman, T. A., Seifert, B., & Martin-Harris, B. J. (2003). Interrater reliability of videofluoroscopic swallow evaluation. *Dysphagia, 18*(1), 53-57.

Strub, R. L., & Black, F. W. (2000). *The mental status examination in neurology* (4th ed.). Philadelphia: F. A. Davis.

Suiter, D. M., Leder, S. B., & Ruark, J. L. (2006). Effects of neuromuscular electrical stimulation on submental muscle activity. *Dysphagia, 21*(1), 56-60.

Sumi, T. (1969). Some properties of cortically-evoked swallowing and chewing in rabbits. *Brain Research, 15*(1), 107-120.

Takahashi, K., Groher, M. E., & Michi, K. (1994). Methodology for detecting swallowing sounds. *Dysphagia, 9*(1), 54-62.

Teasell, R., Foley, N., Fisher, J., & Finestone, H. (2002). The incidence, management, and complications of dysphagia in patients with medullary strokes admitted to a rehabilitation unit. *Dysphagia, 17*(2), 115-120.

Thorvaldsen, P., Asplund, K., Kuulasmaa, K., Rajakangas, A. M., & Schroll, M. (1995). Stroke incidence, case fatality, and mortality in the WHO MONICA project. World Health Organization Monitoring Trends and Determinants in Cardiovascular Disease. *Stroke, 26*(3), 361-367.

Toogood, J. A., Barr, A. M., Stevens, T. K., Gati, J. S., Menon, R. S., & Martin, R. E. (2005). Discrete functional contributions of cerebral cortical foci in voluntary swallowing: A functional magnetic resonance imaging (fMRI) "Go, No-Go" study. *Experimental Brain Research, 161*(1), 81-90.

Tracy, J. F., Logemann, J. A., Kahrilas, P. J., Jacob, P., Kobara, M., & Krugler, C. (1989). Preliminary observations on the effects of age on oropharyngeal deglutition. *Dysphagia, 4*(2), 90-94.

Tsukamoto, Y. (2000). CT study of closure of the hemipharynx with head rotation in a case of lateral medullary syndrome. *Dysphagia, 15*(1), 17-18.

van Herwaarden, M. A., Katz, P. O., Gideon, R. M., Barrett, J., Castell, J. A., Achem, S., et al. (2003). Are manometric parameters of the upper esophageal sphincter and pharynx affected by age and gender? *Dysphagia*, *18*(3), 211–217.

Van Riper, C. (1954). *Speech correction: Principles and methods* (3rd ed.). Englewood Cliffs, NJ: Prentice-Hall.

Veis, S. L., & Logemann, J. A. (1985). Swallowing disorders in persons with cerebrovascular accident. *Archives of Physical Medicine and Rehabilitation*, *66*(6), 372–375.

Wade, D. T., & Hewer, R. L. (1987). Motor loss and swallowing difficulty after stroke: Frequency, recovery, and prognosis. *Acta Neuroogica Scandinavica*, *76*(1), 50–54.

Wang, T. G., Wu, M. C., Chang, Y. C., Hsiao, T. Y., & Lien, I. N. (2006). The effect of nasogastric tubes on swallowing function in persons with dysphagia following stroke. *Archives of Physical Medicine and Rehabilitation*, *87*(9), 1270–1273.

Welch, M. V., Logemann, J. A., Rademaker, A. W., & Kahrilas, P. J. (1993). Changes in pharyngeal dimensions effected by chin tuck. *Archives of Physical Medicine and Rehabilitation*, *74*(2), 178–181.

Wheeler, K. M., Chiara, T., & Sapienza, C. M. (2007). Surface electromyographic activity of the submental muscles during swallow and expiratory pressure threshold training tasks. *Dysphagia*, *22*(2), 108–116.

Widdicombe, J. G. (1986). *Reflexes from the upper respiratory tract (Volume 2: Control of breathing, part 1)*. Bethesda, MD: American Physiological Association.

Wilcox, F., Liss, J. M., & Siegel, G. M. (1996). Interjudge agreement in videofluoroscopic studies of swallowing. *Journal of Speech and Hearing Research*, *39*(1), 144–152.

Wise, S. P., & Strick, R. L. (1984). Anatomical and physiological organization of the non-primary motor cortex. *Trends in Neuroscience*, 7(11), 442–446.

Witte, U., Huckabee, M. L., Doeltgen, S. H., Gumbley, F., & Robb, M. (in press). The effect of effortful swallow on pharyngeal manometric measurements during saliva and water swallowing in healthy participants. *Archives of Physical Medicine and Rehabilitation*.

Wojner, A. W., & Alexandrov, A. V. (2000). Predictors of tube feeding in acute stroke patients with dysphagia. *AACN Clinical Issues*, *11*(4), 531–540.

Wolf, S. L. (1994). Biofeedback. In J. A. Downey, S. J. Myers, E. G. Gonzales, & J. S. Lieberman (Eds.), *The physiological basis of rehabilitation medicine* (2nd ed., pp. 563–572). Stoneham, MA: Butterworth-Heinemann.

Yim, H. B., Kaushik, S. P., Lau, T. C., & Tan, C. C. (2000). An audit of percutaneous endoscopic gastrostomy in a general hospital in Singapore. *European Journal of Gastroenterology and Hepatology*, *12*(2), 183–186.

Zaidi, N. H., Smith, H. A., King, S. C., Park, C., O'Neill, P. A., & Connolly, M. J. (1995). Oxygen desaturation on swallowing as a potential marker of aspiration in acute stroke. *Age and Ageing*, *24*(4), 267–270.

Zald, D. H., & Pardo, J. V. (1999). The functional neuroanatomy of voluntary swallowing. *Annals of Neurology*, *46*(3), 281–286.

Zenner, P. M., Losinski, D. S., & Mills, R. H. (1995). Using cervical auscultation in the clinical dysphagia examination in long-term care. *Dysphagia*, *10*(1), 27–31.

Index

A

Airway protection
  and CN V, 38
  and CN X, 33
  and SA (swallowing apnea), 141
      (*See also under* Swallowing
      respiratory coordination)
  swallowing, normal, 43, 141
Alcohol abuse, 2
Aneurysm, 1. *See also* Stroke
Anterior cingulate, 20, 25, 26
Anterior insula, 26
Antiplatelet agents, 7
Antithrombotic agents, 6-7
ASHA, Instrumental Diagnostic
      Procedures for Swallowing,
      162
Aspiration
  and feeding tubes, 213-214
  and free water, 217-220
  P-A (Penetration-Aspiration)
      Scale, 135, 136, 156-157
  and SAD (swallowing apnea
      duration), 148
  and sensitivity/specificity, 97
  and tracheotomy, 302
Aspiration pneumonia, 70
Aspirin, 6
Assessment. *See* CSE (clinical
      swallowing examination)

Atherosclerosis, 1
Auscultation, cervical, 113-114

B

Basal ganglia, 20, 25, 26
Botulinum toxin, 299-300
Brainstem mechanisms, swallowing
  defined, 29
  dorsal medullary region, 29-30,
      31
  evidential history, 28-29
  NA (nucleus ambiguus), 30-31
  and NTS (nucleus tractus
      solitarius), 20, 29
  pharyngeal swallowing initiation,
      29
  reflexive cough response
      laryngeal control, 30
  sensory feedback absence, 31
  ventral medullary region, 30-31
Brodmann's area, 26

C

Carotid endartectomy (CEA), 7
Case examples
  base of skull traumatic insult,
      78-79
  brainstem stroke, 173-174
  manometric evaluation, 171-174